3rd edition
psychiatry

National Medical Series

In the basic sciences

anatomy, 2nd edition
the behavioral sciences
    in psychiatry, 3rd edition
biochemistry, 3rd edition
clinical epidemiology and
    biostatistics
genetics
hematology
histology and cell biology,
    2nd edition
human developmental anatomy

immunology, 3rd edition
introduction to clinical medicine
microbiology, 2nd edition
neuroanatomy
pathology, 3rd edition
pharmacology, 3rd edition
physiology, 3rd edition
radiographic anatomy

In the clinical sciences

medicine, 2nd edition
obstetrics and gynecology,
    3rd edition
pediatrics, 3rd edition
preventive medicine and
    public health, 2nd edition
psychiatry, 3rd edition
surgery, 3rd edition

In the exam series

review for USMLE Step 1,
    3rd edition
review for USMLE Step 2
geriatrics

The National Medical Series for Independent Study

3rd edition
psychiatry

EDITOR

James H. Scully, M.D.

Clinical Professor of Psychiatry
Georgetown University School of Medicine
Deputy Medical Director
American Psychiatric Association
Washington, District of Columbia

Williams & Wilkins

Philadelphia • Baltimore • Hong Kong • London • Munich • Sydney • Tokyo

A Waverly Company

**Williams
& Wilkins**

Copyright © 1996
Williams & Wilkins
Suite 5025
Rose Tree Corporate Center
Building Two
1400 N. Providence Road
Media, PA 19063 USA

Printed in the United States of America

Diagnostic and Statistical Manual of Mental Disorders, 4th ed. (DSM-IV) diagnostic descriptions and criteria are referred to in, or have been adapted for, this book with permission of the American Psychiatric Association.

96 97 98
10 9 8 7 6 5 4 3 2 1

Contents

Contributors

Donald W. Bechtold, M.D.
Associate Professor of Psychiatry
Director of Training in Child Psychiatry
University of Colorado School of Medicine
Director, Children's Day Psychiatric Hospital
Denver, Colorado

Nancy A. Breslin, M.D.
Assistant Professor of Psychiatry
   and Behavioral Sciences
Director of Psychiatric Clerkship
Department of Psychiatry and Behavioral
   Sciences
George Washington University School
   of Medicine
Attending Psychiatrist
George Washington University Medical
   Center
Washington, District of Columbia

Steven L. Dubovsky, M.D.
Professor of Psychiatry and Medicine
Vice Chairman, Department of Psychiatry
University of Colorado School of Medicine
Denver, Colorado

Gordon L. Neligh, III, M.D.
Associate Professor of Psychiatry
Director, Program for Public Psychiatry
University of Colorado School
   of Medicine
Denver, Colorado

James H. Scully, M.D.
Clinical Professor of Psychiatry
Georgetown University School
   of Medicine
Deputy Medical Director
American Psychiatric Association
Washington, District of Columbia

Roderick Shaner, M.D.
Associate Professor of Clinical
   Psychiatry
Director, Medical Student Education
   in Psychiatry
University of Southern California
   School of Medicine
Los Angeles, California

Preface

This third edition of *NMS Psychiatry* incorporates the diagnostic criteria used in the new *Diagnostic and Statistical Manual of Mental Disorders,* Fourth Edition, commonly known as the DSM-IV. The DSM-IV continues the tradition of phenomenologic, scientifically based diagnosis first begun in DSM-III 15 years ago. Rather than labeling a patient based on a theory of psychopathology, these diagnostic manuals are empirically derived and as free of theoretical bias as possible. There is still much to be learned about the pathophysiology of mental illness, but psychiatry is one of the most exciting frontiers of science. Among the advances since the previous edition are the new serotonin-enhancing medications that have been so successful in treating depression. In addition, these drugs are effective in treating other disorders (such as eating disorders and obsessive-compulsive disorders). New treatments for schizophrenia have also been developed and introduced in recent years.

Despite these advances, stigma still exists, and persons with psychiatric disorders (and those who care for them) continue to deal with reactions fed by fear and ignorance. It is hoped that this book will reduce some of that ignorance. The organization of health care delivery systems is undergoing massive changes, and the shift to generalists and primary care is likely to continue. This will mean that primary care practitioners will need to be more knowledgeable and skilled in diagnosing, treating, and referring persons with mental illness than ever before.

The third edition also introduces new contributors, Drs. Nancy Breslin and Rod Shaner.

James H. Scully, Jr., M.D.

To the Reader

Since 1984, the *National Medical Series for Independent Study (NMS)* has been helping medical students meet the challenge of education and clinical training. In this climate of burgeoning knowledge and complex clinical issues, a medical career is more demanding than ever. Increasingly, medical training must prepare physicians to seek and synthesize necessary information and to apply that information successfully.

The *National Medical Series* is designed to provide a logical framework for organizing, learning, reviewing, and applying the conceptual and factual information covered in basic and clinical studies. Each book includes a concise but comprehensive outline of the essential content of a discipline, with up to 500 study questions. The combination of an outlined text and tools for self-evaluation allows easy retrieval of salient information.

All study questions are accompanied by the correct answer, a paragraph-length explanation, and specific reference to the text where the topic is discussed. Study questions that follow each chapter use current USMLE format to reinforce the chapter content. Study questions appearing at the end of the text in the Comprehensive Exam vary in format depending on the book. Wherever possible, Comprehensive Exam questions are presented as a clinical case or scenario intended to simulate real-life application of medical knowledge. The goal of this exam is to challenge the student to draw from information presented throughout the book.

All of the books in the *National Medical Series* are constantly being updated and revised. The authors and editors devote considerable time and effort to ensure that the information required by all medical school curricula is included. Strict editorial attention is given to accuracy, organization, and consistency. Further shaping of the series occurs in response to biannual discussions held with a panel of medical student advisors drawn from schools throughout the United States. At these meetings, the editorial staff considers the complicated needs of medical students to learn how the *National Medical Series* can better serve them. In this regard, the staff at Williams & Wilkins welcomes all comments and suggestions.

Chapter 1
The Clinical Examination
James H. Scully

I. OVERVIEW

A. Psychiatric evaluation

1. The psychiatric evaluation differs from a routine medical examination in that it includes a **mental status examination** rather than a physical examination, although a physical examination may be included. The examiner asks the patient about his **feelings and relationships,** not just historical facts. The psychiatric evaluation consists of:
   a. **Gathering data** from a careful history of the patient's problems
   b. **Conducting an examination** of the patient
   c. **Developing a differential diagnosis** for further study
   d. **Constructing a treatment plan**

2. A physician who takes psychiatric histories needs special skills because many patients are embarrassed by disclosing emotional problems. Most people are less willing to discuss psychiatric symptoms than physical symptoms.
   a. Most patients are not psychotic, but many patients, especially those who are confused or disorganized, can be helped by the physician to give accurate details of their history.
   b. **Confidentiality** is important in all physician–patient interactions, especially when psychiatric issues are discussed. To maintain confidentiality, physicians should not discuss their patients in hallways or elevators. In teaching programs, case material must be presented. However, it is important to maintain anonymity, and the participants in any conference are bound by confidentiality.
   c. **Exceptions to the rule of confidentiality** are made when the need for safety is paramount, such as in cases of child abuse or when threats are made to harm others.

B. Interview

1. The physician should help the patient to feel comfortable enough to provide personal information.

2. **Nonverbal communication,** such as facial expression and posture, is as important as verbal communication. Also important is how the story is told (i.e., tone of voice, feelings expressed by the patient).

3. During the first few minutes of the interview, the physician should allow the patient to talk about her symptoms.

C. History of the current illness. The interviewer obtains information about:

1. **The onset, duration, or change over time of the symptoms**

2. **Stressful events, especially losses,** including death of a loved one, job loss, and financial problems

3. **The patient's perception of any change in herself** or the perception of change in the patient by another individual (e.g., spouse, friend, supervisor at work)

4. **Past psychiatric illness or treatment,** including medication, hospitalization, or other therapy

5. **Legal issues** with respect to the current illness (e.g., lawsuit, arrest, incarceration) or, if the patient is a student, problems in school (e.g., truancy, suspension, expulsion)

6. **Secondary gain,** which is any benefit that the patient derives from the current problem (e.g., monetary compensation; relief from responsibilities at home, school, or work)

D. **Personal history**

1. **Developmental milestones**
   a. The interviewer obtains information about the patient's **early development,** including details about the patient's mother's pregnancy and delivery of the patient. Information may be obtained from the patient, family members, or hospital records.
   b. The physician determines the patient's **temperament** as a child as well as any important family events (e.g., death, separation, divorce) that may have influenced the development of the patient's temperament.
   c. The interviewer obtains information about the patient's **early experiences and relationships,** including school experiences (i.e., grades, delinquency), friends, family stability, early sexual experiences, and history of neglect or abuse. The patient's early relationships with his parents, siblings, and friends can be important barometers of his development.

2. **Social history**
   a. The physician determines the breadth of the patient's **social life,** such as whether he is a loner and how difficult it is for him to establish friendships.
   b. The interviewer determines whether any **changes in personality** are noted by the patient or by his family or friends.
   c. The interviewer determines the patient's **marital status** and current level of **sexual functioning**.
   d. The physician obtains the patient's **employment history,** including the number of jobs held and the reasons the jobs were terminated. Any problems with alcoholism or antisocial behavior should be noted.
   e. The interviewer obtains the patient's **military service history,** including the highest rank attained and a history of any disciplinary problems or combat experience.

3. **Family history**
   a. The physician asks the patient whether any **family members** have had **psychiatric hospitalization** or any other mental health treatment, suicide attempts, problems with alcohol, or other psychiatric problems. Families often deny significant psychiatric history.
   b. The interviewer determines **genetic risk factors and family attitudes** toward mental illness and treatment.
   c. The physician determines whether any **family member** is successfully using any **psychotropic medication** for the same illness. If so, there is a good chance that the medication will also help the patient.

4. **Psychiatric history. Recurrence of an earlier problem** is noted in the history of the current illness. Episodes of any **other psychiatric illness** are also listed. The physician notes any **previous treatment,** including the name and address of the therapist, medications, and outcome of treatment.

5. **Use and abuse of substances.** The physician asks screening questions for **alcohol and drug problems,** including whether family or friends ever objected to the patient's drinking or drug use and whether the patient ever felt that she had a problem with alcohol or drugs, either legal or illegal. Use of **tobacco** is also listed.

II. **PSYCHIATRIC EXAMINATION.** The assessment of a patient with a psychiatric disorder should always include the psychiatric interview and the mental status examination. It may also include physical examination, laboratory studies, and psychological tests.

A. **Psychiatric interview**

1. **Physician–patient relationship**

   a. Patients are often anxious about a psychiatric evaluation. They may be self-referred, but they are often referred by another health care professional, and may be ambivalent about the psychiatric examination. The physician should be courteous and respectful, and should acknowledge the patient's feelings about being interviewed.

   b. **The environment** can affect the difficulty of the evaluation. The setting of the evaluation can range from a quiet, private office to a busy, noisy intensive care unit in a general hospital.

   c. Family members or others may provide important information. However, the physician should always obtain the patient's **permission to question family members**.

   d. Interruptions should be minimized, and sufficient time should be allowed to complete the interview. Classically, the interview is 50 to 60 minutes long, but 20 minutes may be enough.

   e. The physician should sit so that she is at **eye level** with the patient.

2. **The informal mental status examination** begins immediately. It includes an evaluation of the following characteristics.

   a. Appearance

   b. Manner of relating

   c. Use of language

   d. Mood and affect

   e. Content of discussion

   f. Perceptions

   g. Abstracting ability

   h. Judgment

   i. Insight

3. **Interview technique**

   a. The interviewer leads the interview with the use of both open-ended and direct questions.

      (1) **Open-ended questions** allow the patient to use his own words (e.g., Tell me about your home life. Tell me how your hospital stay has been.).

      (2) **Direct questions** are used to elicit specific information (e.g., Have you ever consulted a mental health professional before? Are you thinking about killing yourself?).

   b. The physician should clearly communicate to the patient that he is listening.

      (1) **Attentive silence.** Allowing the patient to talk is important, but not sufficient. The physician should establish eye contact and convey the message that she is interested in what the patient is saying.

      (2) **Facilitation.** Encouraging comments (e.g., Tell me more about it.) help the patient to focus while relating his history.

      (3) **Summarization.** The interviewer should summarize portions of the patient's story (e.g., So you have been increasingly sad for 3 weeks, during which time you have lost 7 pounds and have been waking up at 4:00 A.M.?). Summarizing the patient's words lets the patient know that the physician is listening and allows the patient to correct any misunderstanding.

      (4) **Clarification.** Clarifying statements are similar to summary statements, but also include connections that the patient may not recognize (e.g., Your difficulty sleeping and your crying spells began in mid-September. Was this after your youngest child left for college?).

B. **Mental status examination.** In contrast to the psychiatric history, which is a record of the patient's entire life, the mental status examination is an evaluation of the patient at one point in time. During the interview, the physician observes the following characteristics.

1. **Appearance.** The interviewer notes the patient's overall appearance, dress, grooming, and any unusual features or gestures.

2. **Attitude.** The physician notes how the patient relates to the interviewer (e.g., hostile, cooperative, evasive).

3. **Behavior and psychomotor activity.** The physician notes the patient's gait, position, and overall level of activity, noting any unusual mannerisms, agitation, or psychomotor retardation. Manic patients may be unable to sit still, whereas schizophrenic patients may adopt bizarre postures or move stiffly and awkwardly.

4. **Speech.** The physician describes how the patient speaks, noting the following:
   a. **Rate of speech** (e.g., rapid, slow, halting)
   b. **Amount of speech** (e.g., taciturn, lacking spontaneity, grandiose)
   c. **Tone of speech** (e.g., monotone, singsong, slurred)
   d. **Speech impairment** (e.g., dysarthria, stuttering, echolalia), accent, dialect, or any other obvious speech pattern
   e. **Aphasia,** which is a disorder of speech and language that is caused by neurologic illness. The patient is either unable to speak normally or unable to comprehend speech properly. The clinician should distinguish aphasia from disorders of speech and language that are caused by psychiatric illness.

5. **Mood and affect.** The emotional state that the patient experiences internally is known as **mood**. The outward expression of the patient's internal emotional state is known as **affect**.
   a. The interviewer notes whether the patient's mood and affect are the same. For example, a patient who has a depressed mood is likely to appear sad and quiet and to speak softly and slowly. However, some depressed patients have an agitated and anxious affect. On the other hand, a schizophrenic individual may act silly or unconcerned while discussing a sad event, such as the death of a loved one. This inappropriate split between affective feeling and thought content led to the use of the term "schizophrenia," or split mind. It does not mean "split personality."
   b. The physician notes the depth and range of emotional expression.
      (1) **Labile affect** describes sudden shifts in emotional state. The patient may laugh one minute and cry the next without a clear stimulus.
      (2) **Flat affect** describes a shallow and blunted emotional state. Facial expression and voice are lacking spontaneity.

6. **Perception.** The presence of a perceptual problem is noted in the mental status examination or in the history. Perceptual abnormalities involve the sensory nervous system and include the following:
   a. **Hallucinations** are false perceptions of a sensory stimulus. Any sensory modality can be involved.
      (1) **Auditory hallucinations** are seen in psychosis. The hallucinations involve voices, not just sounds, that criticize, comment on the patient's actions, or give commands.
      (2) **Visual hallucinations** are often seen with organic psychosis, especially toxic or drug-related states.
      (3) **Gustatory (taste) and olfactory (smell) hallucinations** should alert the physician to a disorder of the temporal lobe.
      (4) **Tactile hallucinations** are also seen in organic states, such as alcohol withdrawal or cocaine and amphetamine abuse. **Formication** is the tactile hallucination of insects crawling over the skin.
      (5) **Kinesthetic hallucinations** include feeling movement when none occurs. "Out-of-body" experiences described in near-death situations may be kinesthetic hallucinations. Individuals usually describe this phenomenon as floating above their bodies and looking down on the scene.
      (6) Hallucinations of any type that occur while falling asleep (**hypnagogic**) or awakening (**hypnopompic**) occur in normal individuals and are not considered serious or pathologic.
   b. **Illusions** are misinterpretations of an actual sensory stimulus. For example, a patient in the hospital may misperceive the movement of the bed curtain as a person and become frightened. Illusions occur in schizophrenia, but are most common in delirium.

c. **Depersonalization and derealization** are alterations in an individual's perception of reality. With depersonalization, the patient feels detached and views herself as strange and unreal. Derealization involves a similar alteration in the patient's sense of reality of the outside world. Objects in the outside world may seem altered in size and shape, and people appear dead or mechanical.

7. **Thought process.** The pattern of a patient's speech allows the examiner to note the quality of the thought process, including its flow, logic, and associations. Abnormalities of the thinking process include:

   a. **Loose associations.** This abnormality involves the shifting of ideas from one to another with no logical connection, accompanied by a lack of awareness on the part of the patient that these ideas are not connected. The patient's thoughts are difficult for the examiner to follow.

   b. **Tangential thinking.** The patient wanders off the subject as new but related words are spoken. The examiner can usually follow the patient's thoughts, but the patient often loses track of the interviewer's question.

   c. **Circumstantiality.** As with tangential thinking, the patient loses the point of what he is saying, but he stays in the general topic area. Irrelevant details cause digressions in conversation. These digressions are mild if the patient is merely anxious, but can be severe if he is delirious and distractible.

   d. **Blocking,** which occurs when the thinking process stops altogether and the mind goes blank, occurs in states of acute anxiety as well as in schizophrenia.

   e. **Perseveration** is the repetition of the same words or phrases despite the interviewer's direction to stop.

   f. **Echolalia** is the direct repetition of the interviewer's words.

   g. **Flight of ideas,** which is seen in mania, involves rapid speech with quick changes of ideas that may be associated, such as by the sound of the words, but may also involve loose associations.

8. **Content of thought.** Disturbances in thought content include:

   a. **Delusions** are fixed, false beliefs that are outside the patient's culture. For example, a patient's belief that his thoughts are being broadcast outside his head is a delusion, but a belief in Santa Claus is not. Delusions can be paranoid (or persecutory), grandiose, nihilistic, somatic, or bizarre. **Delusions of reference** involve the belief by the patient that some person or object has special significance or power (e.g., a disk jockey is sending the patient special commands).

      (1) Because delusions are fixed, false beliefs, they cannot be corrected by the physician. Contradicting the patient's delusional belief may cause the patient to become angry and stop the interview.

      (2) The physician should not pretend to agree with the delusion, but should take a neutral position and continue the examination.

   b. **Obsessions** are persistent, intrusive thoughts, ideas, or impulses. The patient realizes that the ideas do not make sense and are not being imposed from outside (i.e., delusion). An example is a patient who is always fighting an impulse to run down the hall of the office building through a plate glass window at the end. He knows that this action is potentially life threatening, and he does not want to hurt himself, but he cannot stop thinking about it and feeling anxious. Other common obsessions include fears of contamination and unrealistic fears about physical health, as seen in hypochondriasis (see Chapter 7).

   c. **Suicidal and homicidal thoughts.** Every mental status examination should include questions about violence toward the self or others. It is important to exercise judgment and tact in discussing these issues.

9. **Judgment.** The clinician assesses the social judgment of the patient by determining whether she understands the consequences of her actions. The physician may ask the patient a judgment question (e.g., What would you do if you were stranded at Kennedy Airport with only $1.00 in your pocket?) to make this determination. The examiner must recognize differences in cultural values when assessing judgment.

10. **Insight.** The doctor should assess the patient's awareness of his problem, the cause of the problem, and what type of help is needed. Many people with serious mental illness, such as bipolar disorder or schizophrenia, lack insight and refuse needed treatment.

11. **Cognition.** The mental status examination measures the ability of the brain to function. A formal mental status examination, a number of which are available, is necessary to adequately examine the patient's orientation, concentration, and memory. All mental status examinations are limited in scope compared with extensive neuropsychological tests, but the mini-mental state examination shown in Figure 1-1 is a useful bedside clinical examination.

C. **Clinical laboratory studies.** The clinical laboratory is increasingly important in the diagnosis and treatment of psychiatric illness. The three main functions of the laboratory include screening patients for any underlying medical condition that might be causing the psychiatric symptoms, monitoring blood levels of psychotropic medications, and identifying biologic markers as part of the diagnosis and treatment process.

1. **Screening tests for psychiatric illness caused by a general medical condition**
   a. **Nonselective studies**
      (1) Complete blood count (CBC)
      (2) Blood chemistry evaluation
         (a) Serum glucose level
         (b) Electrolyte levels, including calcium and phosphorus
         (c) Liver function tests, serum glutamic-oxaloacetic transaminase (SGOT), serum glutamate pyruvate transaminase (SGPT), and bilirubin
         (d) Renal function tests: blood urea nitrogen level, creatinine clearance
      (3) Urine analysis
      (4) Screening for syphilis
      (5) Electrocardiogram (ECG)
      (6) Thyroid function tests
      (7) Chest x-ray
      (8) Vitamin B_{12} and folate levels
   b. **Selective procedures,** when clinically indicated (i.e., when results of routine laboratory studies are negative but an organic cause is suspected), include:
      (1) Arterial blood gas analysis
      (2) Blood alcohol level
      (3) Urine drug screen
      (4) Lumbar puncture and examination of the cerebrospinal fluid (CSF)
      (5) Special thyroid function tests
      (6) Heavy metal screen
      (7) Antinuclear antibodies
      (8) Serum and urine copper levels
      (9) Porphobilinogen and δ-aminolevulinic acid levels
      (10) Pregnancy test
      (11) Human immunodeficiency virus (HIV) test
      (12) Monospot test for infectious mononucleosis
   c. **Electroencephalography (EEG)**
      (1) EEG is used to diagnose a variety of seizure disorders. The behavior associated with temporal lobe seizure, or partial complex seizure, is sometimes difficult to distinguish from functional psychiatric disorders.
      (2) In delirium that is caused by metabolic problems, EEG results usually show high-voltage, slow-wave activity. These findings can be helpful in the differential diagnosis.
   d. **Neuroendocrine tests**
      (1) **The dexamethasone suppression test** has limited value in diagnosing mental illness, but it can be used to follow the response of a depressed patient to treatment. The patient is given 1 mg dexamethasone orally at 11:00 P.M. Plasma cortisol levels are measured at 8:00 A.M. and 4:00 P.M. (rarely also at 11:00 P.M.). Dexamethasone ordinarily suppresses the patient's cortisol response. Plasma

cortisol levels greater than 5 pg/dl are considered abnormal. Unfortunately, many conditions, such as dehydration, alcohol abuse, hypertension, diabetes, and weight loss give a false-positive result. This test may help the patient to accept diagnosis and treatment.

    (2) Thyrotropin-releasing hormone (TRH) stimulation test. Some depressed patients have a subclinical hypothyroid condition that causes depression. Other patients have lithium-induced hypothyroidism. The TRH stimulation test involves the intravenous injection of 500 μg TRH. Thyroid-stimulating hormone (TSH) is measured after 15, 30, and 90 minutes. Normally, plasma TSH levels rise sharply to 10 to 20 μg/ml above the baseline level. An increase of less than 7 μg/ml is considered suppressed. This finding may correlate with the diagnosis of depression or subclinical hypothyroidism.

  e. Sleep studies: polysomnography. Several medical problems associated with psychiatric symptoms, such as sleep apnea, seizure disorders, headaches, sexual dysfunction, and insomnia, can be evaluated by the sleep laboratory. Patients with major depression also have abnormal sleep patterns. The sleep laboratory uses the EEG, ECG, and electromyogram (EMG) in addition to the penile tumescence plethysmograph, oxygen saturation, and movement-measuring devices. In depression, findings include:

    (1) Hyposomnia

    (2) Rapid eye movement (REM) latency, which is a shortened time between the onset of sleep and the onset of the first REM period (less than 65 minutes)

    (3) Greater proportion of REM sleep early in the night

2. Monitoring plasma levels of psychotropic drugs. The judgment of the clinician is the most important aspect of monitoring therapeutic efficiency. However, it is increasingly useful to monitor blood levels of certain psychotropic agents.

  a. Lithium. Because of the potential toxicity of lithium at blood levels close to therapeutic levels, monitoring lithium levels is mandatory. Plasma samples should be drawn 10 to 12 hours after the last dose.

    (1) Therapeutic levels range from 0.6 to 1.5 mg/L.

    (2) Toxicity usually occurs at levels greater than 2.0 mg/L, but may occur at lower levels.

  b. Cyclic antidepressants. Plasma levels of tricyclic antidepressants can be useful in adjusting dosages, assessing compliance, and minimizing toxic side effects.

    (1) Nortriptyline and amitriptyline have therapeutic windows (i.e., the therapeutic effect increases until an upper limit of the blood level is reached).

    (2) Imipramine and desipramine have a linear dose–response curve. Above certain levels, side effects outweigh therapeutic effects.

  c. Selective serotonin reuptake inhibitors (SSRIs)

  d. Neuroleptics. Therapeutic levels for antipsychotic medications are not as well established as therapeutic levels for antidepressants. Blood levels may be used to evaluate compliance or nonabsorption.

  e. Clozapine use requires a weekly CBC because of potential toxicity.

3. Identifying biologic markers by brain imaging

  a. Computed tomography (CT) scan can visualize lesions larger than 0.5 cm on cross section. It also shows increased ventricle size associated with loss of brain cells. High ventricle:brain ratios (VBRs) are seen in patients with chronic schizophrenia and bipolar disorder.

  b. Magnetic resonance imaging (MRI) is based on measuring radio frequencies emitted by nuclei when a strong magnetic field is applied. Detailed anatomy can be seen. MRI shows white matter lesions that are not seen by CT scan, such as those that occur with demyelinating diseases (e.g., multiple sclerosis).

  c. Positron emission tomography (PET) shows specific areas of brain activity. Organic compounds, such as glucose, are labeled by short-lived, positron-emitting elements of oxygen, carbon, and nitrogen. A cyclotron is required to produce the labeled glucose, which limits widespread use of this technique. The prepared compound can be localized in the brain, showing the biochemical activity of specific brain areas. For

Patient _____

Examiner _____

Date _____

Mini-mental state examination

Maximum score	Score	
		Orientation
5	_____	What is the (year) (season) (date) (day) (month)?
5	_____	Where are we: (state) (country) (town) (hospital) (floor)?
		Registration
3	_____	Name three objects (1 second to say each). Then ask the patient to name all three after you have said them. Give 1 point for each correct answer. Then repeat them until the patient learns all three.
—	_____	Record the number of trials.
		Attention and calculation
5	_____	Serial 7s: Give 1 point for each correct answer. Stop after five answers.
—	_____	Alternatively, spell "world" backward.
		Recall
3	_____	Ask for the patient to name the three objects repeated earlier. Give 1 point for each correct answer.
		Language
9	_____	Name a pencil and wristwatch (2 points).
		Repeat the following: "No ifs, ands, or buts" (1 point).
		Follow a three-step command: "Take a paper in your right hand, fold it in half, and put it on the floor" (3 points).
		Read and obey the following: Close your eyes (1 point).
		Write a sentence (1 point).
		Copy a design (1 point).
_____		Total score

Consciousness

Assess the patient's level of consciousness along a continuum. _____

Alert   Drowsy   Stupor   Coma

Instructions for administration of the mini-mental state examination

Orientation

Date: Ask for the date. Then ask specifically for parts omitted (e.g., Can you also tell me what season it is?). Give 1 point for each correct answer.

Location: Ask in turn, "Can you tell me the name of this hospital?" (town, country, etc.). Give 1 point for each correct answer.

Registration

Ask the patient if you may test her memory. Then state the names of three unrelated objects clearly and slowly (1 second to say each). After you have said all three, ask the patient to repeat them. This first repetition determines the score (0–3), but repeat the names until the patient can repeat all three (up to six trials). If the patient does not eventually learn all three words, recall cannot be meaningfully tested.

Attention and calculation

Ask the patient to begin with 100 and count backward by 7. Stop after five subtractions (93, 86, 79, 72, 65). Score the total number of correct answers.

If the patient cannot or will not perform this task, ask him to spell the word "world" backward. The score is the number of letters in the correct order (e.g., dlrow = 5, dlorw = 3).

Recall

Ask the patient to recall the three words previously given (score 0–3).

Language

Naming: Show the patient a wristwatch and ask what it is. Repeat for a pencil (score 0–2).
Repetition: Ask the patient to repeat the sentence after you. Allow only one trial (score 0 or 1).
Three-step command: Give the patient a sheet of paper and repeat the command. Give 1 point for each part of the command that is correctly executed.
Reading: On a blank sheet of paper, print the sentence, "Close your eyes," in letters large enough for the patient to see clearly. Ask the patient to read the paper and do what it says. Give 1 point if the patient actually closes his eyes.
Writing: Give the patient a blank sheet of paper and ask him to write a sentence. Do not dictate a sentence; it is to be written spontaneously. It must contain a subject and a verb and be sensible. Correct grammar and punctuation are not necessary.
Copying: On a clean sheet of paper, draw two intersecting pentagons (each side about 1 inch), and ask the patient to copy them exactly as they are. All ten angles must be present, and two must intersect to score 1 point. Tremor and rotation are ignored.

Consciousness

Estimate the patient's level of consciousness along a continuum.

FIGURE 1-1. The mini-mental state examination. (Adapted with permission from Folstein MF, Folstein SE, McHugh PR: Mini-mental state: a practical method for grading the cognitive state of patients. *Psych Res* 12:189–198, 1975.)

example, decreased activity in the frontal cortex is seen in patients with schizophrenia. PET does not show detailed anatomy or lesions smaller than 0.5 cm.

D. **Psychological tests.** These tests provide a standardized objective measure of certain patient characteristics, such as intelligence and personality.

1. **Intelligence tests.** Most intelligence tests measure the **intelligence quotient (IQ),** which is arbitrarily defined as mental age divided by chronologic age multiplied by 100. An individual test score is compared with a standard or norm that is established by assigning the same tasks to a large group of people. These tests are influenced by culture, and do not measure the entire intellectual capacity of the individual being tested. By definition, an average IQ is 100 (range 90–110). The **Wechsler Adult Intelligence Scale (WAIS)** is the most widely used intelligence test.
   a. The WAIS has six verbal and five performance subjects, including information, comprehension, arithmetic, similarities, digit span, vocabulary, picture completion, block design, picture arrangement, object assembly, and digit symbol.
   b. This test generates a verbal IQ, a performance IQ, and a full-scale, or combined, IQ. A difference between the verbal and performance IQ scores of greater than 10 points suggests an organic brain syndrome.

2. Personality tests
   a. Minnesota Multiphasic Personality Inventory (MMPI). The MMPI consists of 550 yes-or-no questions. The results are given as scores in 10 scales: hypochondriasis, paranoia, masculinity–femininity, psychopathy, depression, hysteria, psychasthenia, schizophrenia, hypomania, and social introversion. The pattern of scores is interpreted by comparing the patient's score and subscores against standardized data. Although the test is objective, a trained psychologist should interpret the results.
   b. Rorschach test. In this famous inkblot test, 10 standard ambiguous inkblots are shown to the patient in a predetermined order. The interviewer explores the patient's responses. This projective test shows the patient's thinking and association patterns.
   c. Thematic apperception test (TAT). This test is also projective and consists of 30 pictures, not all of which are shown. The psychologist chooses a specific picture, depending on the psychological area to be examined. For example, one picture shows a seated young woman looking up at an older man. The patient is asked to create a story about the picture. This process indirectly reveals the patient's fantasies, fears, and conflicts. The test is not useful in developing a descriptive diagnosis.
   d. Sentence completion test. This test is also used to elicit the patient's associations. It consists of a series of incomplete sentences that the patient is asked to complete (e.g., I am afraid . . ., I feel guilty . . ., My mother is . . .). The psychologist notes the themes and tone of the responses as well as any subject areas that the patient avoids.
   e. Draw-a-Person test. This test was originally used only with children, but it can also be used with adults. The patient is asked to draw a picture of a person. Then the patient is asked to draw a person of the sex opposite from the person in the first drawing. This test assumes that the drawing represents to some degree the patient's view of herself. The test can also be used to detect brain damage.

3. Neuropsychological tests. Specific aspects of brain function are tested by neuropsychological tests, which are usually given in a battery. Expertise is required to conduct these tests. Neuropsychological tests can detect subtle cognitive defects in patients who are not known to be demented and can assess strengths and weaknesses to aid in the rehabilitation of patients with brain damage.
   a. The Halstead-Reitan Neuropsychological Test Battery includes:
      (1) The **trail-making test,** in which the patient is asked to connect alternating numbers and letters. This test assesses the patient's visuomotor perception.
      (2) The **rhythm test,** in which the patient is asked to identify pairs of rhythmic beats. It assesses auditory perception, attention, and concentration.
      (3) Other subtests that allow the neuropsychologist to evaluate a variety of brain functions, such as perception, sensation, concept formation, visuomotor integration, and abstract thought.
   b. The **Luria-Nebraska Neuropsychological Test Battery** and the **Bender-Gestalt Battery** are also used to diagnose brain damage.

III. CLASSIFICATION OF MENTAL DISORDERS

A. **Problems with definitions.** Although the term **"mental disorder"** does not have a precise definition, the *Diagnostic and Statistical Manual of Mental Disorders,* 4th edition (DSM-IV) defines it as a "significant clinical syndrome with behavioral and psychological symptoms, causing distress or impairment in functioning." Historically, mental disorders were dealt with separately from physical disorders. This practice perpetuates the belief of mind–body dualism.

1. Causes of mental illness can be:
   a. Biological
   b. Psychological
   c. Sociocultural-environmental

2. Normal reactions to stressful events, such as the death of a loved one, are not considered mental disorders.

3. **Socially unacceptable behavior,** such as crime, is not necessarily indicative of a mental disorder.

4. Few **diagnostic systems** consider mental disorders to involve both biological and psychological factors, but this split impairs the development of a comprehensive, integrated understanding of mental disorders.

B. **Classification of mental disorders.** The DSM-IV is based on empiric findings from literature reviews of data reanalysis and field trials. It uses a multiaxial assessment.

1. **Diagnostic axes**
   a. **Axis I: clinical syndromes.** These syndromes include organic mental disorders, schizophrenia, depression, substance abuse, and other conditions that may be a focus of clinical attention.
   b. **Axis II: personality disorders.** These disorders include prominent maladaptive personality features and defense mechanisms.
   c. **Axis III: general medical disorders.** These physical disorders are not necessarily causes of the psychiatric symptoms, but they are relevant to the treatment.

2. **Other domains for assessment**
   a. **Axis IV: psychosocial and environmental problems.** These problems include stresses that may affect the context in which the disorder developed. Generally, only psychosocial or environmental stresses that were present during the last year are listed. Stresses that occurred before the previous year are noted if they clearly contribute to the current disorder or treatment [i.e., history of trauma in a patient who is being treated for posttraumatic stress disorder (PTSD)]. Common sources of stress include:
      (1) Change in marital status (e.g., engagement, marriage, separation)
      (2) Parenting stress (e.g., birth, illness of a child, or problem with a child)
      (3) Interpersonal problems (e.g., disagreement with friends, dispute with neighbors)
      (4) Occupational problems (e.g., trouble at school or work, unemployment, retirement)
      (5) Change in living circumstances (e.g., moving)
      (6) Change in financial status, especially loss
      (7) Legal problems (e.g., arrest, lawsuit, trial)
      (8) Developmental milestones (e.g., puberty, menopause)
      (9) Physical illness or injury (when related to the development of an Axis I disorder, it is listed in Axis III)
      (10) Other stresses (e.g., natural disaster, rape, unwanted pregnancy)
   b. **Axis V: global assessment of functioning (GAF)** [Figure 1-2]. The physician rates the patient's level of psychological, social, and occupational functioning at the time of the evaluation. The GAF may also be used to rate the highest level of functioning for at least a few months during the last year.

IV. **PREVALENCE OF PSYCHIATRIC DISORDERS.** The largest study of the prevalence of psychiatric disorders is the **Epidemiologic Catchment Area (ECA)** study (Table 1-1). Fifteen diagnostic categories from the *Diagnostic and Statistical Manual of Mental Disorders,* 3rd edition, revised (DSM-III-R) were studied in five sites and more than 20,000 people. A cross section of the general population was interviewed.

A. In any 1 year, a mental disorder or substance abuse disorder affects 28.1% of the American population older than 18 years of age.

B. Severe mental illness affects 2.8% of the American adult population, or approximately 5 million adults.

Consider psychological, social, and occupational functioning on a hypothethical continuum of mental health and illness. Do not include impairment in functioning caused by physical or environmental limitations.

Code (Note: use intermediate codes when appropriate, e.g., 45, 68, 72.)

100   No symptoms; superior functioning in a wide range of activities; life's problems never seem to get out of hand; patient is sought out by others because of his many positive
91   qualities

90   Absent or minimal symptoms (e.g., mild anxiety before an examination); good functioning in all areas; interested and involved in a wide range of activities; socially effective; generally satisfied with life; no more than everyday problems or concerns (e.g., an
81   occasional argument with family members)

80   Symptoms are transient and predictable reactions to psychosocial stressors (e.g., difficulty concentrating after family argument); no more than slight impairment in social,
71   occupational, or school functioning (e.g., temporarily falling behind in school work)

70   Some mild symptoms (e.g., depressed mood, mild insomnia) or some difficulty in social, occupational, or school functioning (e.g., occasional truancy, theft within the household), but patient is generally functioning well; has some meaningful
61   interpersonal relationships

60   Moderate symptoms (e.g., flat affect, circumstantial speech, occasional panic attacks) or moderate difficulty in social, occupational, or school functioning (e.g., no friends,
51   unable to hold a job)

50   Serious symptoms (e.g., suicidal ideation, severe obsessional rituals, frequent shoplifting) or serious impairment in social, occupational, or school functioning (e.g., no
41   friends, unable to hold a job)

40   Some impairment in reality testing or communication (e.g., speech is sometimes illogical, obscure, or irrelevant) or major impairment in several areas, such as work or school, family relations, judgment, thinking, or mood (e.g., depressed man avoids friends, neglects family, and is unable to work; child frequently bullies younger
31   children, is defiant at home, and is failing at school)

30   Behavior is considerably influenced by delusions or hallucinations or patient has serious impairment in communication or judgment (e.g., sometimes incoherent, grossly inappropriate behavior, suicidal preoccupation) or is unable to function in
21   almost all areas (e.g., stays in bed all day; has no job, home, or friends)

20   Some danger of hurting self or others (e.g., suicide attempts without clear expectation of death, frequent violent behavior, manic excitement) or occasional failure to maintain minimal personal hygiene (e.g., smears feces) or gross impairment in
11   communication (e.g., largely incoherent or mute)

10   Persistent danger of severely hurting self or others (e.g., recurrent violence) or persistent inability to maintain personal hygiene or serious suicidal attempt with clear
1   expectation of death

0   Inadequate information

FIGURE 1-2. The Global Assessment of Functioning (GAF) scale. [Adapted with permission from Endicott J, Spitzer RL, Fleiss, et al: The Global Assessment Scale: A procedure for measuring overall severity of psychiatric disturbance. *Arch Gen Psychiatry* 33:766–771, 1976; Shaffer D, Gould MS, Braic J, et al: Children's Global Assessment Scale (CGAS). *Arch Gen Psychiatry* 40:1228–1231, 1983; and Luborsky L: Clinicians' judgments of mental health. *Arch Gen Psychiatry* 7:407, 1962.]

TABLE 1-1. Results of the Epidemiologic Catchment Area Study

Disorder	1 Month Number in Millions	1 Year Number in Millions
Any mental disorder covered in survey	28.9 (15.7%)	51.7 (28.1%)
Substance abuse disorders	7.0 (3.8%)	17.5 (9.5%)
Alcohol abuse/dependence	5.2 (2.8%)	13.6 (7.4%)
Drug abuse/dependence	2.4 (1.3%)	5.7 (3.1%)
Mood disorders	9.6 (5.2%)	17.5 (9.5%)
Bipolar disorder	1.1 (0.6%)	2.2 (1.2%)
Major depression	3.3 (1.8%)	9.2 (5.0%)
Dysthymia	6.1 (3.3%)	9.9 (5.4%)
Schizophrenia	1.3 (0.7%)	2.0 (1.1%)
Anxiety disorders	13.4 (7.3%)	23.3 (12.6%)
Phobia	11.6 (6.3%)	20.1 (10.9%)
Panic disorder	0.9 (0.5%)	2.4 (1.3%)
Obsessive-compulsive disorder	2.4 (1.3%)	3.9 (2.1%)
Somatization	0.2 (0.1%)	0.4 (0.2%)
Antisocial personality disorder	0.9 (0.5%)	2.8 (1.5%)
Severe cognitive impairment	3.1 (1.7%)	5.0 (2.7%)

C. Overall, the rates for men and women are approximately the same, but rates for men and women differ for specific disorders.

  1. Men have higher rates of substance abuse and antisocial personality disorder.

  2. Women have higher rates of depression, phobia, and dysthymic disorder.

D. By comparison, in 1 year, nearly 50% of Americans have a respiratory illness, and more than 20% have cardiovascular disease.

E. The **National Comorbidity Survey (NCS)** headed by Kessler conducted structured diagnostic interviews on a sample of more than 8000 Americans.

  1. Of respondents 15 to 54 years of age, 48% report at least one lifetime mental disorder, and 29.5% report at least one mental disorder in the previous year.

  2. Fourteen percent report three or more psychiatric disorders in their lifetime. The respondents report 53.9% of the lifetime disorders and 89.5% of the severe disorders in the last year.

  3. Major depression is the most common disorder, with a lifetime incidence of 17.1%. A lifetime history of alcohol dependence is reported by 14.1% of respondents.

F. **Treatment**

  1. Only 42% of respondents with one or more disorders receive any professional care. Only 1 in 4 (26%) receive treatment in the mental health sector. Only 1 in 12 (8%) receive treatment in substance abuse facilities.

  2. Only 58.8% of respondents with three or more disorders (the most severely ill) receive professional care. Of these patients, 41% receive treatment in the mental health specialty sector, and 1 in 7 (14.8%) receive treatment in substance abuse facilities.

V. **EVALUATION AND MANAGEMENT OF PSYCHIATRIC EMERGENCIES. A psychiatric emergency, or crisis,** is a stress-induced pathologic response that physically endangers the affected individual or others or significantly disrupts the functional equilibrium of the individual or her environment. The pathologic response may occur as an acute alteration in the individual's thought, mood, or behavior. The individual, the environment, or both may experience or react to the situation as emergent.

A. **Evolution of a crisis**

1. **Stressors** from any source create a problem for an individual. In a crisis, the normal **coping mechanisms** of the individual are insufficient, and the individual is overwhelmed.

2. **Increased anxiety and disorganization** may follow the stressor, and may further impair the individual's functional integrity and problem-solving capacity.

3. **Failure of adaptation** may cause an increasing sense of helplessness, accompanied by panic, depression, or both, and may result in further disorganization.

4. **Impulsive, maladaptive, and even desperate attempts by the individual to regain equilibrium** are likely in this situation. The new equilibrium may reorganize the individual and reduce dysphoria, but still be maladaptive because it limits the function of the individual or disrupts the environment required to maintain it. For example, an individual may diminish anxiety and reduce the frequency of nightmares after a traumatic event by using alcohol. However, medical, social, and occupational complications may result from excessive use.

5. A **request for help** may occur at any time during this cycle, depending on the individual's response to the crisis and the social context. An individual with any psychiatric diagnosis or an individual with no preexisting disorder can have a psychiatric emergency. A diagnosis of a major mental disorder may be the result of an individual's maladaptive responses.

B. **Components of stress-induced responses.** A dynamic interplay occurs among the stressor, the affected individual, and the social system that influences the individual's response. The severity of the psychopathologic response creates a psychiatric emergency out of a specific crisis.

1. **Stressors** depend on the interplay of individual and social factors, but they are usually either predominantly internal or external.
   a. **Internal stress** occurs when a person faces a normal developmental task for which he is ill equipped or ill prepared. A normal environmental event may have great psychological meaning for the individual, and may cause a disruptive increase in needs, a loss, or a conflict. Examples include an anxious adolescent who becomes disorganized when leaving his family to attend college, and an aging, lonely woman who becomes suicidal after her cat dies.
   b. **External stress** results from a life event that is normally recognized as a significant source of stress, such as the death of a family member, a divorce, or a serious illness.

2. **The affected individual** determines whether a particular stress is major or minor, and whether the response is adaptive or maladaptive.
   a. Healthy individuals may resolve a crisis in an adaptive, growth-promoting fashion.
   b. Healthy individuals may become so overwhelmed by stress that they have a pathologic adaptation. They are then more vulnerable to future stress.
   c. Individuals with significant disorders may decompensate with even minor environmental stress.

3. **Social system.** Individuals have varying needs for external support and structure and varying capacity to adapt to stress. Both the type of stress and the type of response affect the amount of environmental support that is available.

    a. Some individuals have many supportive resources that facilitate an adaptive resolution to a crisis.

    b. Some individuals have sources of support that are insufficient in the face of severe stress.

    c. Some individuals have sources of support that are easily overwhelmed or are even actively intolerant of their attempts to resolve the crisis. For these individuals, the external environment becomes another source of stress.

C. Principles of evaluation

1. Immediate assessment of the condition and the dangerousness of the patient's behavior is essential. This assessment can be made on the basis of the following factors:

    a. Patient's behavior. Loud, agitated, angry, and threatening behavior requires limit setting and control before further evaluation can take place.

    b. Arrival in the emergency department. A patient who is brought in handcuffed or is otherwise restrained should be assessed cautiously despite calm or withdrawn behavior. The patient may be calm as a result of external control, and withdrawing this control prematurely may cause an escalation of the agitated behavior.

    c. Reports on behavior. Reports of dangerousness from family members and others must be investigated, even though the patient's history or behavior may be inconsistent.

2. Thorough evaluation. Secure surroundings that provide safety and comfort for both the evaluator and the patient should be available for a more extensive evaluation.

    a. These steps should be followed for all patients.

        (1) The **physical setting** should be quiet, open, and sparsely furnished. There should be a minimum of objects that may be used as weapons. Both the interviewer and the patient should have an unobstructed exit from the room. A call button to summon immediate help must be easily accessible to the interviewer.

        (2) **Trained assistants** who provide a show of force and can subdue an agitated patient should be readily available. It may be necessary to have help inside or just outside of the interview room.

        (3) **Mental status examination.** The physician should observe the patient's appearance, manner, and behavior during the evaluation.

    b. These steps may not be necessary for patients who are cooperative. However, if indicated by the history or by an escalation of the patient's behavior, **these steps should be initiated before the evaluation can proceed safely**.

        (1) A **search for weapons** may be indicated by the history or the patient's behavior before further evaluation takes place.

        (2) **Verbal and nonverbal expressions of expectation of the patient to control himself** and to be responsible for his behavior may be necessary. The patient may need to be reminded that external control is also available.

        (3) **Physical restraint** in the form of two- or four-point leather restraints is indicated if the patient cannot respond to verbal limit setting and reassurance. The need for safety for all people concerned supersedes the patient's requests, but the clinician should recognize the restrained patient's vulnerability and helplessness and treat her with respect and compassion.

            (a) If the patient arrives in restraints or handcuffs, adequate evaluation must take place before restraints are removed.

            (b) If an unrestrained patient cannot be controlled, she should be placed in leather restraints until the evaluation is completed. A patient should not be restrained supine, but on the side or with the head elevated to prevent aspiration if vomiting occurs. In addition, a patient in restraints requires constant monitoring.

3. Identification of a crisis

    a. Overt. A crisis may be immediately apparent from the patient's behavior or the circumstances surrounding his arrival in the emergency department.

   b. Covert. A patient who is calm and superficially cooperative may still be potentially dangerous to herself or to others. Empathic, detailed history taking with a high level of suspicion often shows the nature of the emergency. The following factors should raise the index of suspicion.

     (1) Risk factors. Certain historical data and mental status findings increase the probability of specific emergencies. Examples include a history of alcoholism, violence, or findings of command hallucinations.

     (2) Vague, evasive, or qualified answers to questions in crucial areas, such as suicide, homicide, and impulse control, must be vigorously pursued. A patient's attempt to minimize or ignore the consequences of observed or reported behavior should not be accepted without investigation. Discrepancies between the patient's history and the reports of others must be explored. The interviewer may need to meet individually with the other people to determine their true concerns.

     (3) Feelings of discomfort on the part of the physician should be examined. An intuitive, experienced physician may detect subtle discrepancies between the patient's affect and her verbal content, and may identify a latent emergent situation.

4. Symptoms and current illness

  a. Patient. The interviewer can establish rapport by allowing the patient to tell his own story as much as possible. The examiner should obtain relevant information with the following questions:

    (1) What symptoms or problems led the patient to seek help?

    (2) Why is the patient requesting help now?

    (3) Why are these symptoms a problem at this particular time?

    (4) What are the patient's normal coping mechanisms in times of stress?

    (5) What is his level of functioning in general?

    (6) How did he cope with similar stresses in the past?

    (7) How is he attempting to resolve the problem?

  b. Others. Family members, friends, employers, and co-workers may be able to answer many of these questions if the patient will not or cannot answer them accurately. Different individuals may accurately describe a particular aspect of the patient's situation or level of function, and the physician can use this information to compose an integrated picture of the patient.

5. Patient history. The level of detail provided in the history affects the accuracy of the picture of the patient. In a crisis, detailed history taking may not be feasible; however, the following areas should be explored.

  a. Previous psychiatric illness. The symptoms, circumstances, treatment, and response to treatment of previous illnesses should be outlined.

  b. Dangerous behavior. Previous episodes of self-destructive or assaultive behavior should be carefully explored because they have significant predictive value.

  c. Medical history

    (1) Significant medical illness may have a direct effect on the current crisis, may color the presentation, or may produce chronic vulnerability to stress.

    (2) Drugs. Prescribed medication, alcohol, and illicit drugs can profoundly affect thinking, feeling, and behavior. They may cause a crisis or significantly impair the patient's adaptive capacity.

6. Physical examination should be thorough, with particular attention paid to evidence of drug intoxication, withdrawal symptoms, and acute or chronic neurologic disease.

7. Laboratory tests should be guided by other findings and by the differential diagnosis. Blood and urine tests for toxic agents may be particularly helpful in an emergency situation.

VI. SPECIFIC PSYCHIATRIC EMERGENCIES

A. Suicide

1. **Clinical presentation**
   a. **Overt**
      (1) **Suicidal behavior.** A patient may ingest drugs or attempt suicide by slashing his wrists, shooting himself, jumping out a window, or otherwise injuring himself. Thus, the patient often requires medical or surgical intervention (e.g., gastric lavage, suturing) before a psychiatric assessment can be completed. The patient should be considered acutely suicidal until proven otherwise. Careful observation is needed to prevent another suicide attempt or to prevent the patient from leaving the emergency department.
      (2) **Suicidal ideation.** The patient may be obviously depressed, expressing concerns with little prompting and experiencing considerable pain and distress. She may ask for help in controlling her suicidal impulses and for relief from depression.
   b. **Covert**
      (1) **Suicidal behavior.** Although the patient may minimize or deny the implications of his behavior, he may have accidents that range from suspiciously to obviously suicidal. The patient who is unconscious of his self-destructive impulses may still be highly suicidal. A similar type of patient is one who appears homicidal or assaultive but whose behavior is primarily an attempt to provoke others, such as the police, to kill him.
      (2) **Suicidal ideation.** The patient may seek medical evaluation of a minor or severe somatic symptom. She may appear depressed or may disguise her distress. Empathic questioning may prompt the patient to reveal her feelings. The patient may show distress that is out of proportion to objective findings or may visit the emergency department many times over a short period. Although hoping to obtain help, the patient may take the medication given for a somatic symptom in a suicide attempt.
   c. **Chronic suicidal ideation and behavior.** The patient repeatedly calls or visits the emergency room with suicidal ideation and attempts. Self-destructive behavior may be a means by which the patient attempts to manipulate the environment or relieve internal discomfort rather than an attempt to die. These patients evoke frustration and hostility in caregivers and are at great risk to be ignored or actively rejected. Because they are also at great risk to kill themselves by design, miscalculation, or impulsiveness, careful evaluation is required.

2. **Risk factors**
   a. **Demographics**
      (1) The suicide rate in men is two to four times greater than that in women. However, women attempt suicide more often.
      (2) Whites and Native Americans have much higher suicide rates than blacks and Hispanics.
      (3) Divorced, widowed, and separated individuals have higher suicide rates than married people.
      (4) White men older than 45 years have the highest suicide rate. There was a significant increase in the suicide rate among adolescent boys in recent years. The elderly account for 10% of the American population and 25% of suicides.
      (5) Suicide rates do not differ significantly by economic status or occupation. Professional women, including physicians, have higher suicide rates than professional men.
   b. **Psychopathology.** Psychiatric illness is present in almost all people who commit suicide. Comorbidity (i.e., multiple psychiatric illnesses) is common.
      (1) **Mood disorder.** Major depression is the most common disorder, and is present in approximately half of people who commit suicide.

    (2) Substance abuse-related disorder. Alcohol is implicated in more than 25% of suicides. Other drugs, such as marijuana and cocaine, are seen in younger victims. Depression and substance-related disorders are present in two-thirds of all suicides.

    (3) Schizophrenia. Approximately 5% of suicide victims have schizophrenia. Individuals with schizophrenia have approximately the same risk as those with major depression.

    (4) Delirium, dementia, and other cognitive disorders. As a primary diagnosis, these disorders are present in 4% of people who commit suicide. Another psychiatric diagnosis is usually present as well.

    (5) Panic disorder. The diagnosis of panic disorder is statistically related to an increased incidence of suicide. Most researchers believe that the presence of comorbid mental disorders, such as depression and substance abuse-related disorder, in patients with panic disorder is more important in suicidal behavior.

    (6) Personality disorders. Borderline and antisocial personality disorders occur in patients with suicidal behavior. Other psychiatric illnesses, especially substance abuse, are usually present as well.

  c. Medical illness. Poor health in the last 6 months increases the risk of suicide. Terminal illness accounts for fewer suicides than publicity suggests. Lack of postmortem examinations makes these risks unknown.

  d. Genetics. Most family studies involve mood disorders in which suicide is a factor, rather than suicide alone.

    (1) In one study of twins, suicides occurred only among monozygotic pairs, not among dizygotic pairs.

    (2) Family studies of an Amish community also show increased suicide rates in families with heavy genetic loading for unipolar, bipolar, and other mood disorders.

    (3) There appears to be a genetic risk of suicide that is independent of the risk of psychiatric illness.

3. Assessment of lethality (suicide risk)

  a. Episodic suicidal ideation and behavior. Suicidal behavior may remit and relapse in response to the patient's changing internal emotional and cognitive states and his environment. The patient, the environment, or both may require intervention to protect the patient.

  b. Ambivalence of the suicidal patient. The balance between the patient's wish to live and her wish to die must be evaluated, including the factors that tip the balance one way or the other. Eight of ten patients who eventually commit suicide give some warning of their intentions.

  c. Risk factors (predictors). In many cases, the patient's ambivalence and the episodic nature of suicidal behavior permit the behavior to be identified and prevented. The following predictors may aid the physician in determining which patients are at risk and to what extent.

    (1) Demographic indicators. Unemployed, divorced white men older than 45 years are at particularly high risk. Any of these factors singly or in combination, should alert the physician to investigate the situation more fully.

    (2) Historical indicators. A recent loss, real or symbolic, or a change in the patient's status may precipitate a crisis, with the patient experiencing anxiety and depression.

      (a) Current illness. Patients who report hopelessness, helplessness, loneliness, and exhaustion are worrisome. An unexpected change in behavior, such as giving away possessions, or an unexpected change in attitude, such as calm or resignation in the midst of a distressing situation, should be investigated. Overt or indirect talk of death should be followed up with specific questions about fantasies, wishes, plans, and means. In a patient who makes an unsuccessful suicide attempt, the following additional issues are important:

        (i) The patient's perception of the lethality of the attempt, his expectations of rescue, and his relief or disappointment at being alive are often more important than the objective dangerousness of the attempt, particularly in cases of apparent minimal danger.

(ii) The extent to which the precipitating crisis is resolved or is being resolved may influence the patient's wish to remain alive and his attitude toward the future.

(b) **A history of suicide attempts** increases the risk of suicide, particularly if many attempts are made. The circumstances and lethality of the previous attempts should be determined.

(c) **Medical history.** A history of chronic illness or an acute change in physical health increases the risk of suicide.

(d) **Family history.** A family history of suicide is important both in terms of the patient's identification with the individual who died and the possibility of inheritance of an affective disorder. The patient may experience stress at the anniversary of the death or when she reaches the age of the person who died.

(3) **Diagnostic indicators** include depression, thought disorder, and impairment of impulse control, especially secondary to alcohol or drug abuse.

(4) **Mental status.** The physician should assess the severity of depression, the presence of psychosis (especially command hallucinations), and any problems with impulse control. In addition, the physician should be aware of the patient's response to the interview (e.g., whether she feels understood, experiences some relief, and expresses more hopefulness or remains angry, pessimistic, and desperate).

(5) **Resources.** The availability and support of family and friends are crucial. The physician should obtain their perceptions of the patient's lethality. They may need to be interviewed away from the patient to feel comfortable stating their concerns. Additionally, in planning for treatment, the physician must be confident of their support and willingness to assume some responsibility for the patient. In particular, the physician must ascertain that there is no collusion with or covert encouragement of the patient's suicidal behavior.

4. **Countertransference reactions to suicidal patients.** Countertransference refers to the physician's emotional reactions to the patient. These reactions may be unconscious or only dimly conscious. They may have a powerful effect on the physician's attitude toward the patient, his approach to the patient, and even his clinical judgment.

a. The **physician** has his own attitudes toward suicide and death, his own set of personal and clinical experiences, and conflicts about his own aggressive or self-destructive impulses. Unless the physician is aware of these reactions, he may minimize or distort clinical data from the patient to accommodate his personal feelings or beliefs. The physician may fear being overwhelmed if the patient admits to suicidal ideation. He may even fear that he will influence the patient to commit suicide by talking about it.

b. The **patient's behavior** may produce **frustration, anger, and helplessness in most caregivers**. A patient may evoke so much hostility that the physician may wish that the patient were dead. This reaction is serious because others in the patient's environment may feel similarly.

5. **Principles of emergency treatment**

a. The patient must be protected.

b. A psychiatric consultation is necessary if there is any question about the patient's lethality.

c. Treatment options include:

(1) **Hospitalization.** A patient should be hospitalized if the lethality of her ideation or behavior is high. Lethality might be high because of the persistence of the patient's wish to die, the severity of her concurrent psychopathology, or the absence of reliable sources of support in her social environment.

(a) A patient can be hospitalized voluntarily if she concurs with the need for inpatient treatment.

(b) A suicidal patient can also be hospitalized involuntarily if she refuses voluntary hospitalization. The length of time that a patient can be held initially for treatment varies from state to state, but it is often in the range of 72 hours. A severely suicidal patient who resists treatment may require one-to-one observation to prevent escape or self-injury.

(2) Outpatient treatment is less restrictive than hospitalization. It is indicated in patients who have some crisis resolution, mild concurrent psychopathology, environmental resources, and a therapeutic response to the interview. It usually involves a follow-up appointment within 48 hours and intensive crisis treatment thereafter. Somatic treatment can be initiated on an outpatient basis, but limited quantities of medication should be dispensed because of the potential for overdose.

B. Violence

1. Etiology. Violent behavior is a result of the interplay between innate psychobiologic factors and the external environment.

a. Biologic factors

(1) Neurotransmitters. Serotonin metabolism appears to be involved in violent behavior in the same way that it is involved in suicidal behavior [i.e., lower levels of 5-hydroxyindoleacetic acid (5-HIAA) are found in the CSF of offenders who kill with unusual cruelty than in the CSF of nonviolent offenders].

(2) Limbic system. The role of partial complex seizures in violent patients is controversial. However, there appears to be no overall difference in the level of violent behavior between patients with psychomotor epilepsy and those without.

(3) Chromosomal abnormalities. Sex chromosome abnormalities, particularly XYY, were believed to influence criminal behavior because there was an increased number of men with that abnormality in prison. However, recent studies do not support this hypothesis. Arrests for violence are more strongly associated with low intelligence than with chromosomal abnormality.

(4) Endocrine abnormalities

(a) Because such a high percentage of violent acts are committed by men, there is speculation that androgens may be involved. However, no studies show this connection. With the exception of pedophilic behavior, antiandrogen treatment is not effective in decreasing violence.

(b) Premenstrual syndrome is implicated in aggressive behavior in women and was even used as a legal defense for violence. However, there is no scientific evidence of a causal link.

(5) Alcohol and drugs. Alcohol decreases impulse control and inhibition and impairs judgment. There is a clear association between alcohol intoxication and violent behavior. Other drugs that have a similar effect on the brain and behavior include amphetamines, cocaine, phencyclidine (PCP), and sedative-hypnotic drugs. The aggressive and criminal behavior that is associated with obtaining these and other illegal drugs is also an indirect cause of violent behavior.

b. Psychosocial factors

(1) Developmental. A patient who was abused as a child is at increased risk of becoming an abusive adult. Witnessing abuse in childhood is also associated with increased violent behavior. Spouse abuse and family violence, even if not directed at the child, can influence the child's later behavior.

(2) Guns. The number of deaths and injuries caused by firearms continues to rise. The risk of gun death among people 15 to 19 years of age rose 77% from 1985 to 1990.

(3) Environment

(a) Crowding appears to be a factor in the increased potential for violence.

(b) Weather also has an effect on violence. Increased ambient temperature to the point of discomfort may produce increased aggression. However, aggressive behavior diminishes in very hot weather.

(4) Socioeconomic factors. Studies of race and violence have contradictory and controversial findings.

    (a) Nonwhite populations experience higher rates of violence, as both victims and aggressors, than white populations.

    (b) The best studies show that race and economic inequality are not related to violence, but that **severe poverty** and **marital disruption** are. The socioeconomic factors that disrupt the family structure also appear to increase the risk of aggression and violence in the children of these families.

2. Differential diagnosis. Any patient is potentially dangerous, but certain diagnoses are more likely to be associated with violence. Further, an accurate diagnosis permits the institution of specific treatment measures.

  a. Psychotic disorders

    (1) Bipolar disorder: manic type. Manic patients are often irritable and angry rather than amusing. They are pressured and hyperactive, and may become aggressive if their grandiose, unrealistic plans are blocked. Their behavior may also be disorganized and unintentionally violent.

    (2) Schizophrenic disorders. These psychotic disorders may be accompanied by considerable panic and agitation as well as deficient reality testing and impulse control. Schizophrenic people who refuse to take medication, who have a history of violence, and who have command hallucinations are particularly at risk of being violent. More commonly seen are patients with paranoid schizophrenia. These individuals are hostile and fearful of attack, and they may act aggressively to defend themselves. Schizophrenic patients may experience command hallucinations that order them to hurt others.

    (3) Paranoid disorders. Patients with paranoid disorders generally have stable, well-developed delusions but better reality testing and impulse control than patients with schizophrenia. However, their overly controlled and often denied hostility may erupt as murderous rage if the patient feels particularly threatened or experiences diminished impulse control.

  b. Nonpsychotic disorders

    (1) Intermittent explosive disorder. This disorder is more common in men than in women. Patients have discrete episodes of loss of control, and they commit serious assaults or destruction of property. Their behavior is grossly out of proportion to any precipitating psychological stressors. They may have genuine remorse about their actions afterward, but many of these patients enter prison or mental hospitals. A family history of violence is common.

    (2) PTSD. Trauma victims who have also committed acts of violence (e.g., combat veterans) often fear a loss of control. Explosions of aggressive behavior may be unpredictable. These episodes may be associated with flashbacks, and are triggered by something in the patient's environment. Drug and alcohol use can complicate the situation, especially in patients with chronic feelings of rage and frustration.

    (3) Personality disorders. Substance abuse increases the likelihood of acting out behavior in people with any type of personality disorder.

      (a) Patients with **borderline personality disorder** have difficulty regulating mood and behavior. Impulsive behavior, including violence, sexual promiscuity, suicidal gestures, and difficult and intense interpersonal relationships are seen with this disorder.

      (b) Patients with **antisocial personality disorder** exhibit outbursts of violence as well as pervasive antisocial behavior, such as lying, stealing, and reckless actions that may endanger others.

      (c) Patients with **paranoid personality disorder** are easily offended and are quick to react to any imagined or real insult. When two people with paranoid personality disorder are placed together, violence can easily result.

  c. Other disorders

    (1) Substance abuse. Alcohol intoxication is the most common cause of violent behavior in American culture. Other drugs that are associated with violence include sedative–hypnotics, such as barbiturates and benzodiazepines, and stimulants, such as cocaine, amphetamines, and PCP. Glue sniffing and steroid use also increase violent behavior. The physician should evaluate the patient for dysarthria, nystagmus, unsteady gait, and tremors. Patients with PCP intoxication often exhibit confusion, disorientation, rage, and violent behavior.

(2) **Central nervous system disorders.** Traumatic injuries to the brain, including birth injury, are associated with violent behavior. Postconcussion syndrome, which can be caused by apparently minor head injury, causes increased irritability and impulsive behavior. Any other organic mental disorder, including infection, degenerative processes, or ingestion of poison, can affect behavior.

(3) **Partial complex seizures.** Temporal lobe epilepsy is considered a cause of violence, although violence during a seizure is rare. Whether violent behavior is increased between seizures is a controversial issue. If the patient shows a repetitive pattern of poorly directed episodes of violence, she should undergo EEG with nasopharyngeal leads, regardless of whether other seizure activity is present.

(4) **Adult attention deficit disorder.** Some patients continue to have symptoms of attention deficit disorder after childhood. The symptoms include hyperactivity, poor concentration, low frustration tolerance, and poor impulse control. Treatment with methylphenidate may be effective for these individuals.

3. **Assessment of dangerousness.** Although an accurate clinical diagnosis is important, it is only one element of an overall assessment of imminent and ongoing dangerousness. Future violent behavior is difficult to predict, but consideration of the following issues is helpful.

a. **Episodic violent behavior.** The fact that violent behavior is an infrequent event for most people increases the difficulty of predicting future occurrences. However, there is always a balance between the individual's internal state, including the degree of tension and the control over expression of aggression, and the environment. Certain combinations of internal and external factors may produce an assaultive crisis. An astute clinician can often identify when a patient is exceeding an acceptable expression of anger and frustration and approaching a loss of control and assaultiveness. Appropriate interventions at various points of this cycle may prevent the crisis or minimize the likelihood of serious injury.

b. **Internal control of violent impulses.** Factors that impair impulse control, either transiently or chronically, may be crucial in determining whether an individual only fears a loss of control or actually acts on his impulses. In addition, violence is more likely to occur in certain contexts. The extent to which the current setting recreates a previous situation that resulted in a loss of control should be examined. The patient's perception of external danger, whether real or imagined, and the need to protect himself are important factors.

c. **Risk factors**

(1) **Demographic indicators.** Boys and men who are 16 to 25 years of age are at particularly high risk for violent behavior. Because domestic violence is so prevalent, parents and spouses are at risk.

(2) **Historic indicators**

(a) A **recent major life change** may place an individual under increased stress and may lead to increased internal tension and frustration. The patient's feelings of internal pressure, frustration, anger, and potential explosiveness should be carefully explored.

(i) Situations and individuals that increase or decrease the feelings of tension should be identified. The patient's attempts to cope with these feelings and the results achieved should be discussed.

(ii) The **patient's level of optimism or pessimism about preventing a violent action** should be noted.

(iii) The patient's **thoughts and fantasies about violence** are also important. Certain sadistic fantasies or violent ruminations may be directed toward a specific individual or group. Specific threats require investigation of the patient's relationship with and access to the threatened individual.

    (iv) **Specific plans and the availability of and familiarity with weapons** increase the danger.

    (v) The **patient's perception of what prevents her from carrying out the violent action** is also important.

    (vi) Current use of **drugs and alcohol** should be explored.

  (b) History of violence

    (i) A history of violent behavior is the most reliable predictor of future violence. This history includes fighting, assaults, arrests, and sanctioned violence (e.g., violent actions by soldiers and police).

    (ii) A history of impulsive or self-destructive behavior, including accidents, arrests for speeding or reckless driving, and self-mutilation, puts the individual at increased risk.

  (c) Childhood history

    (i) A history of witnessing or experiencing neglect or abuse in childhood increases the likelihood of abuse and brutality directed toward the patient's children.

    (ii) A childhood history of cruelty to animals is also associated with continuing aggressiveness.

(3) Diagnostic factors. The common diagnostic denominator is the degree to which the patient's thoughts are impaired in the contexts of hostility, irritability, and distorted perceptions of reality.

(4) Mental status. Fluctuation in the patient's level of agitation throughout the interview should be noted. The patient's impulse control and judgment during the examination may contradict the content of his speech. Command hallucinations to hurt others are particularly worrisome, as are escalating delusional perceptions of external danger because these perceptions may be accompanied by frantic attempts at self-preservation. Sometimes delusional thinking places others in danger in the guise of protecting them. For example, a psychotic mother may believe that she must bathe her child in scalding water to purify her. Any evidence of confusion or an organic mental disorder is significant because it suggests impairment of impulse control and judgment.

(5) Social system. The thoughts of the patient's family and friends concerning his potential for violence should be sought in separate interviews, especially if these individuals are potential victims. The family may provide reliable information about the patient's access to weapons. The clinician should assess whether the potential victim behaves in a challenging or provocative way toward the patient. If the patient appears calm, an interview with both the patient and the potential victim may be necessary to allow the physician to observe their behavior toward each other and to determine whether the crisis is resolved. The use of available community resources beyond those offered by family and friends (e.g., safe houses) should be assessed.

(6) Physician's feelings. Persistent feelings of fear or unease on the part of the physician may be important clues that further investigation and evaluation are necessary.

4. Countertransference reactions to violent patients

  a. Physician's reaction. An angry, agitated, and threatening patient is likely to frighten the physician. The physician's lack of awareness of this fear, previous personal experiences with violence, and conflicts over her own aggressive impulses may affect the physician's response to the patient.

    (1) No reaction. The physician may ignore or minimize the patient's concern with loss of control.

    (2) Anger. In response to her own fears, the physician may become angry and argue with the patient. She may challenge and humiliate the patient, escalating an already dangerous situation.

        (3) Counterphobic reaction. In response to unconscious fear and feelings of lack of control, the physician may act as though she is in control of the situation.

        (4) Overly frightened reaction. The physician may overestimate the patient's violent potential and feel unnecessarily anxious and self-protective.

    b. Consequences. Intense, unacknowledged countertransference reactions can interfere with clinical judgment and treatment. Behavior may range from being overly concerned with control, or even punitive, to releasing the patient prematurely or permitting her to escape to avoid dealing with her. Either way, the patient may receive an inadequate evaluation and inappropriate treatment, and potential victims may remain in considerable danger.

5. Principles of managing the violent patient

    a. Safety

        (1) An adequate number of trained staff members must be available to restrain the patient physically if necessary.

        (2) Staff members should treat the patient firmly, but compassionately.

    b. Behavioral techniques

        (1) It is important to act calmly.

        (2) The clinician and staff members should speak softly in a nonauthoritarian way.

        (3) Both the patient and the examiner should sit during the interview.

        (4) Staff members should check for the presence of weapons and confiscate any that are found.

        (5) There should be immediate access to an exit from the examining room.

        (6) Seclusion and restraint can be used to prevent imminent harm to others.

    c. Psychopharmacologic approach

        (1) Neuroleptics are the most commonly used medications in emergency situations. Haloperidol 5 to 10 mg may be given intramuscularly or orally every 30 minutes until agitation is controlled. The maximum dosage is 100 mg/day. Neuroleptics should be avoided in patients who are experiencing alcohol or drug toxicity or withdrawal.

        (2) Benzodiazepines may be used with neuroleptics and in cases of withdrawal. Lorazepam 2 to 4 mg is given orally or parenterally every 4 to 6 hours. In some patients, benzodiazepines disinhibit violent behavior.

        (3) Phenobarbital in dosages of as much as 640 mg/day orally or amobarbital 200 to 500 mg intravenously (in 10% solution) is effective in managing aggressive behavior in patients with seizures. Side effects include decreased pulse rate and blood pressure.

        (4) Other medications that are useful in managing violent patients include lithium, carbamazepine, phenytoin, and β-blockers such as propranolol.

           (a) Lithium is useful in treating bipolar illness, but it is not effective for treating other conditions.

           (b) Carbamazepine 600 mg/day is effective in decreasing aggressive behavior in some patients with schizophrenia and in those with partial complex seizures.

           (c) Phenytoin is effective in patients with episodic dyscontrol syndrome, although carbamazepine may be more effective.

           (d) Propranolol is effective in the treatment of patients with brain damage.

           (e) Buspirone helps to control aggression in some elderly patients.

    d. Responsibility to warn and protect others

        (1) In American society, an individual is held responsible for his own actions, and information provided to a physician is considered confidential. However, as a result of the *Tarasoff* decision (*Tarasoff v. Regents of University of California,* 1976) and other legal cases involving attacks on third parties, clinicians are now expected to weigh the need for confidentiality against the need to protect others. In the *Tarasoff* case, the clinician was found liable for not warning the plaintiff that the patient had specifically threatened her.

(2) If the patient makes a credible threat to harm a specific person, the clinician has a duty to warn that person. Good medical practice may also require involuntary treatment of the patient.

6. **Spouse abuse.** Violence in the home is pervasive, involving all socioeconomic classes. The most common pattern is husbands battering wives. Surveys indicate that one of four women will be assaulted by a household partner in her lifetime. Sixty percent of female homicide victims are killed by someone they know.

   a. **Clues.** The physician may consider the situation private family business, and therefore avoid involvement. Because the situation may be chronic, with a certain equilibrium, both partners may resist intervention. Also, the distinction between victim and perpetrator is not always clear. The following signs warrant further investigation.

      (1) Unusual or unexplained trauma suggests abuse, especially during pregnancy, which is often a time of particular stress.

      (2) Vague somatic complaints may reflect underlying psychological distress in either partner.

      (3) Threats of violence from either spouse should be investigated.

      (4) Evaluation of any psychiatric symptoms, especially chronic stress and depression, may result in disclosure of abuse at home.

      (5) Overconcern of the patient's spouse or partner, to the extent that the patient is not allowed to be alone or is rushed out of the emergency department, may disguise continuing abuse and a fear of exposure.

      (6) Behavioral problems or psychiatric symptoms in children may reflect chaos and violence in the home.

   b. **Evaluation**

      (1) Victim. After establishing a supportive relationship with the patient, the physician should ask increasingly specific questions about violence, both past and current. The physician should not be deterred by evasive answers or initial denial, but should recognize the vulnerable position of the victim (i.e., she may fear abandonment or retaliation if she is candid and may see no alternatives for herself). A discussion of resources and alternatives (e.g., safe houses) may be helpful early in the interview if the victim is fearful of cooperating.

      (2) Abusive partner. If present, the abusing partner should be evaluated with respect to dangerousness. If he is not present, an assessment of the level of lethality of the situation should still be made. This assessment should include an evaluation of the partner's capacity for impulse control, the availability of weapons, the provocativeness of the victim, and the homicidal potential of both partners.

   c. **Treatment.** The goal of treatment is to prevent further injury to either partner.

      (1) If there is any question about the lethality of the situation or the psychopathology of the partners, **psychiatric consultation** should be requested.

      (2) If lethality or the risk of future injury is high, the battered partner should not return home. Options include staying with friends or family, referral to a safe house, and hospitalization. If the victim refuses treatment, the physician should make her aware of resources and options, but should not pressure her to accept help that she does not want unless she is returning to a life-threatening situation.

      (3) The physician should support the abused partner's decision not to return home, although the physician should not make the decision for the patient, except in the most serious of circumstances. Further treatment is often helpful to the patient during the process of separating from her partner and establishing an independent life. The patient may repeat the pattern of abuse by finding another abusive partner.

      (4) If the lethality of the current situation is low (i.e., the abusive partner wants help to prevent a recurrence), both partners can be referred for treatment, either as a couple or individually. Treatment should always be offered to the abusing spouse.

      (5) The **child welfare agency** should be notified because the children may also be experiencing physical or emotional abuse.

7. Rape is a crime of violence more than a crime of sexuality. It is the most common violent crime in the United States and also one of the most underreported. As many as 70% to 90% of rapes are unreported for a variety of reasons, one of which is continued victimization of affected women by police, courts, hospital staff, and even family and friends.

a. **Characteristics of the crime**

   (1) **Location.** Rape can occur anywhere from a deserted city street at night to a supermarket parking lot at midday to a woman's own home.

   (2) **Violence.** In all rapes, the woman's life is implicitly threatened. Explicit force is used 85% of the time, and victims are struck or choked 50% of the time. Five percent of women are severely beaten.

   (3) **Victims.** Although rape of men occurs, women are usually the victims. In addition, rape is the only violent crime, except perhaps spouse abuse, in which the victim's story is suspect unless she fights back. There is frequently an implication or even an accusation that the victim invited or encouraged the assault.

   (4) **Assailants.** The rapist is usually a man younger than 24 years of age. Most rapists have a police record, and many are sexually impotent before the rape.

b. **Clinical presentation.** The response of a victim to rape is similar to the response to stress in general and the response to other types of assault in particular. However, many issues intensify the conflicts and impair resolution. The following stages are usually observed, and an accurate diagnosis of the patient's stage of recovery can guide treatment.

   (1) **Denial.** The first stage involves shock and disbelief. The woman may describe a feeling of numbness that may last from a few minutes to several hours or days. The victim may appear shaken and drained, but show little overt emotion. The absence of emotional reaction at this stage should not be mistaken for a lack of concern or lack of distress about the assault.

   (2) **Emotional disorganization.** The patient experiences denial, which alternates with periods of intense fear, anger, humiliation, and depression. These feelings may be associated with intrusive memories of the event, nightmares, phobias, hypervigilance, and anxiety. This stage may vary in intensity, and may continue for months or years.

   (3) **Resolution.** The victim naturally attempts to achieve some resolution to her disorganized state, which is distressing and disruptive to normal functioning.

   (a) **Maladaptive resolution.** The victim's attempts at resolution may be maladaptive, and may cause chronic symptoms or new problems that are as bad as or worse than the initial event. Victims may make drastic changes in lifestyle that diffuse their anxiety about future attacks, but may be professionally and socially crippling. Victims may be unable to relate to others, and they often experience a loss of sexual interest. They may abuse drugs or alcohol in an attempt to decrease the level of anxiety and suppress intrusive memories and nightmares. Without active intervention, some victims may commit suicide.

   (b) **Adaptive resolution.** The victim, with or without treatment, gradually integrates the event. There is a decrease in intrusive recollections and feelings as the victim returns to normal functioning in work and relationships. Similar situations or reminders of the attack may trigger transient reemergence of symptoms, but symptoms are usually less intense as time passes.

c. **Evaluation and treatment.** It is difficult to separate evaluation and treatment in cases of rape. The physician, especially if male, must guard against repeating the humiliation by performing an intrusive interview and examination. It is helpful if the victim is treated and counseled by a female practitioner.

   (1) The **rape crisis team** or a psychiatric consultant should be called immediately to help assess the patient's current needs and support her during the examination.

   (2) The **patient's wishes and requests** should be respected. If the patient is alone and wants family or friends contacted, she should be helped in contacting them. If she prefers not to contact anyone, this wish must be honored.

(3) If the patient is experiencing **denial,** her distress should not be underestimated. When she feels safe, the patient may begin to express the feelings and disorganization associated with the next stage of recovery. If she continues to experience denial, the practitioner should explain that it is natural to have feelings and thoughts that may cause considerable distress and that talking about these thoughts will help her to overcome them.

(4) If the patient is **disorganized and upset,** she may feel considerable pressure to review the details of the event and to express her feelings. She may experience guilt, shame, responsibility, vulnerability, and helplessness.

(5) If the patient arrives in the emergency department immediately after a rape, a **medical examination** should be performed after the patient is prepared. Obtaining details of the event is necessary to guide the physical examination. Specimens must be collected in case the patient wants to press charges. There must be discussion, treatment, and follow-up because of the possibility of venereal disease or pregnancy.

(6) The **patient's resources** should be assessed. Meeting with family and friends separately (especially the victim's partner) may help them to express their outrage and conflicting feelings away from the patient and, as a result, to be more supportive of her.

(7) The **patient's decision** about returning home and obtaining subsequent treatment should be respected unless it is clearly unreasonable or dangerous. If the patient appears to be placing herself in jeopardy, physically or emotionally, it may be necessary to insist on further crisis intervention immediately.

(8) **Psychiatric follow-up** should be arranged. If the patient is resistant to treatment, periodic contact with a rape crisis center may be helpful.

C. **Telephone calls**

1. **General issues.** People may call the emergency department for a variety of reasons, some of which may be covert or overt requests for help for any of the crises described. The physician can take limited action over the telephone, but some general principles should be followed.

   a. The patient's name, telephone number, and address should be obtained.

   b. The physician should attempt to establish an alliance with the patient without becoming too involved over the telephone.

   c. The physician should encourage the patient to come to the emergency department as the next step in treatment.

   d. If the patient refuses to come in for evaluation, the physician's assessment of the patient's potential dangerousness dictates how persistently the physician and staff should encourage the patient to come to the hospital.

2. **Covert presentation.** The telephone request may be a subtle clue to a more serious problem. Use of the telephone may reflect the patient's conflict, discomfort, or embarrassment in seeking help. If the patient reveals the underlying reasons for the call, he may feel less isolated and more receptive toward coming to the emergency department or referral to the appropriate resources. The physician should follow up the referral with both the patient and the agency or clinic to verify that contact is made.

3. **Overt presentation**

   a. **The cooperative patient** may describe a crisis overtly and may simply be requesting help to obtain treatment. In other cases, the patient's ambivalence may require the physician to make arrangements with family, friends, or the police to bring the patient to the hospital.

   b. **The uncooperative patient.** If the physician is concerned about imminent danger and the patient refuses to provide information, it may be necessary to trace the call and follow up any leads that the patient gives. Although it can be frustrating, the physician should attempt to build an alliance with the patient, and she should remind the patient of the limitations of telephone contact.

4. **Chronic callers.** Every emergency department has a contingent of chronic callers. Some of these people are lonely and need reassurance. Some are consciously or unconsciously expressing anger by repeatedly frustrating the staff.
   a. **Approach.** Whatever the motivation for the calls, the staff should attempt to place the caller in the appropriate treatment setting.
   b. **Plan.** Regardless of whether the callers go into treatment, a plan for handling them should be established. Identifying information (e.g., name, aliases, content of calls) should be recorded. This process prevents new staff members from becoming tangled in a frustrating situation and minimizes the maladaptive gratification that these individuals receive from making calls.

BIBLIOGRAPHY

American Psychiatric Association: *Diagnostic and Statistical Manual of Mental Disorders,* 4th ed. Washington, DC, American Psychiatric Association, 1994.

Gaw A: *Culture, Ethnicity and Mental Illness.* Washington, DC, American Psychiatric Press, Inc., 1993.

Hales RE, Yudofsky SC, Talbott JA: *Textbook of Psychiatry,* 2nd ed. Washington, DC, American Psychiatric Press, Inc., 1994.

Kessler R, et al: Lifetime and 12-month prevalence of DSM-III-R psychiatric disorders in the United States: Results from the National Comorbidity Survey. *Archives of General Psychiatry.* January, 1994.

Regier DA, et al: The de facto U.S. mental and addictive disorder service system. *Archives of General Psychiatry.* February, 1993.

Stoudemire A, Fogel BS: *Psychiatric Care of the Medical Patient.* New York, Oxford Press, 1993.

Winokur G, Clayton PJ: *The Medical Basis of Psychiatry,* 2nd ed. Philadelphia, WB Saunders, 1994.

STUDY QUESTIONS

DIRECTIONS: Each of the numbered items or incomplete statements in this section is followed by answers or by completions of the statement. Select the ONE lettered answer or completion that is BEST in each case.

1. Special skill is needed in conducting a psychiatric interview because

(A) psychiatric patients usually do not tell the truth
(B) patients may be embarrassed about their symptoms
(C) patients usually cannot remember details
(D) patients may be afraid of the legal consequences of their answers
(E) patients are usually too psychotic to give accurate details

2. The most common drug associated with violent behavior is

(A) phencyclidine (PCP)
(B) cocaine
(C) amphetamines
(D) steroids
(E) alcohol

3. The examination of a patient with a psychiatric disorder should include

(A) a physical examination
(B) laboratory studies
(C) psychological tests
(D) a mental status examination
(E) screening tests for organic illness

4. The psychiatric interview should always be conducted

(A) in a quiet office
(B) with family members
(C) for at least 45 minutes
(D) with complete confidentiality
(E) at eye level

5. The condition in which a person cannot produce normal language because of a neurologic condition is known as

(A) dysarthria
(B) stuttering
(C) echolalia
(D) pressured speech
(E) aphasia

6. Which disorder is most likely to cause violent behavior?

(A) Bipolar disorder: manic type
(B) Anxiety disorder
(C) Major depressive episode
(D) Somatoform disorder
(E) Obsessive-compulsive personality disorder

7. The term for a false perception of a sensory stimulus in the absence of a stimulus is

(A) hallucination
(B) illusion
(C) delusion
(D) derealization
(E) depersonalization

8. A condition in which the patient feels detached from herself is called

(A) derealization
(B) depersonalization
(C) illusion
(D) hallucination
(E) detachment

9. Circumstantiality is a disorder of

(A) mood
(B) affect
(C) speech
(D) behavior
(E) thinking

10. If a patient has a paranoid delusion that the Federal Bureau of Investigation (FBI) is listening to her telephone calls, the physician should

(A) explain to the patient what a delusion is
(B) call the FBI to prove that the idea is false
(C) agree with the patient to establish rapport
(D) listen without agreeing or disagreeing
(E) stop the examination and hospitalize the patient

11. A decrease in rapid eye movement (REM) latency (i.e., the period between the onset of sleep and the onset of the first REM period) is seen in

(A) dementia
(B) delirium
(C) schizophrenia
(D) depression
(E) alcoholism

12. In the National Comorbidity Survey (NCS), the single most common disorder is

(A) schizophrenia
(B) major depression
(C) alcohol dependence
(D) personality disorder
(E) somatization

13. A person who is rated at 50 on the Global Assessment of Functioning (GAF) scale would be expected to have

(A) mild insomnia
(B) difficulty concentrating after an argument
(C) occasional truancy
(D) lack of personal hygiene
(E) suicidal ideation

14. In the clinical examination, questions about parental divorce, early school experiences, or childhood friendships are considered

(A) developmental milestones
(B) social history
(C) informal mental status
(D) history
(E) personality inventory

15. A compound that is found at a decreased level in the cerebrospinal fluid (CSF) of violent offenders is

(A) norepinephrine
(B) acetylcholine
(C) dopamine
(D) lactic acid
(E) 5-hydroxyindoleacetic acid (5-HIAA)

16. Brain activity, rather than structure, is measured by

(A) magnetic resonance imaging (MRI)
(B) positron emission tomography (PET)
(C) computed tomography (CT)
(D) ventricle:brain ratio (VBR)
(E) skull films

17. One finding of the Epidemiologic Catchment Area (ECA) study is that men have higher lifetime rates than women of

(A) schizophrenia
(B) depression
(C) phobia
(D) bipolar disorder
(E) substance abuse

18. Only 42% of persons with one or more mental disorders

(A) are hospitalized in mental facilities
(B) are treated by psychiatrists
(C) receive any professional care
(D) receive medication
(E) have health insurance

19. An example of internal stress is

(A) an episode of mania in a person with bipolar disorder
(B) a myocardial infarction in a 60-year-old man
(C) a divorce after 15 years of marriage in a 40-year-old woman
(D) disorganization in an 18-year-old college student who is away from home for the first time
(E) irritability and loss of impulse control in a 20-year-old man after a minor head injury

20. A person who laughs one minute and cries the next without any clear stimulus has

(A) flat affect
(B) euphoria
(C) labile mood
(D) labile affect
(E) split personality

21. The most reliable predictor of violence is

(A) abuse of alcohol
(B) a history of previous violence
(C) the presence of delirium
(D) the availability of weapons
(E) the presence of psychotic thinking

22. The highest suicide rates occur among

(A) older white women
(B) young black men
(C) older black men
(D) young Asian women
(E) older white men

23. More than half of adult women who are murdered are

(A) killed by someone they know
(B) killed by a stranger
(C) intoxicated by drugs or alcohol
(D) unmarried
(E) killed by a spouse

24. A rape victim who shows a lack of concern and distress shortly after the episode is demonstrating

(A) that the trauma was not severe
(B) some complicity in the event
(C) a stage of denial or numbing
(D) a maladaptive resolution
(E) an incipient psychotic break

DIRECTIONS: Each of the numbered items or incomplete statements in this section is negatively phrased, as indicated by a capitalized word such as NOT, LEAST, or EXCEPT. Select the ONE lettered answer or completion that is BEST in each case.

---

25. The informal mental status examination includes an observation of all of the following factors EXCEPT

(A) the patient's appearance
(B) recent memory
(C) mood and affect
(D) manner of relating
(E) use of language

DIRECTIONS: Each set of matching questions in this section consists of a list of four to twenty-six lettered options (some of which may be in figures) followed by several numbered items. For each numbered item, select the ONE lettered option that is most closely associated with it. To avoid spending too much time on matching sets with large numbers of options, it is generally advisable to begin each set by reading the list of options. Then, for each item in the set, try to generate the correct answer and locate it in the option list, rather than evaluating each option individually. Each lettered option may be selected once, more than once, or not at all.

Questions 26–30

Match each psychological test with its description.

(A) Rorschach test
(B) Minnesota Multiphasic Personality Inventory (MMPI)
(C) Thematic apperception test (TAT)
(D) Wechsler Adult Intelligence Scale (WAIS)
(E) Halstead-Reitan Neuropsychological Test Battery

26. A series of tests, including the rhythm test and the trail-making test, used to study brain function

27. A projective test in which pictures are shown to help the patient to discuss his fantasies and fears

28. A test in which ambiguous forms are shown in a predetermined order

29. A test that generates an intelligence quotient (IQ) score

30. A multiple-question test that measures paranoia, depression, and hysteria

1. The answer is B *[I A 2].* Patients who have psychiatric problems are often embarrassed about disclosing their symptoms to the physician. Stigma regarding psychiatric illness is still prevalent in American society. However, patients do not usually lie when a physician asks questions sensitively. Unless patients have a memory deficit, they can usually give accurate details. Some patients may be afraid of the legal consequences of their answers, but this situation is unusual. Most psychiatric patients are not psychotic, and even many psychotic patients can give accurate details of their history.

2. The answer is E *[VI B 2 c (1)].* Alcohol is the most common precipitating cause of violent behavior in American culture and is the most widely used drug. Cocaine, especially crack cocaine, is associated with a high incidence of violence among users, but together with amphetamines and phencyclidine (PCP), the number of people who use it is much smaller than the number who use alcohol. Steroids can be associated with violent behavior when used medically or when abused by individuals seeking to build their muscle mass, but not with the same frequency as alcohol.

3. The answer is D *[II].* When a patient with a psychiatric disorder is examined for the first time, a mental status examination and a psychiatric interview should always be conducted. Physical examination, psychological tests, and laboratory tests, including screening tests for organic illness, are important, but are not always necessary. For example, a patient who experiences anxiety in addition to headache and tremor should have his blood pressure checked and should undergo laboratory studies of thyroid function.

4. The answer is E *[II A 1 b–e].* The psychiatric interview should always be conducted at eye level with the patient. This practice is especially important when the interview is conducted in a medical setting, such as a general hospital. It is not always possible to conduct an interview in a quiet office. Family members may be interviewed and can often provide helpful information, but issues of confidentiality must be considered. Psychiatric interviews do not have a specific time limit, and although they are generally confidential,

some elements of psychiatric interviews, such as threats against another individual, are not protected by confidentiality.

5. The answer is E *[II B 4 e].* Impaired speech and language because of neurologic illness is called aphasia. The patient cannot speak normally or comprehend speech properly. Aphasia must be distinguished from other psychiatric problems, such as echolalia, pressured speech, or stuttering. Patients with dysarthria have difficulty enunciating, but can produce normal language.

6. The answer is A *[VI B 2 a (1)].* Patients who have bipolar disorder and who are experiencing a manic episode are often irritable and have a low frustration tolerance. They also experience great pressure in their thinking and activity. They may quickly become aggressive if they are slighted or frustrated in their plans. Patients with the other diagnoses may have considerable psychomotor agitation (e.g., those with anxiety disorder or major depressive episodes) or dramatic demands (e.g., those with somatoform disorder), but these patients are far less likely to strike out at others. An individual with obsessive-compulsive personality disorder tends to be overly controlled and avoids direct expression or acknowledgment of anger.

7. The answer is A *[II B 6 a–c, 8 a].* A hallucination is a false perception of a stimulus in the absence of any stimulus. An illusion occurs when there is a misperception of a true stimulus, and a delusion is a fixed, false belief. Depersonalization and derealization are alterations in the perception of reality. They usually occur together. In derealization, the patient perceives her immediate environment as somehow unreal or changed. In depersonalization, the patient feels detached or outside her own body.

8. The answer is B *[II B 6 c].* Depersonalization is the condition in which a patient feels detached from herself and experiences events as though she is an outside observer. The patient's sense of reality is distorted and misperceived. Derealization involves an alteration in the sense of reality of the outside world. Illusion is a misperception of a sensory stimulus, and hallucination is a false perception of a sensory stimulus when one is not present. Detachment is not a technical term used in psychiatry to describe a mental phenomenon.

9. The answer is E *[II B 7 c]*. Circumstantiality is a problem in a patient's thinking that affects the patient's speech pattern. The patient speaks about a given topic, but often loses the point of what he is saying. It is not a disorder of mood or affect. Although this disorder is also called circumstantial speech, it is a problem of thinking rather than a problem of speech.

10. The answer is D *[II B 8 a]*. Because a delusion is a fixed, false belief, it is not useful to attempt to correct the patient's belief, especially during the evaluation interview. It is best to take a neutral stance and continue the interview. Also, it is not helpful for the interviewer to agree with the patient about something that is obviously not true. Although the patient may require hospitalization at some point, it is important to continue the interview to obtain more information.

11. The answer is D *[II C 1 e (2)]*. A decrease in rapid eye movement (REM) latency is seen in the sleep electroencephalograms (EEGs) of depressed patients. This decrease is not found in conditions such as dementia, delirium, schizophrenia, or alcoholism.

12. The answer is B *[IV E 3]*. In structured diagnostic interviews conducted in a national sample of more than 8000 people, major depression is the single most common disorder, with a lifetime incidence of 17.1%; 14.1% report a lifetime history of alcohol dependence. Other disorders are not as prevalent in this study.

13. The answer is E *[III B 2 b; Figure 1-2]*. The Global Assessment of Functioning (GAF) scale is used to rate the highest level of functioning for at least a few months during the last year. It is a 100-point scale, with 100 indicating the highest level of functioning. Suicidal ideation, that is, thoughts of suicide but no action, is listed on example 50 on the GAF. A patient with mild insomnia, occasional truancy, and problems after an argument generally has higher level functioning in the range of 60 to 80. Someone who lacks personal hygiene has a lower rating.

14. The answer is A *[I D 1 a–c]*. The personal history of a patient includes important childhood events. These events are called developmental milestones. The way in which the patient dealt with these events may provide information about his current coping style.

15. The answer is E *[VI B 1 a (1)]*. 5-Hydroxy-indoleacetic acid (5-HIAA) is a metabolite of serotonin. Low levels of this compound in the cerebrospinal fluid (CSF) are associated with increased violent behavior. Causality is not demonstrated.

16. The answer is B *[II C 3 c]*. The positron emission tomography (PET) scan shows specific areas of brain activity (glucose metabolism). The other technologies are used to visualize brain structures.

17. The answer is E *[IV C 1]*. In this study, the overall rates for men and women are approximately the same, but different rates for men and women are reported for certain disorders. Men have higher rates of substance abuse and antisocial personality disorder.

18. The answer is C *[IV F 1]*. Fewer than half of individuals with mental disorders receive professional care. Only 26% receive care in the mental health care sector.

19. The answer is D *[V B 1 a]*. Internal stress may occur in an individual who is faced with a normal developmental task, such as leaving home to attend college. When the individual is unable to accomplish this developmental task, massive psychological disruption may occur, and a psychiatric emergency may result. Although it is appropriate to experience some anxiety on leaving home for college, disorganization in thinking is a result of extreme internal stress. Mania and myocardial infarction are major illnesses and, thus, external stressors. Divorce is an obvious external stress, as is the occurrence of irritability and loss of impulse control after minor closed head trauma.

20. The answer is D *[II B 5 b (1)]*. The person who laughs one minute and cries the next without a clear stimulus from the environment has a labile affect. Mood is considered an emotional state of the patient as experienced by the patient. Because it is unclear what the patient is experiencing, a labile mood is not correct. For example, a patient who is depressed with a depressed mood (i.e., he feels sad inside) may show an anxious affect to the interviewer. Flat affect involves little demonstration of emotion, and split personality is a discrepancy between affective feeling and thought content.

21. The answer is B *[VI B 3 c (2) (b) (i)]*. A history of violence is the most reliable predictor of future violence. It is an indicator that the person previously overcame internal controls against violence. Alcohol is often associated with violence, but it does not cause violent behavior. Delirium is less common. Weapons are readily available in American society, but they do not cause violence. Psychosis is a factor only when the patient has a history of violence.

22. The answer is E *[VI A 2 a (4)]*. Older white men have the highest suicide rate. Although a significant increase is reported in the suicide rates among adolescent boys and among blacks, the overall rates among these groups are lower than that among older white men.

23. The answer is A *[VI B 6]*. Sixty percent of female homicide victims are killed by someone they know, not by a stranger. Battering by a husband or partner is the most common pattern of family violence, but it is not the cause of the majority of homicides in women.

24. The answer is C *[VI B 7 b (1)]*. An early reaction of shock and disbelief can last for days. The reaction is probably an adaptive one, and does not indicate that the trauma was minimal. Feelings of self-blame are common, and are a psychological defense. However, these feelings do not mean that the woman had any role other than victim. Denial is rarely a sign of psychosis.

25. The answer is B *[II A 2 a–i]*. The informal mental status examination begins when the physician first observes the patient. It includes the patient's appearance, manner of relating, use of language, mood and affect, and content of the discussion. Assessment of recent memory requires a formal mental status examination.

26–30. The answers are: 26-E, 27-C, 28-A, 29-D, 30-B *[II D 1, 2 a–c, 3 a (1)–(3)]*. The Halstead-Reitan Battery is a series of subtests, known as neuropsychological tests, that detects cognitive defects and helps in rehabilitation planning.

The thematic apperception test (TAT) is a projective personality test. The patient is shown several pictures and asked to create a story. The patient's response reveals information about the patient.

The famous Rorschach test uses inkblots. It is a projective test that reveals information about the patient's thought patterns.

The Wechsler Adult Intelligence Scale (WAIS) is the most widely used intelligence test. The intelligence quotient (IQ) is arbitrarily defined as mental age/chronologic age $\times$ 100.

The Minnesota Multiphasic Personality Inventory (MMPI) consists of 550 yes-or-no questions. The results are given according to 10 scales, including hysteria, paranoia, and depression.

Chapter 2

Schizophrenic Disorders
Gordon L. Neligh

I. INTRODUCTION

A. | **Definition.** Schizophrenia is a disorder, or a group of disorders, characterized by positive and negative symptoms.

  1. Positive symptoms are those that are added to the clinical picture, including delusions, hallucinations, and agitation.

  2. Negative symptoms are characteristics of the patient that are subtracted from the clinical picture, including affective flattening, social withdrawal, apathy, anhedonia, and poverty of thought and content of speech.

B. | **Diagnosis.** Current criteria for the diagnosis of schizophrenia require that symptoms be present for at least 6 months, although the course varies widely among individuals.

C. | The **etiology** of schizophrenia is **unknown**.

D. | The **prognosis** is **highly variable,** depending at least in part, on the diagnostic criteria used to define the disorder.

E. | Modern **treatment** includes a combination of pharmacologic, psychotherapeutic, and psychosocial interventions, the responses to which are also highly variable.

II. DIAGNOSIS. Established biologic markers or pathognomonic clinical features defining schizophrenia do not exist.

A. | The *Diagnostic and Statistical Manual of Mental Disorders,* 4th edition, (DSM-IV) has been edited so that elements from previous diagnostic systems and from studies of the frequency of symptoms in different populations form the current diagnostic criteria for schizophrenia.

  1. The **diagnostic criteria** of the DSM-IV represent a departure from trends established by the DSM-III and the DSM-III-R in that they are **less specific concerning symptoms** of schizophrenia, and oriented more toward the course of the disorder (Tables 2-1 and 2-2).

  2. The newer criteria are **more inclusive** to include patients who were excluded from the previous criteria.

B. | **The International Pilot Study of Schizophrenia** was an attempt by the World Health Organization to discover reliable methods of diagnosing schizophrenia across different cultures and national boundaries.

TABLE 2-1. DSM-IV Diagnostic Criteria for Schizophrenia

A. Two of the following for most of 1 month:
  1. Delusions
  2. Hallucinations
  3. Disorganized speech
  4. Grossly disorganized or catatonic behavior
  5. Negative symptoms

  (Note: Only one of these is required if delusions are bizarre or if hallucinations consist of a voice keeping up a running commentary on the person's behavior or thoughts, or if there are two or more voices conversing with each other.)

B. Marked social or occupational dysfunction

C. Duration of at least 6 months of persistent symptoms such as attenuated forms of Group A symptoms (above) or negative symptoms. At least 1 month of this must include a Group A symptom.

D. Symptoms of schizoaffective and mood disorder are ruled out.

E. Substance abuse and medical conditions are ruled out as etiological.

---

   1. Using psychiatric interviews and the Present State Examination (PSE), the **most common symptoms** were noted (Table 2-3). However, the most common symptoms are also commonly found in other disorders, such as organic mental disorders and mood disorders.

   2. Disadvantages. This diagnostic approach is of limited use with individual patients because it does not propose minimal or threshold criteria for the diagnosis in individual cases. Rather, it has been a basis for other diagnostic systems, such as the DSM-III-R and to a lesser extent the DSM-IV.

III. EPIDEMIOLOGY. Because of problems in defining the diagnosis of schizophrenia and difficulties in sampling methods, precise epidemiologic data on schizophrenia have been difficult to obtain.

A. Incidence, prevalence, and costs

   1. The **incidence of schizophrenia** has been reported to range from 0.030%–0.120% a year for individuals older than 15 years, with the greatest rates appearing among the industrialized nations and among groups suffering from high levels of cultural disruption. Although the common wisdom holds that men and women develop schizophrenia at the same rate, recent Canadian data suggest that men in a large city develop schizophrenia at a rate two to three times that of women.

   2. Prevalence. As with the incidence of schizophrenia, developing countries generally have lower prevalence rates of schizophrenia, which reflects lower incidence rates and better prognostic expectations than in the industrialized world (e.g., schizophrenic patients in developing countries tend to recover from their illness at a higher rate than do schizophrenic patients in industrialized nations).
     a. Point prevalence (i.e., the number of cases at one moment in time) of schizophrenia has been estimated to range from less than 0.010% to as high as 3.0% in different populations, as a result of both varying diagnostic criteria and true differences.
     b. Lifetime prevalence of schizophrenia in the United States is estimated to be somewhat less than 1.0%.

   3. Costs. In the United States, the indirect costs of schizophrenia have been estimated to be between $10 and $20 billion annually.

TABLE 2-2. Schizophrenia Subtypes

In all of the following subtypes of schizophrenia, the diagnostic criteria for schizophrenia must be met first, particularly criterion A symptoms:

Paranoid type

A. Preoccupation with one or more delusions or frequent auditory hallucinations

B. Does not have prominent disorganized speech, disorganized behavior, flat or inappropriate affect, or catatonic behavior

Disorganized type

A. All of the following are prominent:

   1. Disorganized speech

   2. Disorganized behavior

   3. Flat or inappropriate affect

B. Does not meet criteria for catatonic type

Catatonic type. Clinical picture is dominated by at least two of the following:

A. Motoric immobility as evidenced by catalepsy or stupor

B. Excessive motor activity (apparently purposeless and not influenced by external stimuli)

C. Extreme negativism or mutism

D. Peculiarities of voluntary movement, such as posturing, stereotyped movements, prominent mannerisms, or prominent grimacing

E. Ecolalia or echopraxia

Undifferentiated type. Symptoms of schizophrenia criterion A are present, but the criteria are not met for paranoid, catatonic or disorganized types.

Residual type

A. Criterion A for schizophrenia is no longer met, and criteria for other subtypes of schizophrenia are not met.

B. Evidence of the disturbance (evidenced by negative symptoms or two or more criterion A symptoms) is present in an attenuated form.

B. The sex ratio of schizophrenia is roughly equal in the Western world; however, men tend to develop schizophrenia earlier than women. In developing countries, men appear to suffer from schizophrenia at a rate that may be several times that of women. Perhaps because of the difference in age of onset, men with schizophrenia tend to never have been married, whereas women with schizophrenia tend to be divorced or separated. Perhaps because of a later onset, women tend to have a better prognosis for schizophrenia in many parts of the world.

C. Onset

1. **Onset tends to be earlier for men than women.** Schizophrenia usually occurs in late adolescence or early adulthood, although cases continue to appear with decreasing frequency throughout adult life.

2. **Patients with early onset** tend to have more disorganized features and a worse prognosis for recovery and preservation of function than do patients with late onset.

3. **Patients with late onset** tend to have more paranoid features and a better prognosis and preservation of function than do patients with early onset.

D. **Course and prognosis** vary widely depending on a variety of social, economic, and treatment factors as well as the diagnostic criteria used to define the population.

1. **Social recovery** (i.e., return to independent living and social and occupational functioning) is often more common than is complete remission of symptoms. Several studies

TABLE 2-3. Symptoms of Schizophrenia

Most Frequently Found Symptoms*	Highest Reliability of Symptoms	Lowest Reliability of Symptoms
Lack of insight	Suicidal ideation	Negativism
Auditory hallucinations	Elated thoughts	Perseveration
Verbal hallucinations	Ideas of reference	Stereotyped behavior (e.g., lip smacking, chewing)
Ideas of reference	Delusions of grandeur	
Suspiciousness	Hearing thoughts aloud	
Flatness of affect	Derealization	
Voices speaking to the patient	Lack of concentration	
Delusional mood	Hopelessness	
Delusions of persecution	Delusions of persecution and reference	
Inadequate description of problems		
Thought alienation		
Thoughts spoken aloud		

*In descending order.

    suggest that over a period of 15 years or longer, more than two-thirds of schizophrenic patients experience complete, or "social," recovery with adequate treatment.

    2. Recovery rates are better for the following schizophrenic patients: those with a late onset of illness, those from developing countries, and those recovering in times of economic prosperity.

E. **Socioeconomic status** is correlated with the prevalence and incidence of schizophrenia as well as its course.

    1. In the United States, the highest rates of schizophrenia are found in the lower socioeconomic classes, suggesting that either socioeconomic factors produce or precipitate schizophrenia or that schizophrenic patients tend to drift downward in socioeconomic status (i.e., **drift hypothesis**).

    2. In India, the highest rates of schizophrenia occur in the upper castes, suggesting that social stress on a class of people, rather than drift, may be a major factor in precipitating schizophrenia.

    3. During the **depression of the 1930s,** the outcome of schizophrenia in the United States and Great Britain was worse than either before or after that period of time.

    4. In cities with populations of more than 100,000, the incidence of schizophrenia increases in proportion to the size of the city, although this relationship does not hold true in rural areas and smaller cities.

F. **Familial patterns** of incidence of schizophrenia reveal that biologic relatives of schizophrenics have an increased risk for developing this illness. However, recent studies with narrower diagnostic criteria than used previously suggest lower rates of risk among biologic relatives of schizophrenics than was found in earlier studies.

    1. Twins. Monozygotic twins raised together have a concordance rate of 91%, whereas monozygotic twins raised apart are concordant at a 78% rate in one study. Other studies of twins reveal a concordance rate of 40%–50% for monozygotic twins and about 10%–14% for dizygotic twins.

    2. Parents. If both parents are schizophrenic, the child's risk for developing schizophrenia ranges between 15%–55%.

3. **Relatives.** Some studies show high rates of mental illness (not necessarily schizophrenia) or, in some cases, positive traits, such as creativity, in relatives of schizophrenics.

4. **Genetics.** Patterns of transmission of schizophrenia in families do not fit any known pattern of pure genetic transmission, and current theories suggest a pattern of transmission that may be activated through as yet unknown biologic, social, and psychological factors.

   a. Reports of a gene location on **chromosome 5** associated with some patterns of familial transmission of schizophrenia have failed to replicate in later studies.

   b. **Defects in smooth pursuit eye movements** have also been associated with some familial patterns of transmission of schizophrenia. Although the association cannot explain all of the smooth pursuit ocular motor dysfunction in schizophrenia, it may prove to be a tool in future studies of the genetic transmission of schizophrenia.

G. **Season of birth** appears to be correlated with the risk for developing schizophrenia. In both the Northern and Southern Hemispheres, the risk for developing schizophrenia is greatest for individuals born in the late winter and early spring.

H. The risk of **mortality** for young schizophrenic patients is several times higher than that of the general population. As schizophrenic individuals become older, their risk of mortality approaches that of the general population. The risk of mortality is significantly increased among schizophrenic patients by suicide, accidents, and a number of medical illnesses.

IV. **CLINICAL FEATURES** of schizophrenia vary according to diagnostic criteria used to define the population and, to some extent, the etiologic models of the clinician or researcher. In general, features of schizophrenia reported by patients (e.g., hallucinations) tend to be more reliable than those observed by clinicians (e.g., poverty of thought content). Symptoms of schizophrenia usually include disruptions in areas of psychological and social functioning. However, even in cases of severe disruption, some areas of functioning may be reserved (e.g., a hospitalized patient with chronic schizophrenia who exhibits bizarre behavior and severe disruptions of speech and thinking may retain the skills of a concert pianist). **Symptoms of schizophrenia may change and become less severe over the course of the illness.**

A. **Form of thought** refers to the structure of thought as experienced by the patient and displayed through verbal communication. Disturbances in the form of thought are defined as **formal thought disorder,** which may manifest as the following.

1. **Loosening of associations** is observed in speech when connections among the patient's ideas are absent or obscure. The listener may feel as if his understanding of the patient's thought had been suddenly lost. (This symptom may be contrasted with tangentiality and flight of ideas typical of mania and anxiety disorders, in which ideas are coherent but the patient may lose the point of a string of ideas.) **Examples** of loosening of associations follow.

   a. **Word use may be highly idiosyncratic and individualized.** Words may be created (**neologism**) or selected by the patient according to an internal logic and special symbolism that are the patient's own.

   b. **Abnormal concept formation is a perceptual defect** in which schizophrenic patients are unable to exclude irrelevant or competing ideas from their consciousness; thinking becomes overinclusive. Extraneous items and details that have specific meaning to the patient are incorporated into the patient's communication but are difficult for the listener to follow.

   c. **Logic in schizophrenia may follow a primitive pattern** (in the piagetian sense). Illogical reasoning occurs in schizophrenic patients, as does exclusion of important information from the reasoning process and frank distortion of logical connections. Causal connections are assumed to exist by the patient when no connections can be perceived by others. Symbols may be treated as if they were actual objects or may be inappropriately substituted for other logical elements.

   d. **Concreteness may substitute for abstraction.** The ability to form abstract ideas may be severely impaired. The ability to discern abstractions within ideas may become limited, and concrete interpretations of abstract ideas may become predominant. The ability to understand metaphors and similes may be lost. In general, patients with early-onset schizophrenia may experience greater deterioration of abstraction ability than patients with late-onset disease, as measured by psychological tests. Simultaneous preoccupation with symbols and abstractions, and the loss of the ability to process these, are features commonly seen among schizophrenic patients.

   e. **Language structural problems** are seen in schizophrenia, but many of these problems are rare; however, unusual, stilted language is common. Examples include:

   (1) **Neologisms**

   (2) **Verbigeration** (the persistent repetition of words or phrases)

   (3) **Echolalia** (a repetition of the words or phrases of the examiner, which is seen in severely disorganized psychotic states)

   (4) **Mutism** (a functional inhibition of speech and vocalization, which is seen in a variety of nonpsychotic and psychotic illnesses)

   (5) **Word salad** (a complete lack of language, which is seen in patients with psychosis and several very specific central nervous system lesions)

2. **Poverty of content and speech** is seen in several of the schizophrenic spectrum disorders. Speech may be complex, concrete, or limited in overall productivity, but generally lacks specific information content.

3. **Thought blocking** is an internal interruption in a patient's speech and flow of thought. It may appear that the patient is being interrupted by a hallucination, although the patient may not be able to identify the interruption.

B. **Content of thought.** Among the most characteristic features of schizophrenia are **delusions,** which are defined as fixed, false beliefs. Delusions cannot be changed by reasoning and are inconsistent with the beliefs of the patient's cultural group. However, they may have a culturally based content (e.g., Americans believing that they are the targets of influence by the Central Intelligence Agency). In some cases, delusions may be so individualistic that no cultural connections can be made. Delusions may be relatively circumscribed or may pervade all aspects of the patient's life and thinking. In some cases, delusions may appear relatively trivial to the patient but, more commonly, they become an organizing force in the patient's life. Delusions may be simple in their organization or may be highly complex and systematized. Sexual, religious, and philosophical content of delusions are common.

1. **Delusions of persecution** are ideas that others are trying to harm, spy on, influence, humiliate or interfere with the patient's affairs. Persecutory delusions are frequently pervasive and actively incorporate features of the patient's life.

2. **Delusions of reference** occur when the patient believes that random events in the environment have special meaning and are directed specifically at the patient (e.g., strangers, the television, or the radio are talking about the patient, or random events, such as accidents, have been designed to harm or influence the patient). **Ideas of reference** differ from delusions of reference in intensity rather than form.

3. **Delusions of influence** occur when patients believe that their thoughts and actions are controlled by outside forces. In extreme cases, patients feel as if they were robots without thoughts and actions of their own. Patients may feel that body parts, frequently the genitals, are manipulated by unseen forces. Likewise, patients may feel as if their thoughts have been removed and replaced by alien thoughts.

4. **Thought broadcasting** is experienced by patients as thoughts leaving their head and going directly to objects in the environment. This may be experienced by patients as a physical sensation. For those who have not experienced this phenomenon, thought broadcasting is a symptom that is difficult to understand.

5. **Grandiose delusions** are more common in patients with mania than in those with schizophrenia. However, schizophrenic patients may feel as if they are central figures in the complex delusional systems in the environment. The patient's feelings of having special knowledge, special relationships with important figures, or of posing a threat to conspiracies may all be considered grandiose. These grandiose delusions are differentiated from the expansive and positive grandiose delusions that are typical of mania.

6. **Somatic delusions** in schizophrenic patients typically include feelings that the body has been manipulated or altered by outside forces. These somatic delusions must be differentiated from the somatic delusions of other disorders, such as delusions of having cancer or a decaying body, which are typical of major depression with melancholic features. Patients with somatic delusions may feel that:
   a. An electronic device has been placed in their body.
   b. Their body is under the control of others.
   c. Portions of their body are not their own.

C. **Perceptual disorders** in patients with schizophrenia include a variety of distortions of sensory experiences and their interpretation. **Recent data suggest that a fundamental perceptual defect in schizophrenia is the inability to habituate and suppress extraneous environmental stimuli or internal thought processes.** However, it must be emphasized that **no perceptual disturbance is pathognomonic of schizophrenia.** Perceptual distortions may occur in healthy people as well as in patients with mood disorders or organic mental syndromes.

1. **Hallucinations** are sensory experiences that occur without corresponding environmental stimuli.
   a. **Auditory hallucinations** range from unformed buzzing sounds to complex voices holding conversations. The most characteristic auditory hallucinations of schizophrenia include hearing voices speaking about the patient in the third person, hearing voices making derogatory comments about the patient, and hearing a single voice telling the patient to commit some action. The voices may be muffled or distinct, familiar or unfamiliar, single or multiple, and of either sex. Patients may hear their own voice spoken aloud.
   b. **Command hallucinations** are a special form of auditory hallucination in which voices tell the patient to commit some action. In some patients, these hallucinations are so persistent that they become difficult to resist. When the patient hears command hallucinations telling him to harm himself or someone else, the patient must be considered dangerous.
   c. **Visual hallucinations.** Although more common in other disorders, particularly organic mental disorders, visual hallucinations are also experienced by schizophrenic patients. These hallucinations may be simple, but they are most characteristic of schizophrenia when they are complex and related to the patient's delusional system (e.g., a visit from aliens).
   d. **Other hallucinations may be tactile, gustatory, olfactory** (frequently an unpleasant and indescribable odor), or **somatic.** Like the visual hallucinations, these hallucinatory experiences also occur in other disorders (e.g., olfactory hallucinations in complex partial seizures). In schizophrenic patients, they are frequently connected to delusional systems.

2. **Illusions** are misperceptions or misidentifications of identifiable environmental events or objects that may occur in any sensory modality. Illusions are common in a variety of disorders and occur in normal individuals as well. In schizophrenic patients, illusions may be variants of a normal experience given a delusional explanation.
   a. **Déjà vu** feelings are defined as those in which unfamiliar situations feel strangely familiar. These illusions also occur as a normal phenomenon and in several forms of epilepsy.
   b. **Jamais vu** feelings are defined as those in which familiar situations are experienced as novel and unfamiliar. These illusions also occur in epilepsy.

    c. Hypersensitivity to light, sound, or smell is common in schizophrenia and to other disorders, such as migraine headaches.

    d. Distorted perceptions of time also occur in a variety of conditions, such as dissociative states and anxiety.

    e. Misperceptions of movement, perspective, and size, which are typical of organic conditions and anxiety, also occur in schizophrenia.

    f. Changes in body perception of one's own body or the body of others also occur.

D. **Affect** is defined as the observable manifestations of mood and emotion. Affective findings in patients with schizophrenia may be, in some cases, unreliable due to the parkinsonian effects of the neuroleptic drugs and to cultural differences in body language. Affective disturbances in schizophrenia include **blunted affect, flat affect,** and **inappropriate affect** (see Chapter 1).

E. **Sense of self** is the perception of one's individuality, separateness from others, and continuity in space and time. The erosion of the sense of self may lead to the delusions of reference and influence found in schizophrenia.

    1. In normal individuals, a solid sense of self is thought to be the basis of good self-esteem and an ability of the individual to weather losses, disappointments, and slights from others.

    2. In schizophrenia, as well as in other conditions, a disrupted sense of self may manifest as:
      a. Loss of self-esteem
      b. Confusion about sexual identity
      c. An inability to separate oneself from events in the environment (i.e., feeling that one's thoughts have harmed another person)
      d. Projection of one's own fears or suspicions onto others
      e. Experiencing the self and others as dichotomous opposites (i.e., all good or all bad) with little integration of the opposing features

F. **Volitional symptoms** of schizophrenia are among the most persistent and intractable. Difficulties initiating and maintaining purposeful and goal-directed activity and interest in the environment may account for the difficulties many patients with schizophrenia experience in maintaining stable work and living situations.

    1. Interest in the environment may be difficult to generate and maintain for schizophrenic patients. This difficulty may be related to ambivalence, resulting from conflicting wishes or desires, or to an inability to generate interest internally.

    2. Initiative, or the ability to begin a goal-directed activity, is often lacking in advanced cases of schizophrenia. Patients may experience difficulty finding housing, financial support, and other needs as a consequence of this symptom. They also may be unable to initiate spontaneous movement without direction from others.

    3. Drive is the ability to pursue a goal-directed activity after it has been started. Difficulties in maintaining goal-directed behavior appear to be common in, although not unique to, schizophrenia. These difficulties may be a result of the cognitive symptoms experienced by these patients or the inability to sustain thoughts amid the perceptual and cognitive disturbances of schizophrenia.

    4. Ambition may be preserved in the absence of drive and initiative, as in patients whose grandiose wishes are to be film or music stars, or it may be absent. Unrealistic ambitions combined with the patient's delusions may be an organizing principle for complex dysfunctional patterns of behavior.

G. **Relationship to the external world.** The tendency for patients to become increasingly preoccupied with internal events and decreasingly influenced by external events is characteristic of schizophrenia. Preoccupation with delusional and hallucinatory symptoms and difficulty in communicating with others may lead to withdrawal from the world, which in its extreme form is called **autism.**

H. **Motor activity.** Some alterations in motor activity and behavior may be associated with the pharmacologic treatment of schizophrenia.

1. **Quantitative changes.** The amount of activity and its "driven" quality ranges from the extremes of agitation in excited catatonic states and acute psychotic exacerbations to the withdrawn and inactive states associated with catatonic stupor and chronic institutionalization. **Akathisia, bradykinesia,** and **tardive dyskinesia** are commonly associated with the effects of neuroleptic medications rather than with schizophrenia.

   a. **Catatonic stupor** is a state of dramatic motor inactivity in which patients may, if untreated, be immobile for weeks or months at a time. Patients may be unable to initiate eating, drinking, or elimination functions. As patients recover, it is clear that they have been aware of events in the environment. Patients in this state may require aggressive medical care to avoid dehydration, electrolyte disturbances, and infections. Catatonic stupor may change abruptly to catatonic excitement in some cases. Medical illnesses and affective disorders are the most common causes of catatonia.

   b. **Catatonic excitement,** a hypermetabolic state, is a psychiatric emergency. The patient's activity and speech may be excessive, driven, and purposeless. Patients in this state may be violent. Before pharmacologic and electroconvulsive treatments were available, patients in this state frequently died of acute hyperthermia. Catatonic excitement may also be caused by organic conditions (e.g., use of phencyclidine) and mania.

2. **Qualitative changes.** Psychopharmacologic interventions frequently confuse the clinical picture of movement abnormalities by adding features of parkinsonian movement difficulties and the choreoathetotic movements of tardive dyskinesia. Even without pharmacologic treatment, patients with schizophrenia may show a variety of movement abnormalities (e.g., increased flexor muscle tone, unusual mannerisms, bizarre gestures).

   a. **Catatonic posturing** is demonstrated by patients who assume strange postures and hold them for long periods.

      (1) **Catatonic rigidity** is demonstrated by patients who resist being moved from their unusual rigid postures.

      (2) **Waxy flexibility.** Patients' limbs may be moved like wax, and they will hold the newly assumed position for long periods of time.

   b. **Echopraxia** is the behavioral equivalent of echolalia. Patients involuntarily mimic the movements of another person.

   c. **Automatic obedience** refers to the following of directives in an unquestioning, robot-like manner.

   d. **Mannerisms and grimacing.** The manner of schizophrenic individuals may appear artificial and stilted. Inappropriate silliness is seen, particularly in hebephrenic patients and patients with frontal lobe damage, and is frequently accompanied by unusual mannerisms. Particular mannerisms may have special meanings that are connected to delusions or hallucinations. Grimacing movements may be subtle or pronounced but may be mistaken for the orofacial dystonias of tardive dyskinesia.

   e. **Stereotyped behaviors** (stereotypy). Purposeless repetitive movements (or verbalizations) are seen in a variety of conditions. These movements may involve the entire body, such as rocking, or may involve repetition of complex gestures. The movements may have magical significance or may be purposeless to the patient.

   f. **Perseveration** is involuntary repetition of a task. For example, patients who are asked to copy a series of circles may continue to copy the figures until they run off the page. Patients may repeat an answer to a question until asked to stop. Perseveration is also seen in patients with organic mental syndromes, particularly in those with damage to premotor areas.

I. **Social behavior.** In early and severe cases of schizophrenia, there may be a loss of the social skills, body language, and empathic abilities that permit people to interact successfully with others and to pursue social and vocational functioning. Schizophrenic individuals frequently are perceived by others as bizarre, hostile, or socially inappropriate. Impairment of social skills; disturbances of thought, perception, speech, and behavior; or long-term institutionalization can result in schizophrenic patients who are severely socially debilitated and who may live on the fringe of society as severely dysfunctional "street people." In the past, these same individuals may have been long-term institutionalized patients.

V. **PATHOGENESIS.** The course of schizophrenia may be highly variable, ranging from the presence or absence of a prodromal phase, remission or lack of between episodes, a downward deteriorating course, or full or social recovery.

A. **Premorbid personality.** Although certain personality features seem to antedate the development of schizophrenia in about 25% of cases, research has not demonstrated specific personality features that reliably predict the development of schizophrenia. A study of home movies suggests that preschizophrenic children showed greater negative affect than did normal siblings, and female preschizophrenic children consistently showed less joy in their facial expressions.

B. **Family interactional patterns** are thought by some investigators to be potential predisposing factors to the development of schizophrenia. Whatever the premorbid interactive pattern is between children who develop schizophrenia and their parents, the relationship between the initial onset of schizophrenia and parental interactive styles is unclear. Any premorbid pattern should not be confused with findings that expressed emotionality (EE) in families may precipitate relapses in schizophrenic patients.

1. Some studies suggest that children predisposed to schizophrenia do not exhibit the same responsiveness to mothers as do other children, and mothers of these children react to this lack of responsiveness with frustration and disappointment.

2. Other studies suggest that mothers of schizophrenic patients are overly anxious, rejecting, aggressive, and indifferent.

3. Recent studies suggest that parents' relatively normal reactions to certain cognitive and interactive patterns of preschizophrenic children may be associated with the eventual development of schizophrenia. For example, social awkwardness in a child may be met with overprotection and disappointment by the parents.

C. **Initiating factors** do not appear to be specific to schizophrenia but represent specific stresses that interact with a predisposing trait to precipitate schizophrenia.

1. **Time of onset.** The peak time of onset of schizophrenia is in late adolescence and early adulthood. This is a time of multiple stresses related to leaving home, choosing a career, and developing relationships. A smaller peak occurs in the fourth decade, particularly among women.
   a. It has been proposed that separation from parents unmasks psychotic features that have been present since childhood.
   b. Other studies suggest that these intense stresses are responsible for activating the processes that result in schizophrenia.

2. **Precipitating events**
   a. **Psychosocial stressors.** Cultures experiencing social and economic stress are associated with high rates of schizophrenia. However, it cannot yet be determined which stressors produce schizophrenia in vulnerable individuals and which do not.
   b. **Traumatic events.** On a case-by-case basis, specific traumatic events that appear to precipitate schizophrenic symptoms can be isolated. It is not clear, however, that either the level of stress or loss for the schizophrenic individual is different than might be experienced by a normal individual.
   c. **Drug and alcohol abuse.** Certain drugs (e.g., amphetamines, cocaine, hallucinogens, phencyclidine, anticholinergics) and alcohol may precipitate schizophrenic symptoms. It is not clear whether these drugs cause syndromes that resemble

schizophrenia or whether these drugs precipitate schizophrenia in vulnerable individuals. In some cases, use of these drugs may represent an attempt at self-treatment
in individuals who are developing schizophrenia.

D. **Clinical course**

    1. Onset. The onset of schizophrenia is variable and has prognostic significance.

        a. Acute. Schizophrenia may present abruptly with confusion, agitation, affective
involvement, hallucinations, and delusions, following an identifiable stressor. This
clinical picture may develop in a period as short as 1 or 2 days; however, relatively
few of these patients develop schizophrenia with the chronic course required for a
DSM-IV diagnosis. Instead, they meet the criteria for **brief reactive psychosis** or
schizophreniform disorder, which has a less than 6-month course.

        b. Trema (German for "stage fright") is characterized by anxious, irritable, and
depressed feelings that may last from a few days to 1 month or longer. These feelings may be a reaction to perceptions that something is going wrong. As this condition progresses, the patient may feel as though the environment is odd and
ominous.

        c. An insidious prodromal phase portends a bad prognosis when psychotic features
eventually appear. In general, the prognosis is worse if the patient experiences substantial deterioration in functioning without ever having achieved a high level of
psychosocial functioning before the onset of psychotic symptoms. This course may
be associated with subsequent high levels of negative symptoms. Symptoms
observed in patients with this pattern of onset include:

        (1) Social withdrawal

        (2) Impairment in role functioning (e.g., as a student, parent, spouse)

        (3) Peculiar behavior

        (4) Neglect of grooming and personal hygiene

        (5) Blunted or inappropriate affect

        (6) Vague, digressive, overelaborative, or circumstantial speech, or poverty of
speech or content of speech

        (7) Odd beliefs that are inconsistent with the cultural group of which the patient is a
member, or magical thinking that influences behavior

        (8) Unusual perceptual experiences, such as recurrent illusions, "telepathy," or
recurrent déjà vu experiences

        (9) Marked lack of initiative, drive, ambition, interest, or energy

    (10) Diminished ability to correctly perceive social cues, particularly abstract social
cues

    2. Active phase. Schizophrenia cannot be diagnosed without an active phase, involving
active hallucinations, delusions, catatonic behavior, or grossly inappropriate affect and
behavior. This phase may remit in part or completely or continue as the central feature
of the clinical course.

    3. Residual phase. Symptoms of the residual phase are largely those of the prodromal
phase. Negative symptoms of schizophrenia may be prominent, and difficulty
recovering previous levels of psychosocial functioning may be a major part of the
clinical picture. A variety of different lifetime courses have been described, and
recovery of social function is more common than is complete recovery from residual
symptoms.

    4. Duration. Symptoms of schizophrenia must be present for at least 6 months for a diag-
nosis of schizophrenia to be made.

        a. For patients without symptoms for 6 months, a variety of other diagnoses may be
appropriate, including schizophreniform disorder, brief reactive psychosis, and atypical psychosis.

        b. If there is **no episode of acute psychosis,** diagnoses of schizoid or schizotypal per-
sonality disorder, delusional disorder, paranoid personality disorder, or borderline
personality disorder may be appropriate.

5. Deterioration from a previous level of functioning is a key feature. Role performance in relationships, work, self-care, or school performance is impaired, and residual symptoms may interfere with social functioning. However, recent studies challenge the assumption that this deterioration is uniform and lifelong.

    a. Patterns of long-term courses. A large number of courses for individual schizophrenic patients has been described. Onset may be acute or insidious. The course may involve a single continuous episode of symptoms, may be episodic, or may evolve from an episodic to a continuous course. Outcome may range from eventual severe impairment to complete recovery. Almost all combinations of these elements are possible. About 25% of schizophrenic patients experience the insidious onset of symptoms, continuous course, and eventual severe impairment.

    b. Patterns of recovery. Different measures of recovery produce very different outcome estimates.

        (1) Social recovery is often defined as economic and residential independence with low disruption in social relationships. Errors in this measurement are possible because it is tied to the status of the economy and to the level of tolerance for social deviance in the culture. These rates tend to be higher than those for complete recovery.

        (2) Complete recovery implies complete remission of psychotic symptoms and return to previous levels of social and occupational functioning.

        (3) Hospitalization rates have been used to measure failures in recovery. Although easiest to measure, it is probably the least accurate measure of the course of schizophrenia. Rates of rehospitalization may depend on a variety of factors, ranging from the available health care resources and service delivery systems to the community acceptance of deviant behavior.

E. **Prognosis.** Much of the data on the prognosis of schizophrenia is based on observations of the disease courses of less than 10 years or of patients whose behaviors may represent adaptations to institutionalized life. In addition, the prognosis of schizophrenia may depend on socioeconomic factors and the availability of adequate psychosocial interventions. Many of the factors following may be seen as intermediate-term prognostic factors.

    1. Statistics

        a. Modern treatment methods in the United States make it possible for about 90% of schizophrenic patients to recover sufficiently to live outside the hospital most of the time.

        b. Some studies suggest that about 75% of individuals who meet the diagnostic criteria for schizophrenia will experience substantial or complete recovery 20 to 25 years (or longer) after the onset of illness.

    2. Prognostic variables in schizophrenia fall into several groups. Early in the course of schizophrenia, a number of variables have been identified that predict a short-to-intermediate course in schizophrenia. Long-term prognostic factors have not been identified. Positive symptoms (see I A 1) carry much less ominous prognostic implications than do negative symptoms (see I A 2).

        a. Separation of good from poor prognostic factors. Patients currently fitting DSM-IV diagnostic criteria for schizophrenia are a group that has been selected for poor prognostic features in the short or intermediate term.

            (1) Acute psychotic disorders are now considered to be **schizophreniform disorder** or **brief reactive psychosis** if they do not continue for the 6-month course required for a diagnosis of schizophrenia.

            (2) Patients with mood disorders in addition to psychotic symptoms are now diagnosed as having **schizoaffective disorder, major depression with psychotic features,** or **bipolar mood disorder**.

            (3) Many patients previously considered to be schizophrenic are now included in diagnostic categories of **delusional disorder** and **borderline personality disorder**.

b. Poor prognostic factors. Patients with a predominance of negative symptoms, poor cognitive performance on neuropsychological testing, and abnormalities on computed tomography (CT) and positron emission tomography (PET) scans are reported to have poor outcomes.

F. **Complications**

1. **Social network.** Compared with normal individuals, chronic schizophrenic patients tend to have small social networks. Whereas the social networks of normal individuals may be composed of 20 to 30 individuals, chronic schizophrenic patients may have networks as small as three to five people. The networks of people with chronic mental illnesses also tend to be highly interconnected.
   a. Before the onset of illness, schizophrenic patients have fewer and less satisfactory social relationships than do those with affective disorders or than do normal subjects.
   b. Social connections outside the family are associated with a good prognosis.
   c. In contrast to affective psychosis, family involvement in one study had a negative prognostic significance.

2. **Impaired educational achievement.** Despite normal or high intelligence, many schizophrenic patients are unable to complete educational plans after the onset of illness.

3. **Impaired work performance.** Employment appears to improve the prognosis of schizophrenic patients. However, these patients may have significant difficulties finding employment, particularly during economic depressions. Schizophrenic patients often are employed at jobs requiring lower skill than their educations and intelligence suggest they have.

4. **Sexual relationships.** Marriage rates for those with schizophrenia are lower than rates for the general population. Schizophrenic men tend to be married less frequently than schizophrenic women. Some reports suggest that sexual dysfunction is common in schizophrenic men and women.

5. **Crime.** Schizophrenic patients are not more violent than the average person in the population, despite the frequent publicity of bizarre and violent crimes committed by schizophrenic people. There is evidence that when services are not provided to schizophrenic patients through the mental health service delivery system, they may enter the criminal justice system, often for relatively minor crimes. This process is often referred to as the **criminalization of the mentally ill**.

6. **Premature death.** Schizophrenic patients risk premature death from suicide, homicide, and medical illnesses (e.g., cardiovascular disease, infectious diseases, cancer). A particular risk factor for people with schizophrenia is smoking. Some evidence suggests that smoking briefly "normalizes" some average evoked potential abnormalities associated with schizophrenia, leading to the hypothesis that schizophrenic patients may smoke heavily as a form of self-treatment of symptoms. Neoplasms that are common in patients with schizophrenia are those associated with smoking.

7. **Poverty.** According to the Epidemiologic Catchment Area studies, people in the lowest socioeconomic quartile had an eightfold increase in their risk of schizophrenia over those in the highest quartile.

8. **Homelessness.** An estimated 5%–8% of people with schizophrenia are homeless. Many more live in substandard housing or depend on relatives to maintain their standard of living, including housing.

9. **Psychiatric comorbidity.** Patients with schizophrenia are reported to suffer from other psychiatric symptoms, including anxiety, depression, and obsessive-compulsive symptoms. It is not clear in all cases that these reports represent carefully screened populations (e.g., excluding autistic people from the sample) or that depressive symptoms have been differentiated from deficit symptoms.

VI. **DIFFERENTIAL DIAGNOSIS.** The diagnosis of schizophrenia is made after a complete clinical and historical evaluation of the patient. Patients who fit the current diagnostic criteria for schizophrenia are unlikely to be confused with other diagnostic groups. However, symptoms suggestive of schizophrenia may be found in a number of conditions, which must be ruled out (Table 2-4).

A. **Organic mental disorders and syndromes (psychotic symptoms attributable to a medical condition)**

1. An acute medical illness affecting the brain, which may present with psychotic symptoms, is called a **delirium**.

2. Long-term, supposedly irreversible medical or neurologic syndromes with cognitive and psychiatric features are called **dementias**. Dementias often mimic the negative symptoms of schizophrenia.

3. **Differentiation.** To differentiate schizophrenia from organic mental syndromes, the psychiatrist must rely on a high index of suspicion, an exacting mental status examination, physical and neurologic examinations and, sometimes, a neuropsychological examination.
   a. Localized brain illnesses and injuries may produce **focal abnormalities,** resulting primarily from localized damage to the brain that can mimic a variety of cognitive, behavioral, and even linguistic findings found in schizophrenia.
   b. **Nonfocal,** or generalized, **alterations** in brain function can present with acute confusion and psychotic symptoms suggestive of schizophrenia. Visual hallucinations are somewhat more common, and auditory hallucinations are less common in organic mental syndromes.

4. **Medical disorders** known to cause psychiatric symptoms should be considered when evaluating patients (see Table 2-4).

B. **Mood disorders** are often accompanied by symptoms that are confused with those of other psychotic illnesses, including schizophrenia. For example, depression with severe melancholic features is, in some studies, a more common cause of the catatonic syndrome than schizophrenia. Mood-congruent delusions and hallucinations are a common feature of severe mood disorders.

1. **Manic episodes.** Manic patients who present with irritability, suspicions of persecution, delusions, and hallucinations may be indistinguishable from patients with schizophrenia. At the height of a manic episode, the patient may demonstrate bizarre behaviors, incoherence, and other features thought to be pathognomonic of schizophrenia. Careful family histories and longitudinal observations may be required to differentiate these conditions.
   a. If organic causes for the manic syndrome and personality disorder have been ruled out, a manic episode by definition implies that the patient suffers from **bipolar disorder**.
      (1) Patients with bipolar disorder usually suffer from both manic and depressive episodes at some time in their lives. However, in some patients only mania is present.
      (2) The typical patient with bipolar mood disorder suffers more from manic episodes early in life and from depression in later years.
   b. In many cases, there may be two or more mood cycles per year, including mania and major depression. In extreme cases, patients may experience over four episodes of illness per year and up to several per day. These patients are called **rapid cycling bipolar disorder** patients.

2. **Major depressive episodes** (including those associated with bipolar disorder). Patients with severe depression may present with paranoid symptoms, social withdrawal, and severely restricted affect, all of which are suggestive of schizophrenia. Patients who develop melancholic features and delusions concerning cancer, a rotting body, guilt, and other mood-congruent delusions particularly resemble schizophrenic

TABLE 2-4. Medical Disorders That Can Mimic Schizophrenia

Disorders	Comments
Vascular disorders	Vascular disorders must be considered in older patients. Cerebral vasculitis is particularly apt to mimic schizophrenia.
Autoimmune diseases	SLE is notorious for mimicking schizophrenia. Steroids used in treatment of autoimmune disease may cause organic mental syndromes.
Nutritional deficiencies	Overdoses of vitamins are also part of the differential diagnosis.
Metabolic disturbances	
Alcoholism	Delirium tremens and alcoholic hallucinations are frequently mistaken for acute schizophrenia.

Sleep disorders
   Sleep apnea
   Kleine-Levin syndrome
   Narcolepsy
	Narcolepsy is more likely to present with symptoms of depression than schizophrenia.

Hydrocephalus
   Obstructive hydrocephalus
   Normal-pressure hydrocephalus	

Epilepsy
   Complex partial seizures
   Absence seizures	

Degenerative diseases	Degenerative diseases occur more often in older people, who have a low probability of developing schizophrenia.

Congenital disorders
   A subclinical form of PKU
   Smaller twin
   Minimal brain dysfunction
	The development of schizophrenia is associated with the smaller of a pair of twins who has poor motor function and slow development, theoretically as a result of intrauterine insult. Children and adolescents who demonstrate symptoms of minimal brain dysfunction may develop schizophrenia.

Infections
   Bacteria
   Fungi
   Viruses
   Parasites
	Bacterial infection, particularly associated with meningitis, may be the cause of an organic mental syndrome. Although rare, parasitic infection can result in a dramatic organic mental syndrome.

Toxicity
   Drug abuse
   Abuse of gasoline and toulene-based inhalants
   Carbon monoxide
   Lead
   Agricultural and industrial chemicals
   Prescribed medication
      Digitalis
      Anticholinergics
      Antihypertensives
      CNS depressants
      Steroids	

Traumatic insults to the brain
   Acute subdural hematomas
   Chronic subdural hematomas
   Direct trauma
   Postconcussion syndrome
   Left temporal lobe damage
	Left temporal lobe damage is particularly likely to produce schizophrenia-like symptoms.

Endocrine disorders
   Thyroid problems
   Parathyroid problems
   Pituitary adenomas
   Pheochromocytoma	

Neoplasms	In addition to primary and metastatic tumors of the brain, tumors in other parts of the body can cause psychiatric symptoms and cognitive deficits through paraneoplastic effects.

CNS = central nervous system; PKU = phenylketonuria; SLE = systemic lupus erythematosus.

individuals. Likewise, indecisiveness, slowing of thoughts, and lack of spontaneity in speech and behavior may resemble the negative symptoms of schizophrenia. Recent studies suggest that depression, at least in the first episode of psychosis, may be part of the overall illness pattern, which remits along with other acute symptoms and without additional treatment. This implies that separating depressive symptoms from acute psychotic symptoms may be unwarranted.

3. **Postpsychotic depression.** There is some controversy as to whether postpsychotic depression represents a true depression with the same biologic features as a major depressive episode, or if it represents a phase of predominant negative symptoms of schizophrenia. Likewise, oversedation and parkinsonian symptoms may resemble the clinical picture of depression. During a first psychotic episode, different criteria reveal that up to 75% of patients suffer from depressive symptoms. However, 98% of these symptoms remitted with the resolution of psychosis. This suggests that antidepressant treatment should not be initiated except in patients for whom depression persists after the resolution of psychotic symptoms.

4. **Schizophreniform disorder** (Table 2-5). This diagnostic category was created to differentiate those who were previously regarded as "good prognosis" schizophrenic patients from "poor prognosis" schizophrenic patients. Patients with symptoms suggestive of schizophrenia for whom no organic cause for psychotic symptoms has been found and who meet the diagnostic criteria for schizophrenia, except that their symptoms have lasted less than 6 months, are appropriately diagnosed as having schizophreniform disorder. A few patients with schizophreniform disorder eventually meet the criteria for schizophrenia. However, the majority of patients with schizophreniform disorder recover without ever having met the diagnostic criteria for schizophrenia.

5. **Schizoaffective disorder** (Table 2-6). Patients present with either a manic episode or a major depressive episode with acute psychotic symptoms suggestive of schizophrenia or as an episode of psychotic symptoms without mood symptoms (in an individual in whom a mood disorder has been previously diagnosed). Criteria for diagnosing this disorder are as follows.
   a. The patient has a family history that is more positive for mood disorder than for schizophrenia.
   b. The patient has a prognosis intermediate between mood disorders and schizophrenia.
   c. The patient frequently responds to combinations of medications and treatments used for both schizophrenia and mood disorders.

6. **Delusional disorder** (Table 2-7). This relatively rare disorder may be mistaken for schizophrenia, unless a careful history is taken and corroborated as much as possible. These patients often have prominent delusions of a nonbizarre nature, but have not met criterion A for schizophrenia for more than a few hours. Also, these patients lack the global functional deterioration that is common in patients with schizophrenia. Delusions may be plausible (e.g., being followed, being poisoned, having a serious disease).

TABLE 2-5. DSM-IV Diagnostic Criteria for Schizophreniform Disorder

A. Meets criteria A, D, and E of schizophrenia

B. An episode of the disorder lasts at least 1 month but less than 6 months.

Prognostic features should be specified in the diagnosis:
   With good prognostic features (at least two of the following):
   1. Onset of prominent psychotic symptoms within 4 weeks of the first noticeable change in usual behavior or functioning
   2. Confusion or perplexity at the height of the psychotic episode
   3. Good premorbid social and occupational functioning
   4. Absence of blunted or flat affect

Without good prognostic features:
   Should be specified if good prognostic features are absent

TABLE 2-6. DSM-IV Diagnostic Criteria for Schizoaffective Disorder

A. An uninterrupted period of illness during which there is either a major depressive episode or manic episode concurrent with symptoms that meet criterion A for schizophrenia

B. During the same period of illness, there have been delusions or hallucinations for at least 2 weeks in the absence of prominent mood symptoms.

C. Symptoms meeting criteria for a mood episode are present for a substantial portion of the total duration of the active and residual periods of the illness.

D. Not due to direct effects of substance abuse

Specify type:
　Bipolar type: if manic episode or both manic and major depressive episodes
　Depressive type: if major depressive episode only

7. **Brief psychotic disorder** (Table 2-8). Like schizophreniform disorder, this diagnostic category describes patients who were considered schizophrenic under previous diagnostic criteria but whose good prognosis differentiates them from the patients diagnosed as schizophrenic under current criteria. The illness of a brief psychotic disorder lasts **between 1 day and 1 month**. Clearly, the differential diagnosis for an acutely psychotic person is very large, with a need to rule out medical conditions, substance abuse, and mood disorders.

8. **Atypical psychosis** is a diagnosis of exclusion. This category is reserved for patients who have some diagnostic features of schizophrenia but who do not fit all the criteria for schizophrenia. This diagnosis is appropriate for patients with nonorganic psychotic presentations, which, after exhaustive examination, do not fit another diagnostic criterion for classification of psychotic symptoms.

9. **Personality disorders.** With the decline of the use of such terms as "process schizophrenia" and "pseudoneurotic schizophrenia," there has been less diagnostic confusion

TABLE 2-7. DSM-IV Diagnostic Criteria for Delusional Disorder

A. Nonbizarre delusions (i.e., involving situations that could occur in real life such as being followed, poisoned, infected, having a disease, loved at a distance) of at least 1 month's duration

B. Has never met criterion A for schizophrenia (for more than a few hours)

C. Apart from the impact of the delusion(s) or its ramifications, functioning is not markedly impaired and behavior is not obviously odd or bizarre

D. If mood episodes have occurred concurrently with delusions, total duration has been brief relative to the duration of the delusional periods

E. Not due to the direct effects of a substance (e.g., drugs of abuse, medication) or a general medical condition

Specify type:
　Erotomanic type: delusions that another person, usually of higher status, is in love with the individual

　Grandiose type: delusions of inflated worth, power, knowledge, identity, or special relationship to a deity or famous person

　Jealous type: delusions that one's sexual partner is unfaithful

　Persecutory type: delusions that one (or someone to whom one is close) is being malevolently treated in some way

　Somatic type: delusions that the person has some physical defect or general condition

　Mixed type: delusions characteristic of more than one of the above types but no one theme predominates

　Unspecified type

TABLE 2-8. DSM-IV Diagnostic Criteria for Brief Psychotic Disorder

A. Presence of at least one of the following symptoms:
  1. Delusions
  2. Hallucinations
  3. Disorganized speech (e.g., frequent derailment or incoherence)
  4. Grossly disorganized or catatonic behavior
B. Duration of an episode of the disturbance is at least 1 day and no more than 1 month, with eventual return to premorbid level of functioning. (When the diagnosis must be made without waiting for the expected recovery, it should be qualified as "provisional.")
C. Not better accounted for by a mood disorder (i.e., no full mood syndrome is present) or schizophrenia, and not due to the direct effects of a substance or general medical condition
Specify if:
  With marked stressor(s) (brief reactive): if symptoms occur shortly after and apparently in response to events that, singly or together, would be markedly stressful to almost anyone in similar circumstances in the person's culture

  Without marked stressor(s): if psychotic symptoms do not occur shortly after or are not apparently in response to events that, singly or together, would be markedly stressful to almost anyone in similar circumstances in the person's culture

  With postpartum onset: if onset within 4 weeks' postpartum

between schizophrenia and personality disorders. However, in the case of several specific personality disorders, features of the clinical presentation may be confused with those of schizophrenia. Personality disorders most likely to be confused with schizophrenia include the following (using DSM-IV nomenclature):

  a. **Paranoid personality disorder.** People suffering from this disorder interpret the actions of others as deliberately demeaning or threatening. Behavior is characterized by questioning the loyalty of others, holding grudges about insults or slights, and lacking trust in others. This disorder can be differentiated from paranoid schizophrenia in that it lacks acute psychotic episodes and extreme deterioration.

  b. **Schizoid personality disorder** is often found among biologic relatives of schizophrenic patients, suggesting that these disorders share some undetermined genetic commonality. The lack of social interests of these patients results in a restricted lifestyle, which may be confused with the social deterioration of schizophrenia. However, the lack of hallucinations and delusions differentiates these patients from schizophrenic patients.

  c. **Schizotypal personality disorder** is also frequently found among biologic relatives of schizophrenics. Because of the odd beliefs, magical ideation, and eccentric behavior and appearance of these patients, this disorder may be confused with schizophrenia. However, it can be differentiated from schizophrenia because of the lack of a history of an active phase (see V D 2).

   (1) Phenomenologic investigations suggest that extreme social anxiety may, in fact, be the genetic link between schizophrenia and schizotypal relatives.

   (2) Further refinements of this diagnosis and its relationship to genetic factors in schizophrenia may involve differentiation of affective versus nonaffective subtypes of this disorder (which may be more appropriately assigned to borderline personality disorder).

   (3) There is evidence that people who suffer from schizotypal personality disorder may suffer from similar sensory gating problems as do people with schizophrenia.

  d. **Borderline personality disorder.** People with this personality disorder suffer from a lifelong pattern of identity instability and disturbance (e.g., confusion regarding sexual identity, career choice, self-image; chaotic social networks). In severe cases, psychotic features may appear in response to stress, but they may not be of sufficient duration or intensity to warrant a diagnosis of schizophrenia.

e. Other personality disorders exhibit symptoms of sufficient severity that they may sometimes be misdiagnosed by the incautious clinician as schizophrenia.

    (1) Dependent personality disorder may be mistaken for exhibiting schizophrenic ambivalence, lack of drive, and fear of being alone.

    (2) Obsessive-compulsive personality disorder may demonstrate such restrictions of affective expression that it is mistaken for the flattened affect described in former diagnostic systems for schizophrenia. In addition, ambivalence, circumstantial speech, and other features may give the impression of schizophrenia without a diagnostic evaluation.

10. Autism, particularly Asperger syndrome (a high-functioning form of autism), may be mistaken for schizophrenia if DSM-IV criteria are not used. Patients suffering from this disorder are often eccentric, emotionally labile, and anxious, and they demonstrate poor social functioning, repetitive behavior, and fixed habits. Affect may be interpreted as bizarre or flat. Social interactions are severely impaired by a lack of empathy or understanding of other people, and motor performance is clumsy and ill coordinated. Because these patients do not generally have positive symptoms, they may be most easily mistaken for "simple schizophrenics" by the casual diagnostician.

C. **Religious and cultural subgroups.** Diagnosticians from one culture may confuse culturally based beliefs and behavior patterns with symptoms of schizophrenia. Religious beliefs, if held by a group of people of which the patient is a member, cannot be considered psychotic by members of another group or culture. Likewise, cultural differences in body language and acceptable affective expression may be interpreted as bizarre by physicians from other cultures. This diagnostic confusion is best avoided by consulting a physician from the same culture as the patient or a physician experienced with that culture.

VII. ETIOLOGIC THEORIES

A. **Genetic theories.** Evidence for genetic transmission of risk for schizophrenia is widely accepted and seems substantial. However, the nature of this genetic transmission remains elusive.

1. Possible mechanisms. As early as the 1920s, simple mendelian models for the transmission of a gene for schizophrenia were found to be inapplicable. Since then, several models for the possible genetic transmission of schizophrenia have been developed.

    a. A single gene with variable penetrance. This model proposes that a single gene may transmit the schizophrenic genotype that may be expressed as a result of environmental, social, or psychological factors. Such a monogenetic mechanism was hypothesized to be:

        (1) An inherited biochemical or metabolic disorder

        (2) An immunologic defect that makes the individual prone to infection by unknown viral pathogens

        (3) A defect in a specific protein or enzyme

        (4) A defect in personality organization, which predisposes the individual to the eventual development of schizophrenia

    b. A single gene whose expression is modulated by polygenes. This model proposes that the basic gene for schizophrenia is transmitted in a simple, known pattern and that a combination of other genes regulate the expression of the schizophrenic phenotype. This hypothesis is at least partially supported by the following findings in relatives of schizophrenic patients:

        (1) Increased saccadic eye movements and smooth pursuit ocular movement deficits

        (2) Schizophrenic spectrum personality organization

        (3) High levels of creativity in biologic relatives of schizophrenic patients

    c. Polygenes. This model supposes that the development of schizophrenia is the result of the expression of multiple genes, which produce the schizophrenic phenotype. Although evidence for this model is good, isolation of these combinations of genes requires sophisticated mapping of human DNA and techniques of frequency analysis. This model appears to account for the differences in severity of the disease, the variable rates of pathology in families, and other puzzling findings.

  2. Evidence. A variety of study designs have been used to gather evidence of genetic transmission of schizophrenia or of a risk factor that predisposes a person to the development of schizophrenia.

    a. Family studies

      (1) Associations of schizophrenic family pedigrees with abnormal average evoked potentials and with defects in eye movement pursuit patterns are currently promising.

      (2) The most common research method used in family studies compares the prevalence of schizophrenia in families of schizophrenic patients with control families, which consist of both normal controls and controls with other psychiatric disorders. In studies completed since the establishment of modern diagnostic criteria, the risk of relatives of schizophrenic patients developing schizophrenia ranges from 3.5%–6.0% (compared with previous rates of 0.2%–1.7%). These studies do not, however, establish the mode of transmission (i.e., whether or not the increased risk in these families is caused by environmental or genetic factors).

    b. Twin studies compare the rates of concordance for monozygotic and dizygotic twins in which one member of the pair is diagnosed with schizophrenia. An assumption is made in these studies that the twins experience an equal environment, which may not be true. Also, these studies have not used raters who are blind to the diagnosis of schizophrenia in one twin. Therefore, these studies cannot claim to answer absolutely the question of genetic transmission of schizophrenia.

      (1) Recent twin studies demonstrate concordance rates of schizophrenia for monozygotic twins to be between 33%–60%.

      (2) The same studies demonstrate a same-sex dizygotic twin concordance rate of 6% and 21%.

      (3) Studies that show low rates of concordance for monozygotic twins demonstrate low rates of concordance for dizygotic twin pairs.

      (4) Dizygotic twin pairs and nontwin siblings both show a concordance rate of 10%–12%.

      (5) Other factors in monozygotic, twin pairs discordant for schizophrenia include differences in finger ridge counts, left hippocampal volume, and left hippocampal activation during the Wisconsin Card Sort Test.

    c. Adoption studies seek to separate social and environmental factors from genetic factors that might cause schizophrenia. These studies find no role for "vertical cultural transmission" of schizophrenia in families, no increased rate of schizophrenia in nonbiologic relatives of schizophrenic patients, but an increased rate of schizophrenia and schizophrenia spectrum disorders in biologic relatives of schizophrenic adoptees.

B. **Biochemical theories.** It is clear that neurotransmitters in the brain are involved in the pathophysiology of schizophrenia. However, their specific role is undetermined. Schizophrenia may be caused by alterations in specific neurochemical systems, as a result of some other more fundamental pathophysiologic process in the brain.

  1. Neurotransmitter systems

    a. Dopamine. One of the oldest biochemical theories of the etiology of schizophrenia is that dopamine and dopaminergic receptors are involved in the pathophysiology of this disorder.

      (1) Theories

        (a) Current theories suggest that dopamine receptors, particularly the D-1 and, more significantly, the D-2 receptor, are involved in schizophrenia. Areas of the brain suspected to be involved include the mesolimbic, prefrontal, and striatal dopaminergic systems. In contrast to the D-2 receptor, there is evidence that the D-3 receptor is not involved in schizophrenia. D-4 and D-5 receptors have also been identified but the possible roles of these receptors in schizophrenia is unknown.

(b) Hypodopaminergic and hyperdopaminergic schizophrenic conditions (measured by receptor density and receptor sensitivity) may represent different syndromes, in which negative or positive symptoms predominate.

(c) Other theories suggest that dopaminergic autoreceptors (i.e., presynaptic receptors that provide feedback regulation to the dopaminergic neurons) may be involved in schizophrenia or, at least, in the treatment of symptoms.

(d) Some theories suggest that dopamine systems reflect only a link in chains of neurons involving multiple neurotransmitters, and problems with other types of neurons are reflected in dopaminergic systems as a secondary effect.

(e) The combination of low prefrontal dopamine activity may be associated with negative symptoms, and increased dopamine activity in mesolimbic areas may be associated with positive symptoms. This combination of dopamine effects might explain previously contradictory evidence about the role of dopamine in schizophrenia.

(2) Evidence for the dopamine hypothesis

(a) The most convincing evidence for the role of dopamine in schizophrenia is pharmacologic. Neuroleptic medications appear to exert their primary effect of alleviating the positive symptoms of schizophrenia through the blockage of dopamine receptors. However, although this evidence appears suggestive, it is indirect evidence that could be accounted for in other ways. The widespread use of neuroleptics, which may alter dopamine receptor density and sensitivity, has confounded more direct evidence.

(b) Postmortem examination of the brains of schizophrenic people show increased D-2 receptor density.

(c) Cerebrospinal fluid (CSF) examination for dopamine-related compounds demonstrates equivocal results.

(d) Discriminating between subtypes in which positive and negative symptoms predominate may clarify two different patterns of dopamine receptor increases and decreases.

(e) Studies of schizophrenic patients who have never received neuroleptic treatment report that many of these patients had substantial parkinsonian symptoms.

(3) Evidence against the dopamine hypothesis. Perhaps the strongest evidence against the dopamine hypothesis is that the newer neuroleptics (e.g., clozapine) do not interfere with dopamine binding at the D-1 and D-2 receptors. Yet, the neuroleptics show a substantial antipsychotic effect in some patients meeting the diagnostic criteria for schizophrenia.

b. Neuropeptides. Over 40 neuropeptides with possible CNS activity have been identified.

(1) Biochemistry. Unlike monoamines, neuropeptides are synthesized in the soma of the cell, packaged, and transported to the synapse. They are inactivated by peptidases in the synapse and are not reabsorbed into the presynaptic neuron. In contrast to the monoamine neurotransmitters, the action of the neuropeptides is long acting. They have unique anatomic localization in the brain and are correlated with behavioral, pharmacologic, and electrophysiologic findings that make it clear that they play significant roles in behavior.

(2) Theories. Studies of the possible roles of specific neuropeptides in schizophrenia are in their infancy and are plagued by methodologic problems. Nevertheless, the overlapping distribution of neuropeptide systems, such as cholecystokinin with dopaminergic systems in the brain, are typical of the enticing findings.

(3) Evidence suggesting roles for specific neuropeptides has been gathered through postmortem examination of the brain and CSF (for comparisons of receptor and peptide levels) and through the administration of peptides and peptide receptor antagonists.

(a) Although assays for opioid peptides have not provided significant results, administration of destyrosine-γ-endorphin has produced neuroleptic-like activity.

(b) Preliminary findings suggest that cholecystokinin, neurotensin, and δ-sleep–inducing peptide systems may be altered in schizophrenia.

(c) Reports of the ability of naloxone to transiently reverse schizophrenic symptomatology in some patients are inconclusive.

c. Norepinephrine

    (1) Theories. Few theories of the role of norepinephrine in schizophrenia suggest that norepinephrine acts alone in the pathogenesis of this illness. Rather, current models suggest that norepinephrine dysregulation exposes fundamental defects in the functioning of dopamine or other neurotransmitter systems. Acutely paranoid psychotic states may be accompanied by increased levels, whereas chronic schizophrenic patients appear to show state-dependent fluctuations, depending on the transient variation in emotional and arousal states. Individual theories focus on the increased, decreased, and defective metabolism of norepinephrine.

    (2) Evidence. There is a great deal of evidence that norepinephrine is involved in the pathophysiologic process of schizophrenia, but there is little evidence about its precise role.

        (a) Low dopamine-β-hydroxylase levels in the CSF appear to be correlated with better psychosocial functioning in schizophrenic patients.

        (b) In autopsied brain tissue, decreased levels of dopamine-β-hydroxylase and 3-methoxy-4-hydroxyphenylglycol (MHPG) were found in schizophrenic patients with brain atrophy.

        (c) Increased norepinephrine and MHPG have been found in some areas of the brain, and increased norepinephrine has been found in the plasma and CSF of schizophrenic patients.

d. Serotonin has long been of interest in the pathogenesis of schizophrenia because of findings that hallucinogens with psychotomimetic properties appear to be active in the serotonin systems of the brain.

    (1) It may be that serotonin is active in the pathophysiology of schizophrenia as a modulator of other systems, such as dopamine.

    (2) Like norepinephrine, abnormalities of the serotonin systems in schizophrenia are manifested by increased levels of serotonin itself and its metabolite (5-hydroxyindoleacetic acid) in CSF.

    (3) Serotonin and its metabolites appear to be:

        (a) Increased in patients with chronic schizophrenia

        (b) Decreased in paranoid and acute patients

        (c) Correlated with agitation

        (d) Affected by antipsychotic medications, especially newer medications like clozapine and risperidone

    (4) When fenfluramine, a serotonin antagonist, was administered to several patients and then withdrawn, the negative symptoms of these patients improved. This finding suggests a possible role for this medication in receptor upregulation.

e. γ-Aminobutyric acid (GABA). Interest in GABA has been generated by the hypothesis that GABA may be inversely related to dopamine activity in the brain.

    (1) The best studies report that there are no significant differences in GABA levels in the CSF of medicated and drug-free schizophrenic patients and healthy control subjects. On the other hand, low levels of GABA are found early in the course of schizophrenia and increase with the duration of the illness.

    (2) Baclofen is a $GABA_B$ receptor agonist that produces exacerbations of schizophrenic symptoms.

    (3) Benzodiazepines, which work in part as GABA agonists, alleviate both positive and negative psychotic symptoms in some patients.

    (4) Low levels of GABA have been found in patients with a number of psychiatric disorders, most significantly depression.

    (5) In addition to GABA, dopaminergic systems also interact with acetylcholine and glutamate.

f. Prostaglandins (PGs) have been of interest in schizophrenia, particularly the PGEs, because they are thought to have effects in modulating catecholamine systems in the brain.

  (1) PGE_1 can produce catalepsy in animals, and high levels of PGE are found in endotoxin-induced cataleptic states.

  (2) Stimulation of PGE_1 production in platelets results in increased synthesis of PGE in healthy individuals but not in schizophrenic patients.

  (3) Quantitative measures of PG levels in CSF demonstrated that PGE_2 and PGFs were absent in schizophrenic patients in contrast to patients with mood disorders who had demonstrable levels of both compounds.

g. Phospholipids are constituents of membranes of all cells, including neurons. The possibility that phospholipids may have a role in mental illness, and in schizophrenia in particular, is fairly recent.

  (1) Phosphatidylcholine, phosphatidylserine, and **phosphatidylethanolamine** have attracted interest for their potential roles in schizophrenia.

    (a) Phosphatidylserine has been found to be significantly increased in the neuronal cell membranes of schizophrenic patients.

    (b) Phosphatidylserine is found in high concentrations in neuronal tissue. It may have a role in catecholamine neurotransmission and a possible role as a second messenger across cell membranes.

  (2) Recent studies have focused on the positive lithium response in some schizophrenic patients as predicted by the theories concerning the methylation of phospholipids and phosphatidylserine.

h. G proteins. Guanosine-triphosphate–binding proteins (G proteins) serve to transmit a wide variety of extracellular receptor-generated signals to intracellular effector systems, including the adenylate cyclase system, several phospholipidase channels, and several ion channels. These proteins are known to be coupled to catecholamine, serotonin, acetylcholine, peptide, and other extracellular messengers. Both direct and indirect evidence has been found for altered levels of G proteins in several areas of the brain thought to be affected by schizophrenia, including the putamen and parahippocampal gyrus.

i. Acetylcholine has attracted attention in schizophrenia research because of its role in initiation of REM sleep and its role in dementing diseases (e.g., Alzheimer dementia), as well as the psychotomimetic characteristics of anticholinergic agents.

  (1) Choline acetyltransferase, an enzyme involved in the synthesis of acetylcholine, has been reported to be reduced in the pontine tegmentum of patients with schizophrenia and increased in the septum, hippocampus, basal ganglia, and nucleus accumbens.

  (2) Acetylcholinesterase has been reported to be increased in the thalamus and septum of people with schizophrenia.

j. Endogenous hallucinogens. There has long been interest in possible endogenous hallucinogens in the brain that might act to produce schizophrenia either as a result of increases from a normal level of a particular neurotransmitter or as a result of alterations of a normal neurotransmitter molecule. Interest has increased following the discovery of what appears to be a phencyclidine (PCP) receptor in the brain, associated with N-methyl-D-aspartate (NMDA) excitatory amino acid receptors.

2. Enzymes, as part of the neuronal systems that may have a role in schizophrenia, are involved in the synthesis, transportation, inactivation, and degradation of neurotransmitters.

  a. Monoamine oxidase (MAO)

    (1) Theory. MAO has a role in the catabolism of amine neurotransmitters, including norepinephrine, dopamine, and serotonin. Decreased levels of MAO could make more of these neurotransmitters available within the synapse, potentially causing or exacerbating schizophrenia.

    (2) Evidence. Platelet MAO activity has been found to be lower in schizophrenic patients than in healthy control subjects in some studies. However, reduced platelet MAO has also been found in association with other psychiatric illnesses. Recently, MAO-B plasma levels have been found to vary with ventricular enlargement in schizophrenia, suggesting cerebral atrophy.

b. Catechol-O-methyltransferase (COMT)

(1) Theory. When *l*-methionine was given to chronic schizophrenic patients in one series of experiments, some of these patients developed an exacerbation of schizophrenic symptoms. Because COMT is a major extracellular route for catecholamine metabolism, interest in methylation possibly producing aberrant neurotransmitters focused attention on COMT.

(2) Evidence. No consistent decreases or increases in levels of COMT have been found in schizophrenia. Other amino acids have been found to exacerbate symptoms of schizophrenia, possibly as a result of nonspecific amino acid toxicity.

c. Creatine phosphokinase (CPK)

(1) Theory. CPK catalyzes the reaction by which creatine phosphate and adenosine diphosphate form creatine and adenosine triphosphate. Three isoenzyme forms of CPK exist in the brain and in cardiac and skeletal muscle. Levels of CPK in skeletal muscle (not brain) have been found to be increased in the sera of acutely psychotic patients. CPK is also increased in nonpsychotic relatives of schizophrenics.

(2) Evidence. CPK increases are not specific for schizophrenia and may be artifacts of increased motor activity.

d. Dopamine-β-hydroxylase (DBH)

(1) Theory. DBH catalyzes the transformation of dopamine to norepinephrine in noradrenergic neurons. DBH is reduced in schizophrenic patients with increased ventricular size. Some studies correlate low DBH with "reactive" schizophrenia, and high DBH with "process" schizophrenia.

(2) Evidence. These findings (atrophy levels and "process" levels) appear to be contradictory, and the significance of DBH in schizophrenia remains unclear.

3. Viruses

a. Theories

(1) Postviral encephalitic conditions with symptoms resembling those of schizophrenia have been reported after known infections with influenza, mononucleosis, Epstein-Barr virus, and human immunodeficiency virus (HIV).

(2) The possibility of a neurotropic slow virus, acting on individuals with specific immune deficiencies, has also been proposed.

b. Evidence for the role of viruses causing schizophrenia remains inconclusive.

(1) The observation that rates of schizophrenia are higher in individuals born in the late winter and early spring fits the seasonal patterns of certain viruses, suggesting a possible infection at birth or close to birth that results in schizophrenia.

(2) Increased amounts of interferon in the CSF of schizophrenic patients have been detected in some studies, but other studies and attempts to treat schizophrenia with interferon have not been encouraging.

4. Immunologic models

a. Theory. Defects in the immune system of patients with schizophrenia have attracted interest on the theories that:

(1) An autoimmune illness might have a role in the pathogenesis of schizophrenia.

(2) An immune deficiency might predispose the individual to schizophrenogenic viral infections.

(3) Schizophrenic patients might suffer immunologic compromise as a result of neurohumoral effects of schizophrenia on the immune system.

b. Evidence

(1) Studies show elevated levels of immunoglobulin G, immunoglobulin M, and immunoglobulin A in subgroups of schizophrenic patients.

(2) For years, there has been a search for a humoral factor (i.e., taraxein) that is responsible for schizophrenia. Interest in taraxein has been engendered by a lipid precipitate of brain extract from schizophrenic patients, which has focused attention on the possibility that taraxein is an autoantibody.

(3) Other studies have focused on delayed hypersensitivity and on other indicators of autoimmune disease.

(4) Recent literature suggests that CSF interleukin-2 may be elevated in schizophrenia. Interleukin-2 is a T-cell–produced factor that promotes cell growth in tissues, including the brain. It is elevated in viral illnesses and some autoimmune disorders.

C. **Neurophysiologic theories.** Pathophysiologic studies of schizophrenia focus on the identification of both **trait-specific** and **state-dependent markers** for schizophrenia and the significance of these physiologic mechanisms once they are identified.

1. **Electrodermal activity.** Changes in skin conductance have been used as a measure of emotional arousal in a variety of situations, such as in industrial and criminal polygraphy, and in a variety of psychiatric conditions.

   a. Increased skin conductance recovery in response to a standard stimulus may be a trait marker for high-risk children who later develop schizophrenia.

   b. Poor-prognosis schizophrenic patients do not habituate to repeated stimuli as do healthy individuals and good-prognosis schizophrenic patients.

2. **Cardiovascular activity.** Both tonic (or resting) levels of heart rate and phasic heart rate responses to stimuli appear to have the most significant relationship to schizophrenia of all the cardiovascular physiologic parameters.

   a. **Tonic heart rate** appears to be elevated in schizophrenic patients and does not appear to be affected by neuroleptic medications. This finding may reflect hyperarousal and increased adrenergic tone. However, it is a nonspecific finding that could be affected by the inactive lifestyles of most schizophrenic patients.

   b. **Phasic heart response studies.** Findings of increased phasic responses have been less consistent than findings of increased tonic heart rates.

3. **Smooth pursuit eye movements** are the slow-tracking lateral eye movements seen when an individual watches a swinging pendulum. Normally, the eyes move in a smooth back-and-forth sinusoidal pattern, but in some schizophrenic and other psychotic patients, this smooth pursuit is interrupted by multiple arrests in which the eye comes to a complete stop, resulting in an irregular pattern.

   a. **Findings**

      (1) This eye movement pattern is found in 45% of first-degree relatives of schizophrenic patients and in 10% of relatives of nonschizophrenic control subjects.

      (2) The concordance rate of this characteristic is higher in monozygotic than dizygotic twins.

      (3) This characteristic is seen in healthy individuals as well as schizophrenic patients, and it may be related to the darting eye movements seen in some schizophrenic patients in clinical settings.

   b. **Evidence.** This finding deserves further investigation as a potential genetic trait associated with a risk for schizophrenia. It may be that the inability of schizophrenic patients to follow a pendulum represents an inability to separate a specific stimulus from extraneous background stimuli. The finding of this abnormality in nonpsychotic relatives of schizophrenic patients suggests a possible linkage of these eye movement patterns and a gene (or genes) causing susceptibility for schizophrenia.

4. **Electroencephalogram (EEG).** To date, no psychiatric disease can be diagnosed definitively on the basis of an EEG alone. The EEG findings in schizophrenia may be more specific to states of emotional arousal, cerebral insufficiency, diffuse neuronal impairment, and other nonspecific states than to schizophrenia. On the other hand, seizure-like phenomena in schizophrenia might represent a new insight into the pathophysiology of schizophrenia. A number of EEG findings in schizophrenia are of interest.

a. Patients with chronic schizophrenia have less power in the fast alpha range (11–13 Hz), more power in the fast beta range (20–40 Hz), and more power in the slow theta and delta bands (0.5–8 Hz) than healthy individuals. These nonspecific findings are also found in users of LSD, demented patients, and alcoholics.

b. Brain electrical activity mapping (BEAM), which generates color maps of EEGs and evoked potential data, has demonstrated bilateral increases in delta activity in schizophrenic patients (particularly in frontal areas) and increased fast beta activity (especially in the left temporal–parietal area). However, because these studies are still plagued with artifacts from eyeblinks and muscle activity, these data must be interpreted with caution.

c. Multivariate analysis techniques are able to solve some of the artifact problems. It may be possible for these techniques to separate different psychiatric disorders, including schizophrenic subtypes, from each other and from healthy presentations.

d. Some investigators have reported spike phenomena reminiscent of partial complex seizures from depth electrodes in certain patients with psychiatric symptoms, such as auditory hallucinations.

5. Evoked potentials. Whereas power spectral analysis deals with the spatial distribution of electrical activity in the brain, evoked potentials deal with the time dimension of specific electrical events. Although there has been a wide range of findings in evoked potential research on schizophrenia, most of these findings are not specific to schizophrenia and can occur in other patients, such as alcoholics and patients with dementia. Waves vary in shape, latency, and amplitude, depending on sensory modality and location.

a. Early evoked potentials are reported to have shortened latencies in patients with chronic schizophrenia as compared with healthy control subjects. The persistent nonsuppression of an early auditory P50 wave in patients with chronic schizophrenia, despite clinical status or medication level, is reported to be a stable trait as compared with healthy control subjects. The central-gating deficits are noted to be most pronounced in frontal, central, and parietal electrode placement sites. Interestingly, it is reported that cigarette smoking produces a brief but substantial improvement in the P50 wave sensory-gating abnormality associated with schizophrenia immediately after smoking (see V F 6).

b. Middle evoked potentials are reported to be reduced in amplitude between 75 msec and 250 msec in people with schizophrenia. Painful electrical shocks were recorded as producing less absolute amplitude in the N120 wave, accompanied by reduced reports of pain in schizophrenic patients. These effects are reversed by naloxone, suggesting possible endorphin mediation of this phenomenon.

c. Late evoked potentials. Of all the findings of the evoked potential research in schizophrenia, the reduction of the P300 wave in patients with schizophrenia is perhaps the most widely replicated. This wave form appears to be related to the presentation of stimuli that are task-related and surprising. It can be evoked by loud noises but has been studied in relation to reaction time to complex task-oriented stimuli.

d. Adaptation. With repeated auditory stimuli, schizophrenic patients fail to suppress a P50 wave, and this suppression failure has been reported commonly among biologic relatives of schizophrenic patients, suggesting that this is a possible genetic trait associated with schizophrenia.

(1) With increasing levels of stimulus intensity, schizophrenic patients are reported to show an **augmenting (increasing) response** as opposed to the **reducing response** of healthy individuals. These findings have prompted speculation about the failure of the evoked potentials of schizophrenic patients to return to normal and the possible inability of persons with schizophrenia to suppress extraneous perceptual and cognitive stimuli.

(2) An inverse relationship has been found between augmenting and reducing responses in schizophrenia and levels of MAO in platelets. Patients with chronic schizophrenia appear to have low levels of MAO activity as well as an augmenting evoked potential response (see VII B 2 a).

6. **Cerebral blood flow and brain metabolism** as measured by oxygen and glucose consumption have become a focus of investigation in schizophrenia in recent years, as a result of advances in measurement techniques.

   a. **Techniques using xenon 133 gas inhalation and scanning** have provided new insights into cerebral blood flow and brain metabolism in schizophrenia.

      (1) One type of PET study uses 2-deoxyglucose, which is not metabolized completely in the brain, labeled with positron-emitting isotopes, such as carbon 11. By assigning the patient a particular cognitive task, activity associated with the specific task can be assessed.

      (2) Other PET techniques use other compounds, such as ^{11}C chlorpromazine, which bind to specific receptor groups, giving an estimation of receptor density in illness. Other compounds labeled for the study of receptor distribution include haloperidol, bromspiperone, sulpiride, and raclopride.

   b. **Findings.** Because of the small numbers of patients in many xenon and PET studies of schizophrenia and because of concerns about diagnostic criteria used to identify schizophrenic patients for these studies, questions exist about which groups of schizophrenic patients demonstrate these abnormalities.

      (1) Xenon 133 studies of schizophrenic patients demonstrated reduced blood flow in the frontal region as compared with posterior brain regions in the resting state.

      (2) There are also reports of increased blood flow in the left hemisphere of schizophrenic patients compared with healthy individuals, who show relatively even distribution in the resting state.

      (3) Schizophrenic patients showed increased left hemispheric blood flow while engaged in spatial cognitive tasks compared with healthy individuals, who demonstrated increased blood flow to the right hemisphere. Neuroleptics were found to increase right cerebral blood flow in these schizophrenic patients.

      (4) Other studies demonstrated that with a standard attention-holding task (e.g., the Wisconsin Card Sort Test), schizophrenic patients failed to demonstrate the increased blood flow to the dorsolateral prefrontal cortex as demonstrated by healthy control subjects.

      (5) Several PET studies demonstrated low metabolic rates in the basal ganglia of schizophrenic patients. Metabolic rates appear to be increased by neuroleptics. This finding has also been replicated in patients with mood disorders.

      (6) Tests of attention administered to schizophrenic patients and healthy control subjects during PET measurements demonstrated that the right superior frontal gyrus may be involved in attention. The tests also demonstrated that people with schizophrenia who have attention problems show relative hypometabolism in this area. Neuroleptics appear to normalize this problem.

      (7) More recent work suggests that relative hypofrontality may be the result of increased occipital activity, rather than reduced frontal metabolism. As with other trends in schizophrenia research, medial frontal and thalamic inactivity correlate with schizophrenia symptom scores and with positive and negative symptom scores. These data support the current popularity of the cortico-striatal-thalamic pathway as a major focus of interest in the pathogenesis of schizophrenia. In addition, the new studies suggest a loss of left–right differentiation in schizophrenia.

      (8) PET scans of neuroleptic-free patients demonstrated that patients who experienced auditory hallucinations had lower relative metabolism in auditory and Broca's areas and higher metabolism in the right hemisphere homologue of Broca's area. This study also found that activity in the striatum correlated with hallucinations.

D. **Neurologic and neuropathologic theories**

1. **Neurologic findings.** Minor nonlocalizing neurologic abnormalities have been detected in 60%–70% of schizophrenic patients. These neurologic "soft signs" include defects in stereognosis, graphesthesia, coordination, balance, gait, and tremor. Some examiners maintain that, particularly in patients with chronic schizophrenia, soft frontal signs

(e.g., snout, suck, and grasp reflexes) are found with increased frequency. Attenuation of glabellar tap-induced blinking is also reported to be reduced in some unmedicated schizophrenic patients, as well as being a parkinsonian symptom in patients taking neuroleptic drugs.

2. **Neuroradiologic findings**
   a. **Increased ventricular size.** The most frequently reported finding in CT scans of the brains of schizophrenic patients is an increase in the size of the lateral ventricles. This finding implies a decrease in the volume of brain tissue and is reported as the ventricle–brain ratio.
   (1) **Methodologic problems** (e.g., patient selection, age adjustment of samples, and technical problems in imaging) continue to obscure findings of increased lateral ventricle size. Several studies have failed to replicate this otherwise frequently positive finding.
   (2) Preliminary studies of third ventricle size suggest that it may also be enlarged. Despite the methodologic problems, increases in lateral ventricle size have been correlated with such factors as poor neuroleptic response, poor premorbid adjustment, a predominance of negative symptoms over positive symptoms, and a possible pattern of familial transmission identified in monozygotic twins.
   (3) A number of studies correlate ventricular enlargement with various neurotransmitter abnormalities, particularly dopamine system abnormalities (see VII B 1 a).
   b. **Cortical surface abnormalities.** Dilation of fissures and sulci on the cortical surface demonstrates loss of brain tissue and, like the enlargement of the lateral ventricles, is increased with age and a variety of neurologic conditions. CT scans demonstrate a range of findings, but the most reliable currently available data suggest that increases in the sylvian fissure, prefrontal cortex, and frontal areas may be the most characteristic patterns of atrophy in schizophrenia, suggesting possible temporal and frontal pathology. The degree of severity of symptomatology has yet to be correlated definitively with cortical abnormalities in schizophrenia.
   c. **Cerebellar abnormalities.** Although cerebellar atrophy (particularly atrophy of the vermis) has been associated with schizophrenia, its presence in schizophrenia is obscured by its presence in a number of other psychiatric and neurologic conditions.
   d. **Magnetic resonance imaging (MRI).** Much of the literature focusing on MRI and schizophrenia deals with neuroanatomic changes associated with negative or deficit symptoms.
   (1) Some studies have suggested that negative symptoms are associated with frontal and parietal cortical atrophy.
   (2) Some studies report enlarged lateral ventricles associated with negative symptoms, although replication of this finding has been inconsistent.
   (3) Other studies report that changes in prefrontal areas were not correlated with negative symptoms, but that structural changes in the right caudate were associated with negative symptoms.

3. **Postmortem findings.** Recent controlled postmortem studies appear to confirm data from CT scans of patients with schizophrenia. Evidence has been found of decreased brain volume, increased ventricular size, decreased width, and more histopathologic changes consistent with cell loss and deterioration. In addition, studies of the brains of unmedicated schizophrenic patients demonstrate reductions in the size of parahippocampal gyri, substantia nigra, amygdala, hippocampal formation, and the medial pallidum. Cell studies demonstrate loss of cells in prefrontal associative areas and a general loss of neurons in relation to glial cells.

E. **Psychological theories**

1. **Routine psychological tests** (see Chapter 1) **and research-oriented psychological tests** demonstrate abnormalities in schizophrenia. Although many of these instruments have been valuable in investigating the neuropathology of schizophrenia, **no psychological test is pathognomonic for schizophrenia.**

    a. The Rorschach test. Schizophrenic patients demonstrate abnormal responses to the overall form of the ink blot, which healthy individuals tend to see in consistent ways. In contrast to healthy individuals, schizophrenic patients tend to see few people and little movement in the ink blot, and responses tend to be crudely formed. Contrary to popular belief, people with chronic schizophrenia tend to show primarily a lack of imagination and creativity on these tests.

    b. The Thematic Apperception Test (TAT) is used less for diagnostic purposes than it is to clarify themes specific to the patient. Interpretations of drawings by schizophrenic patients tend to be distorted and demonstrate a lack of creativity.

    c. The Minnesota Multiphasic Personality Inventory (MMPI). Valid interpretations require specific training, and a diagnosis of schizophrenia on the basis of an MMPI alone cannot be made.

    d. The Wechsler Adult Intelligence Scale (WAIS) measures intellectual performance. In schizophrenic patients, it is typical to see verbal intelligence preserved, while performance scores are low. Specific subtests demonstrate characteristic "scattering" of unusually low and normal scores.

2. Attention deficits are common in patients with schizophrenia. Tasks that require sustained attention, focused attention (e.g., to separate a specific pattern or stimulus from background stimuli), or quick reaction times are difficult for individuals with schizophrenia. This difficulty may persist after the resolution of positive symptoms. They are also found in relatives of schizophrenic patients. Possible explanations for these findings follow.

    a. Patients with schizophrenia may inadequately filter distracting stimuli.

    b. Patients with schizophrenia tend to perform better on tasks with more external control and fewer opportunities for autonomous decisions.

    c. Another theory proposes a **sensory input dysfunction,** which causes a stimulus overload and hyperarousal states.

3. Cognition and information processing. In addition to attention deficits, problems with registration, integration, and retrieval of information have been noted in many schizophrenic patients. The mechanisms for memory storage may be overwhelmed by a flood of information, or there may be an inability to form integrating constructs that help to organize data. Conceptual overinclusiveness diminishes with clinical improvement, whereas idiosyncratic and bizarre thinking persist, suggesting that the latter two reflect a more primary defect. Many of these information processing difficulties are present in the first acute episode of schizophreniform illness, rather than being the result of a chronic, deteriorating process.

4. Generalized deficits. Recent literature suggests that the neuropsychological function of a patient is nonspecific and may reflect generalized brain dysfunction, rather than a localized lesion or a group of characteristic lesions.

F. | **Family interaction theories**

1. Current studies suggest that family communication styles influence the course, and possibly the development, of schizophrenia but can be modified through education to reduce the exacerbatory effects of harmful communication patterns on relapse in schizophrenic patients.

    a. Expressed emotionality, one of the topics in family research receiving a lot of attention, suggests that attributing negative characteristics to the patient by family members is detrimental to the course of schizophrenia.

    b. Current findings suggest that noncritical attitudes of family members toward the patient may even improve the outcome in schizophrenia.

    c. Patients returning to families with high expressed emotion (i.e., highly critical, emotional overinvolvement) were found to have a relapse rate four times higher than that of patients returning to families with low expressed emotion. Maintenance treatment with neuroleptic drugs and reduction in total weekly face-to-face contact had a protective value for patients returning to families with high expressed emotion. The relapse rate was 92% for patients coming from families with high expressed emotion who were not on neuroleptic drugs and who did not reduce time spent with these relatives.

2. **Older studies** that affix blame for the development of schizophrenia on family members, particularly "schizophrenogenic mothers," have caused more harm than good in the treatment of schizophrenia.

3. **Political groups,** such as the Alliance for the Mentally Ill, have attempted to **destigmatize people with schizophrenia** and their families and to **promote biologic and social research** on schizophrenia rather than affixing blame for schizophrenia on the family of the patient.

4. Constant exposure to **double-bind communications** in the family have been hypothesized as being etiologic in schizophrenia. Double-bind communications have the following characteristics:
   a. The communication takes place in an important and intense relationship from which the child cannot flee and in which a response is required.
   b. The two messages, which are expressed on different levels (e.g., verbal and nonverbal), conflict with or deny each other.
   c. The child is forbidden from commenting on the conflicting messages, which would clarify his response; thus, no matter what the child says or does, he is wrong on one level or another. According to this theory, psychosis develops as an attempt to deal with such situations. Double-bind communications occur frequently in daily life, but according to this model, vulnerable individuals in schizophrenic families are at a particular risk from this style of communication.

5. The concept of **familial homeostasis** was elaborated to be a situation in which the identified patient's illness is necessary for the maintenance of family equilibrium. Change or improvement in one individual results in pathologic consequences for other family members as the family attempts to reestablish a new equilibrium.

6. **Pseudomutuality** in family relationships of schizophrenic patients describes the situation when rigid roles are assigned to members at the expense of individuality. Superficial relatedness is maintained at the expense of genuine intimacy, which naturally requires the acknowledgment of individual differences.

7. A **transactional thought disorder** was identified to be predominantly amorphous or fragmented in any given family and can be present in both parents and offspring. The thought disorder can be documented by psychological tests.

8. **Family interaction research**
   a. Factors studied for possible effects on the **development of schizophrenia spectrum disorders** include the following.
      (1) **Communication deviance** was derived from transcripts of parents' responses to seven TAT cards and reflected a communication style with difficulty maintaining a clear focus of attention and meaning. Communication deviance predicted the development of schizophrenia spectrum disorders in some family members. However, it was not clear whether this was a sole effect of communication deviance or whether communication deviance and schizophrenia spectrum disorders were parts of a larger phenomenon.
      (2) **Affective style** was measured from the transcripts of parents' speech in interactions with the child while focused on a family problem and reflected personal criticism, guilt induction, or intrusiveness. Negative affective style was a better predictor of the development of schizophrenia spectrum disorders than high expressed emotion when considered along with communication deviance.
   b. **The Finnish Adoptive Study** is a prospective longitudinal study of children of schizophrenic mothers adopted away into families without a history of schizophrenia. Preliminary data appear to support the contention that children of schizophrenic mothers bear a genetic vulnerability to disordered interactions in the rearing environment.

c. **Family attitudes** are thought by many current family interaction researchers to be the driving force behind expressed emotionality and as such should be amenable to change. Current research demonstrates that participation of the family in a **psychoeducational intervention program** is able to reverse the negative effect of high expressed emotionality on the course of the patient's illness. Other research interventions stress helping families to understand schizophrenia as a chronic illness rather than as a matter of the patient's choice or weakness, thereby reducing blame in these situations.

d. **Transcultural variations** have been found to exist in expressed emotion in families. Those who extend the construct of expressed emotionality to the presumed existence of a "schizophrenogenic" family style have been criticized. Instead, high expressed emotion may reflect a generally overstimulating environment. High expressed emotion may be a response to acute symptomatology. It may also be that current research has ignored the protective effects of low expressed emotion, focusing on the presumed pathology of high expressed emotion.

VIII. TREATMENT

A. **Overview.** Treatment programs for people with schizophrenia must be individualized and comprehensive, taking into account the biologic, psychological, and social needs of the patient. Attention must also be paid to the continuity of care. The care setting should be as nonrestrictive as possible, and every attempt should be made to reintegrate the patient into the community.

B. **Hospitalization**

1. **Indications.** Hospitalization is indicated because of specific problems associated with the person's illness (Table 2-9) rather than because of the appearance of symptoms. Current trends are toward reduction in length and frequency of hospitalization in favor of community treatment, if it is adequate.
   a. First episodes of psychosis and unusual presentations of psychotic conditions in a patient with a more chronic form of schizophrenia may warrant hospitalization.
   b. Hospitalization is not necessarily indicated for an exacerbation of psychotic symptoms if adequate community alternatives are available.

2. **Goals**
   a. **Protection.** The hospital should be a safe environment where physical needs are met, stresses are minimized, and impulses are controlled.

TABLE 2-9. Hospitalization of Patients with Schizophrenia

Problems Requiring Short-term Hospital Care	Problems Requiring Long-term Hospital Care
Risk of suicidal and homicidal ideation	Lack of appropriate community mental health resources
Command hallucinations of a threatening nature, with the clinician's assessment that the patient may act on these hallucinations	Provision of rehabilitative services before discharge to community programs
Extreme fear	Care for a severely debilitated schizophrenic patient
Significant confusion	Treatment of significant comorbidity from medical illnesses, substance abuse, medication complications
Inability of patient to plan and care for himself	Protection from self-inflicted harm or danger to others

    b. Diagnosis. Twenty-four-hour care allows for extensive observation and evaluation of the patient's problems, strengths, history, supports, and responses to treatment. In addition, access to sophisticated diagnostic laboratory and neuroradiologic tests provides the opportunity to differentiate schizophrenia from psychotic conditions resulting from medical conditions.

    c. Therapy. Treatments of various types can be started in the hospital, including neuroleptic medication, vocational and psychosocial rehabilitation, and family education, which are designed to return the patient to the community. Negative symptoms may be helped by cognitive and behavioral treatments and structured schedules. There is no evidence that inpatient psychotherapy without medication is of any benefit in this illness.

3. Side effects associated with hospitalization include the patient possibly experiencing a loss of self-esteem and social stigmatization as a result of being on a "mental ward." In addition, social supports in the community may be lost. With prolonged hospitalization, the patient risks the loss of social and living skills required to live in the world outside the hospital (i.e., institutionalism).

4. The changing role of the hospital in the treatment of schizophrenia results from economic pressures and increasing beliefs about the superiority of community treatment over hospitalization.

    a. Current trends include major reductions in length of stay, a focus on acute stabilization and discharge, and an emphasis on diagnostic clarification rather than on psychotherapeutic treatment. Where adequate community treatment systems exist, it is presumed that the community programs will take over many of the treatment functions of the inpatient unit.

    b. Alternatives to hospitalization. Particularly in the public sector, attempts are being made to provide community-based alternatives to hospitalization. Some of these alternatives involve houses in the community where physicians, nurses, and others provide acute stabilization of psychotic symptoms and rapid reintegration into the community. In other cases, motels and therapeutic foster homes have been used for these purposes.

        (1) In general, these settings are not as well set up to handle violence and to deal with a medical evaluation as a hospital, but they provide less disruption for shorter periods of time in the patient's life than do hospitals.

        (2) These facilities are probably most appropriate for patients whose illnesses are well known by the treatment system, not for first-episode psychotic patients.

C. **Milieu treatment.** The therapeutic environment of the inpatient ward is called the **therapeutic milieu.** Inpatient psychiatric wards frequently use the therapeutic milieu as a major treatment modality for schizophrenic patients. Formal milieu therapy depends on attention to the social structure of the ward and depends on adequate numbers of well-trained staff. Interactions between staff, patients, and formal social organizations (e.g., the patient's ward government) are tools regularly used in milieu therapy. Trends are away from emphasis on milieu therapy because of decreasing lengths of hospital stay and a change of the focus of the hospital stay to diagnosis, rehabilitation programs, and psychoeducational activities.

1. Structure. One aspect of the staff's role in the therapeutic milieu is to support the patient's impaired reality testing, impulse control, and modulation of environmental stimulation. The staff works to reduce the patient's anxiety and control injurious behavior. The structure of the ward should contain regular, structured activities, time alone, and help with personal hygiene and self-care. Milieu therapy avoids intense probing and anxiety-provoking psychotherapeutic interventions, which can be overwhelming for psychotic patients.

2. Flexibility. The milieu should be flexible enough to respond to the changing needs of individuals with regard to length of stay, extent of restrictions, contact with family, group involvement, and activity levels. For example, as the patient's positive symptoms resolve, efforts may be initiated to increase the patient's socialization with other patients, engage the patient in structured recreational and vocational activities, and encourage the patient's participation in the ward government.

3. **Ward community.** The other patients, as individuals and as a group, are used as therapeutic agents in the therapeutic milieu. Open, direct communication and individual responsibility are encouraged. The more organized and improved patients can provide hope and act as models for sicker patients. The patients are encouraged as a group to make decisions about daily activities of the ward and to help change maladaptive behavior of patients through open feedback.

4. **Side effects.** Target-symptom–oriented treatment plans and posthospitalization care plans that involve all of the staff, including staff from programs outside the hospital, may remedy the side effects of milieu treatment.
   a. Premature and harsh confrontation from staff and other patients or too much pressure for recovery may exacerbate psychotic symptoms or delay recovery.
   b. A structured and tolerant atmosphere may promote dependence on the ward, making it difficult to return to the community.
   c. Excessive demands for participation may cause overstimulation and disorganization.
   d. Less ill patients may take advantage of sicker patients, unless the interactions are monitored carefully.
   e. Staff may retain patients in the ward milieu longer than is desirable, creating a tendency for patients to return prematurely to the ward without ever developing a relationship with community services. This appears to be a problem with neophyte therapists who become enmeshed with the patient and her social network, believing that only they really understand the patient. This may result in a fragmentation of team efforts and poor communication with outpatient therapists. Good supervision can reduce this risk to the continuity of care.

5. **Organizational continuity.** With shorter lengths of stay and an increasing reliance of treatment systems on community-based treatment, hospitals need to be a more highly integrated member of the overall mental health treatment system. Case managers from the community are increasingly involved in ward treatment. Diagnostic and treatment information must be relayed between community and hospital staff, and inpatient treatment objectives must be jointly negotiated between systems. Survival of inpatient, hospital-based treatment programs for patients with schizophrenia may depend increasingly on the ability of the inpatient units to respond to needs of the community mental health system.

D. **Group therapy** has long been a mainstay of the treatment of schizophrenic patients in both inpatient and outpatient settings. It is best used in conjunction with other forms of therapy, particularly medications. Although there is a paucity of well-controlled studies of group therapy in schizophrenia, those that exist support the contention that group therapy focused on communication, alleviation of symptoms, and social skills produces improvements in social integration. Patients in this type of group therapy also have fewer readmissions to the hospital than do patients who receive only social skills training. There is little evidence that open-ended, insight-oriented group therapy is effective in the treatment of schizophrenic patients, and some physicians believe that unstructured, confrontational group techniques may exacerbate psychotic symptomatology.

E. **Individual psychotherapy** should be supportive and oriented to helping the patient adapt to the details of daily life. Supportive and adaptive therapeutic techniques are far more effective in the management of schizophrenic patients than are insight-oriented techniques that focus on the patient's inner experience. Cognitive and behavioral therapies may reduce deficit symptoms in schizophrenia.

1. **Therapeutic relationship**
   a. Attempts by therapists to establish a **close or intense therapeutic relationship** may exacerbate symptoms in patients who are highly suspicious or who feel overwhelmed by interpersonal relationships.

    b. Nondirective and affectively restricted therapeutic styles may also cause patients to experience anxiety and exacerbations of symptoms. Insight-oriented psychotherapy alone has not proved to be effective in schizophrenia.

    c. Supportive psychotherapy is characterized by a warm, open relationship, which focuses on promoting the patient's self-esteem and helping the patient learn about his real strengths and limitations. Effective therapy focuses on practical and concrete issues.

  2. Therapeutic techniques. The principles of psychotherapy of schizophrenic patients are as follows:

    a. Education. One of the main techniques of the therapist of a schizophrenic patient is to teach the patient about his illness. Techniques of managing stress, understanding symptoms, and the value of compliance with pharmacologic treatments should be taught. This approach encourages the patient to assume responsibility for treatment.

    b. Focusing on problem solving. The therapist focuses on helping the patient solve concrete problems that arise in daily life. The therapist may offer possible solutions to problems presented by the patient, including an analysis of possible positive and negative outcomes of each solution. The therapist attempts to develop problem-solving skills for the patient in financial, interpersonal, residential, and other areas of the patient's daily life.

    c. Setting reasonable expectations for change. Therapists who have unreasonable expectations for a "cure" may convey these expectations to the patient in a counterproductive manner. Therapists who have generally positive expectations for improving functioning and life satisfaction appear to be correlated with good patient outcomes.

    d. Expressing emotions effectively. Therapies that encourage expression of emotion for its own sake or for "cathartic" value may trigger exacerbations in some schizophrenic patients. The therapist should encourage a discussion of private feelings and how to deal with these feelings but not encourage full-blown expressions of anger and hostility.

    e. Crisis intervention. The therapist may be able to intervene in crises in the patient's life to prevent serious escalations. Unlike the passive roles in other forms of therapy, the therapist may need to become active in working with the patient's family, landlord, or social agencies to reduce the escalation of crises into psychotic episodes.

    f. Concrete limit-setting. The therapist may need to set concrete limits on the patient, such as avoiding substance abuse and violence. These discussions frequently include discussions of consequences of harmful behaviors.

    g. Managing dependence. One of the functions of the therapy of the schizophrenic patient is to increase the patient's appropriate socialization with other people in the community. In meeting this goal, the therapist encourages the patient to rely on a large network of people in the community rather than on only the therapist.

    h. Illness self-management. The therapist and the patient construct "experimental" designs intended to help the patient observe factors that may make both positive and negative symptoms of illness better or worse. The patient may learn how to initiate activity, reduce social isolation, control symptoms with medications, and many other self-management skills.

F. **Case management.** Because of the diverse and changing needs of the schizophrenic patient throughout the course of her illness, a variety of providers and agencies become involved in the person's care in the hospital and community. This can create conflicting treatment expectations and plans. To facilitate the solution of this problem, the role of the individual therapist is giving way to that of the case manager in many mental health systems. The case manager is not confined to the hospital or clinic and may visit the schizophrenic patient in the community or in the home. Roles of the case manager include:

  1. Evaluation. The case manager is responsible for collecting other assessments of the patient's medical, psychiatric, social, and financial needs and compiling these into an overall coordinated plan.

  2. Planning. The overall treatment plan must coordinate diverse service and care providers and attend to the overall continuity of care for the schizophrenic patient. In addition, the case manager must share the overall treatment planning process with other members of the service delivery network.

3. **Linking.** Because of the difficulty that many schizophrenic patients have in gaining access to services required for comprehensive care, the case manager works to link the patient with all elements of the service delivery network. For example, the case manager may help the patient make appointments and even find transportation to these services. The case manager also links different service providers and agencies to solve problems of service delivery.

4. **Advocacy.** The case manager may need to seek resources and services for schizophrenic patients. This may either take the form of **case-specific advocacy,** which is aimed at gaining resources for the individual patient, or **class-specific advocacy,** which is aimed at gaining services, resources, or access to services for a group of patients.

G. **Psychosocial rehabilitation** has become a significant part of treatment programs for schizophrenic patients because returning patients to productive lives in the community has become a priority. Goals of these programs are to reduce symptoms, remediate disabilities, and overcome handicaps associated with schizophrenia. In the past, patients who left inpatient institutions were found to have insufficient skills necessary for independent living; that is, they lacked the skills in social interactions required to gain or retain employment and required to form social support networks needed for survival. Preliminary data suggest that patients who participate in psychosocial rehabilitation programs experience recidivism at about half the rate of control subjects. These programs focus on the following issues:

1. **Social skills training** involves skills required to communicate with strangers and familiar people and to reduce the frequency of symptom-based communication and socially inappropriate behaviors.

2. **Nutrition and food preparation.** Patients who have lived in institutions for much of their lives may be unable to shop, prepare food, and plan a balanced diet.

3. **Residential skills.** Many schizophrenic patients have difficulty finding and maintaining housing. Many community mental health programs offer supervised housing for the transition between inpatient hospitalization and independent community living, in addition to skills training.

4. **Managing finances.** Managing money, even if it is received monthly, may pose substantial problems. In extreme cases, patients may spend their monthly checks in a few days or weeks; thus, the patient is often without food for many days and, in extreme cases, may return to the hospital.

5. **Managing the illness.** Patients are taught to manage medication administration, to watch for side effects, and to report potentially dangerous developments to the treatment system in an appropriate and assertive manner.

6. **Recreational activities.** Patients are taught to pursue recreational and physical activities to reduce stress and to promote general health.

H. **Consumer movement.** Self-help groups of schizophrenic and other chronically mentally ill people are increasingly prominent on the national scene. Clubs for mentally ill people, such as the internationally known Fountain House, are a source of support and improved self-esteem for people suffering from schizophrenia. Current activities associated with the consumer movement include: well-functioning mentally ill patients working in the mental health system with less well-functioning patients, client-operated businesses, and other innovative approaches.

I. **Illness self-management.** The objective of this treatment method is to train patients with persistent schizophrenic symptoms to manage their own illnesses to a greater extent than previously encouraged by the mental health treatment system. Several forms of this training exist, but most encourage the development of skills in several specific areas.

1. **Symptom control** includes learning to recognize and respond to signs of relapse, differentiating relapse from medication side effects, and working with persistent symptoms.

2. **Substance avoidance** focuses on avoiding alcohol abuse and the use of street drugs.

3. **Medication management** requires an understanding of how medications work, how they are taken, and how different side effects should be managed, including when to seek medical help.

4. **Working with the health care system.** Education of how to communicate with health care providers, navigate through the service delivery system, and related skills are taught.

J. **Cognitive remediation.** In contrast to rehabilitation, which focuses on relearning concrete social and functional skills, cognitive remediation attempts to reverse specific neuropsychological performance deficits that are characteristic of schizophrenia. This approach uses behavioral techniques and education to attempt to reverse deficits in performance on instruments such as the Wisconsin Card Sort Test. This approach has produced improvements in patients with brain injury and autism, but is new in its application to patients with schizophrenia.

K. **Pharmacologic treatment and electroconvulsive therapy (ECT)**

1. **Neuroleptic medications** (Table 2-10)
   a. **Mechanism of action.** Traditional neuroleptics have differential effects on D-1 and D-2 dopamine receptors. All traditional neuroleptics exert therapeutic effects by blocking the dopamine system.
   b. **Efficacy**
      (1) **Acute psychosis.** Neuroleptics are effective in alleviating the positive symptoms of schizophrenia, such as hallucinations, delusions, and agitation. They tend to be less effective in treating negative and social symptoms of schizophrenia, such as blunted affect, apathy, anhedonia, and grandiose and persecutory delusions, especially if they are chronic and well organized.

TABLE 2-10. Neuroleptic Medications

Generic Name	Trade Name(s)	Approximate Equivalent Oral Dosages (mg)	Usual Inpatient Oral Dosage Range (mg/day)
Phenothiazines			
Aliphatic			
Chlorpromazine	Thorazine	100	50–1500
Piperidine			
Thioridazine	Mellaril	100	50–800
Piperazine			
Fluphenazine	Prolixin, Permitil	2–4	2–60
Trifluoperazine	Stelazine	5	5–80
Perphenazine	Trilafon	10	16–64
Butyrophenones			
Haloperidol	Haldol	2–4	2–60
Thioxanthenes			
Thiothixene	Navane	5	5–80
Dihydroindolones			
Molindone	Moban, Lidone	10	20–225
Dibenzoxazepines			
Loxapine	Loxitane, Daxolin	10	20–225

(2) Maintenance. Neuroleptics have well-established roles in preventing relapse in schizophrenia, particularly when used in conjunction with a comprehensive treatment plan.

   (a) Recent neuroleptic research shows that too low a dose and poor compliance may lead to relapse, whereas too high a dose risks noncompliance and tardive dyskinesia without appreciable benefit.

   (i) Within 6 to 8 months after discontinuation of neuroleptics, 50% of patients relapse.

   (ii) After 18 months, nearly 75% of medication-free patients relapse.

   (iii) About 25% of patients currently taking medication relapse.

   (b) Two groups of schizophrenic patients may not be effectively treated with maintenance neuroleptics:

   (i) Patients who have had a single acute psychotic episode

   (ii) Very deteriorated chronic schizophrenic patients who may be refractory to treatment

c. Choice of agent. Although there is no evidence that certain subtypes of patients can be chosen prospectively to respond to certain medications, an individual patient may respond well to a particular drug and not to others. Initially, the choice of drug may depend upon side effect profile (e.g., sedation, β-adrenergic blockade, or parkinsonian effects) and the familiarity of the clinician with the particular medication. After an adequate initial trial, if there is not an adequate therapeutic response, trying a neuroleptic from another group, which may have different pharmacologic properties, is justified.

d. Dosage

   (1) Acute psychosis. Recent studies demonstrate that a moderate initial dose (400 to 1200 mg) of chlorpromazine (or the equivalent drug) is usually adequate for the control of psychotic symptoms.

   (a) Massive doses used acutely for rapid modification of psychotic behavior in the past have been shown to be no more effective than moderate doses. In addition, they carry added risks from side effects. However, there does appear to be a number of schizophrenic patients who benefit from very high doses of neuroleptics.

   (b) Whatever the dose, the acute effects of the medication on reducing psychotic symptoms usually occur in 3 to 10 days. In a small number of schizophrenic patients, a much longer time for neuroleptic response may be needed (up to several months).

   (2) Stabilization phase. Following initial control of symptoms, the daily dose of neuroleptics should be reduced gradually to a maintenance level. Eventual tapering of the medication to the point of discontinuation may be indicated.

   (3) Maintenance phase. The goal is to keep the patient relatively symptom-free and with the highest functional level on the lowest possible dose of neuroleptics with the fewest side effects. Higher doses of neuroleptics improve treatment of positive symptoms and may lower the death rate in schizophrenia, but higher doses appear to reduce functioning levels, interfere with socialization, and harm the quality of the patient's life.

   (a) In practice, striking a balance between these poles may be difficult. Absolute protection from risk and reduction of positive symptoms at the expense of quality of life is not acceptable.

   (b) A single daily dose is adequate for maintaining blood levels of the medication. Some protocols require that the medication dose be adjusted on a daily or weekly basis, depending on the presence of positive symptoms versus functional impairment.

   (4) Nonresponse. With neuroleptics, acute agitation that appears to be increasing with increases in medication may be related to akathisia, a parkinsonian side effect of medication. In addition, movement disorders (e.g., severe parkinsonian symptoms, tardive dyskinesia) may preclude the use of neuroleptics at therapeutic doses. Even adequate doses of neuroleptics may be ineffective in treating symptoms of schizophrenia in 20%–30% of people with schizophrenia. In these cases, use of a novel antipsychotic agent (e.g., clozapine or rispiridone) or an augmentation strategy with a medication such as lithium may be indicated.

    (a) Evidence also suggests that obtaining neuroleptic levels in plasma and **adjusting doses** accordingly may be another strategy for treating resistant patients.

    (b) In situations where there are adequate levels of neuroleptic but no response to treatment, **waiting several months** before altering treatment again may be beneficial in some cases.

    (c) **Shifting medications from one class to another** may also be beneficial for reasons that are currently unproved. This strategy may take advantage of variations in affinities of different neuroleptics for different D-1 and D-2 receptors.

    (d) There is little rationale for adding **multiple neuroleptics** to a treatment regimen.

    (e) Administration of **lithium carbonate** or **carbamazepine** in addition to the neuroleptic may benefit some patients with manic-like features of agitation and increased psychomotor activity.

        (i) There is also evidence for a population of schizophrenic patients without agitated or manic-like features who may benefit from lithium.

        (ii) Carbamazepine has proved less effective than lithium, producing modest symptom improvement that often does not last beyond 1 month of treatment.

    (f) **Propranolol** produces a modest improvement in some patients as an adjunctive treatment. This effect may be related to reduction in akathisia and increasing blood levels of the neuroleptic.

e. Route of administration

    (1) Oral. Neuroleptics are routinely administered as tablets, capsules, or oral elixirs. The main problem with the oral route of administration is patient compliance.

    (2) Intramuscular injection. Most neuroleptics are available in injectable form. This route of administration is used with uncooperative patients in acute treatment settings and in cases in which an adequate plasma level cannot be obtained with the oral route.

    (3) Long-acting injections. Both haloperidol and fluphenazine are available as long-acting injections. Such injections provide neuroleptic medication for 1 week to several weeks and have proved valuable for patients who have difficulty complying with oral medications.

f. Adverse effects

    (1) Extrapyramidal syndromes result from blockade of dopamine receptors in the basal ganglia and occur more commonly with the high-potency neuroleptics.

    (a) Acute dystonic reactions, which are more common in young male patients early in treatment, involve sudden tonic contractions of the muscles of the tongue, neck (**torticollis**), back (**opisthotonos**), mouth, and eyes (**oculogyric crises**). As well as being extremely frightening, such reactions can be dangerous if the patient's airway is compromised. These patients can be effectively treated with benztropine (1 to 2 mg intramuscularly) or diphenhydramine (25 to 50 mg intramuscularly or intravenously). Prophylaxis is accomplished with regular, orally administered anticholinergic medication.

    (b) Drug-induced parkinsonism is characterized by cogwheel rigidity, bradykinesia, tremor, loss of postural reflexes, mask-like facies, and drooling. It is more common in elderly patients, and although it usually occurs in the first weeks of treatment, it may appear at varying times with varying doses. It can be effectively treated with any of the antiparkinsonian medications (Table 2-11) and may also respond to a decrease in neuroleptic dosage. Antiparkinsonian agents can generally be tapered and discontinued after 3 to 4 weeks of treatment in most patients. If the extrapyramidal syndrome remains unresponsive, a change to a different class of neuroleptics, usually one of lower potency, is required.

TABLE 2-11. Antiparkinsonian Medications

Generic Name	Trade Name(s)	Usual Oral Dosage Range (mg/day)
Benztropine	Cogentin	1–8
Trihexyphenidyl	Artane, Tremin	2–10
Biperiden	Akineton	2–6
Amantadine	Symmetrel	100–300
Diphenhydramine	Benadryl	25–200

(c) **Akathisia** is a syndrome of motor restlessness, which may involve the entire body but is often most obvious in the patient's inability to keep her legs and feet still. It can be mistaken for anxiety, agitation, or an increase in psychotic symptomatology. The akathisia may respond to antiparkinsonian agents, but if the patient responds poorly, a decrease in dosage or change to another neuroleptic is indicated. In some cases, akathisia can be successfully treated with propranolol, benzodiazepines, or vitamin E.

(d) **Neuroleptic-induced catatonia** occurs more commonly with the high-potency agents and is characterized by withdrawal, mutism, and motor abnormalities, including rigidity, immobility, and waxy flexibility. Although it can be mistaken for a worsening of the patient's psychotic symptoms, it is a complication of neuroleptic therapy. It may represent a variant of the neuroleptic malignant syndrome [see VIII K 1 f (2)]. It should be treated by temporarily discontinuing neuroleptic therapy and, on resolution, changing to a different class of neuroleptic. Amantadine, administered in an oral dose of 100 mg three times daily, may also be helpful.

(e) **Tardive dyskinesia** is a late-onset movement disorder that is thought to result from a disturbance in the dopamine–acetylcholine balance in the basal ganglia. Mechanisms theorized to account for this phenomenon include an increase in the numbers or sensitivity of dopamine receptors in certain parts of the brain following chronic blockade with neuroleptics. However, these theories do not fit all the data about the physiology of this condition.

    (i) **Fasciculations of the tongue** may be the earliest symptom, followed by **lingual–facial hyperkinesias,** which are persistent involuntary chewing, smacking, or grimacing movements.

    (ii) **Choreoathetotic movements of the extremities and trunk,** including the respiratory muscles, can be extremely disabling in severe cases. The symptoms are often noticeable when there is a dosage reduction or discontinuation of neuroleptic medication, but they can usually be detected by close examination between neuroleptic doses.

    (iii) The syndrome can usually be reversed if it is detected early, and neuroleptics are discontinued.

    (iv) In severe cases, tardive dyskinesia may be irreversible and can progress with continued neuroleptic treatment.

    (v) Symptoms are worsened by anticholinergic medication, which should be discontinued if possible.

    (vi) Increased doses of neuroleptics may cause apparent temporary improvement by increasing the dopamine-receptor blockade. However, this ultimately causes further progression of the movement disorder.

    (vii) Patients should be screened every 6 months for early signs and should be maintained on the lowest possible dose to minimize this serious complication of long-term neuroleptic use.

    (viii) Patients withdrawn abruptly from neuroleptics sometimes demonstrate a **withdrawal-emergent dyskinesia** with transient features of tardive dyskinesia that lasts for several days. It is unclear whether this syndrome is an early form of tardive dyskinesia or has another pathophysiologic mechanism.

(2) Neuroleptic malignant syndrome is a potentially life-threatening complication of neuroleptic therapy and is characterized by muscular rigidity, fever, autonomic instability, and an altered level of consciousness. Onset of the full-blown syndrome is rapid over 1 to 2 days after a period of gradual progressive rigidity. Treatment involves immediate discontinuation of the neuroleptic medication and support of respiratory, renal, and cardiovascular functioning and possibly treatment with dantrolene or bromocriptine.

(3) Anticholinergic effects occur with low-potency neuroleptics at a higher rate than with the high-potency neuroleptics. Anticholinergic effects are often seen as a direct result of treatment with a combination of drugs, including neuroleptics, anticholinergic agents used to treat parkinsonian side effects of the neuroleptics, and the inappropriate use of medications for other classes, such as the tricyclic antidepressants. In extreme cases of polypharmacy, combinations (e.g., a low-potency neuroleptic, a tricyclic antidepressant, and one or more anticholinergic agents) may produce a **life-threatening anticholinergic delirium**. Clinicians must watch for the development of increasing psychotic symptoms with the addition of more or different medications to the patient's treatment plan and should suspect anticholinergic delirium in these circumstances. **Levels of anticholinergic side effects include the following:**

  (a) Anticholinergic effects of medication at low doses include blurred vision when changing from close to distant objects, dry mouth, urinary retention in men with enlarged prostate glands, and constipation.

  (b) Anticholinergic poisoning includes restless agitation; confusion; disorientation; hallucinations; delusions; skin that is hot, flushed, and dry; dilation of the pupils; tachycardia; decreased bowel sounds; and urinary retention. Central anticholinergic poisoning may occur without obvious physiologic signs, making iatrogenic anticholinergic poisoning a particularly insidious risk of polypharmacy.

  (c) Anticholinergic abuse. Because of the ability of anticholinergic agents to alter consciousness, patients sometimes abuse prescriptions for anticholinergic agents. Clinicians should treat parkinsonian symptoms with drugs with low antimuscarinic effects (e.g., amantadine) in patients at risk for anticholinergic abuse.

(4) Cardiovascular effects of neuroleptics most commonly include orthostatic hypotension, particularly in elderly patients, which results from adrenergic blockade. This symptom is most commonly associated with the low-potency neuroleptics. In rare cases, neuroleptics may be associated with serious ventricular arrhythmias with electrocardiographic abnormalities (i.e., T-wave changes, prolonged QT intervals) and with cardiac repolarization abnormalities. Risks of all cardiovascular complications are greatest with the low-potency neuroleptics.

(5) Hypothalamic effects include changes in libido, appetite, and temperature regulation. Because of dopamine's mediation of prolactin secretion in the hypothalamus, hyperprolactinemia may be found, resulting in breast enlargement and galactorrhea.

(6) Jaundice of an allergic cholestatic type occurs most commonly with chlorpromazine and usually resolves following withdrawal of the medication.

(7) Agranulocytosis is a rare, unpredictable reaction to the more common neuroleptics and is probably related to interference of DNA synthesis by certain neuroleptics. It is reversible if detected early but may otherwise prove fatal. With the increased use of clozapine in the United States, agranulocytosis may be seen more frequently.

(8) Dermatologic effects include allergic rashes, which respond to discontinuation of the drug, and photosensitivity, which can be treated with sunscreen.

(9) Ophthalmologic effects include a pigmentary retinopathy associated with thioridazine in doses greater than 800 mg/day. Rarely, lens and corneal pigmentation have been reported with chlorpromazine, thioridazine, and thiothixene after long-term treatment, but this is rare. Blurred vision and worsening of narrow-angle glaucoma secondary to anticholinergic effects are more common.

2. **Clozapine, risperidone, pimozide, and other unreleased novel antipsychotics** offer promise of treatment for patients who do not respond to neuroleptics or who suffer serious side effects from the traditional neuroleptics.

   a. **General mechanism of action.** The novel antipsychotics appear to exert their therapeutic effects not by general D-1 and D-2 receptor antagonism but by either selective D-2 receptor blockade or by serotonin receptor blockade in parts of the brain, especially in the mesolimbic system. The antipsychotic effects of the pharmacologic model based on receptor affinity cannot be definitively predicted. A more coherent model of the dopamine and serotonin effects of neuroleptics is needed to fully understand their antipsychotic properties.

   b. **Clozapine** was the first novel antipsychotic in general use in the United States.

      (1) Cost and special issues. Because of potentially lethal side effects [see VIII K 2 b (4)], clozapine is available under a unique prescribing arrangement in the United States. The medication is prescribed as a part of a system of care that includes mandatory weekly blood counts and other monitoring. Initially, this blood work was required to be performed by a specific laboratory system, which drove the cost of the prescription to between $8000 and $9000 per year per patient. It was found that about 30% of treatment-resistant schizophrenic patients benefited significantly from clozapine, but the high cost of the prescription has limited the clinical use of the medication to between 5%–10% of the population that might benefit from it. Studies have shown cost savings for many patients even with the high cost of the medication (e.g., via reduced hospitalization). Clozapine offers substantial hope for patients who suffer significant side effects, such as tardive dyskinesia, from traditional neuroleptics.

      (2) Pharmacology. Clozapine is a dibenzodiazepine that is structurally similar to the neuroleptic loxapine. The mechanism of action for clozapine is not yet understood. It blocks D-1 receptors to a small extent in the mesolimbic and cortical areas of the brain, but has little effect on dopamine receptors in the striatum, possibly accounting for some of its unique properties. Clozapine also has effects on serotonergic, adrenergic, histaminergic, and cholinergic pathways, any one of which could possibly account for antipsychotic properties (see VII B).

      (3) Clinical effects of clozapine are significantly different from those of other antipsychotic agents. In addition to effects on positive symptoms of schizophrenia, clozapine exhibits some effects of reducing negative or deficit symptoms in some patients. It appears to have a markedly reduced propensity to produce neuroleptic malignant syndrome, extrapyramidal symptoms, and tardive dyskinesia (although a very small group of reports of each of these conditions exists).

      (4) Side effects are significant with clozapine.

         (a) Clearly the risk for life-threatening **agranulocytosis** requires the intensive monitoring of the patient's complete blood cell count and state of health. **Febrile conditions** in a patient taking clozapine occur in the first few weeks following initiation of the course of the drug. However, febrile conditions may represent infections secondary to agranulocytosis. Therefore, any fever in a patient on clozapine must receive an aggressive and expert work-up.

         (b) Sedation can be excessive in patients, particularly in early stages of treatment. Some investigators have suggested caffeine, methylphenidate, and other stimulants to alleviate this problem. However, the use of stimulants such as amphetamines and methylphenidate may clearly exacerbate psychotic symptoms. Use of stimulants should be cautious at best, and should be discontinued as the patient adapts to the sedation.

        (c) **Excessive salivation** may be a serious problem for some patients, especially at night. Unlike sedation, the excessive salivation seems to be a more persistent side effect. Although some treatments (e.g., anticholinergic drugs) are available for this side effect, each treatment carries its own risks.

        (d) **Hypotension, dizziness, vertigo.** Some of these symptoms may be related to the adrenergic effects of clozapine. Encouraging patients to flex and extend their feet several times before standing up may reduce blood pooling and thereby reduce orthostatic hypotension.

        (e) **Other side effects.** Clozapine fairly commonly produces nausea and gastrointestinal disturbances. Headache is also fairly common. Many other side effects are found with lesser frequency. Patients who have experienced therapeutic benefit from clozapine often prefer to live with the substantial side effects.

    (5) Prescribing clozapine is not easy. The physician must register with the drug company and must be a part of the system of care, which includes a pharmacist and someone to perform monitoring functions. The weekly blood tests must be performed, and the patient must be located if he fails to report for tests. Clearly, the patient must be informed of the risks very carefully, both before starting the medication (if he can legally give consent) and after starting the medication (if he regains the ability to consent to the treatment as a result of the clozapine).

    (6) Dose and administration. Clozapine is recommended to be initiated at 12.5 mg once or twice a day, increasing to an average dose of 300 to 450 mg per day over a 2-week period. Doses may be gradually titrated upward to up to 900 mg per day. It should be emphasized that some patients will not respond to clozapine. After an adequate therapeutic trial, maintaining nonresponsive patients on clozapine makes little sense.

  c. Risperidone has recently been released for nonexperimental use. Like clozapine, early data suggest that risperidone may have positive effects on negative or deficit symptoms of schizophrenia.

    (1) Pharmacology. Risperidone is a benzisoxazole derivative, and it appears to exert its effects on D-2 and serotonin type 2 (5-HT$_2$) receptors.

    (2) Side effects. Risperidone appears to lack the risk of agranulocytosis that clozapine carries. Unfortunately, it **produces extrapyramidal symptoms** like a neuroleptic agent and probably has a higher risk for producing tardive dyskinesia and dystonia than does clozapine.

        (a) **Other side effects** include insomnia, agitation, dizziness, and constipation.

        (b) Because **increased prolactin secretion** is common (as with other dopamine-blocking agents), galactorrhea, gynecomastia, and amenorrhea can be expected in some patients.

        (c) Single reports each of **thrombotic thrombocytopenic purpura** and **priapism** have caused some concern.

    (3) Dose and administration. Usually risperidone is administered in twice-daily doses, starting at 1 mg twice daily and increasing to 3 mg twice daily over the first few days. Titration up to 16 mg per day is possible, and reduction of doses in some patients, particularly elderly patients, is advised.

  d. Other novel neuroleptic agents

    (1) Pimozide may have a future role in treating schizophrenic patients. Early data suggest that it is helpful in treating negative symptoms. Unfortunately, in the United States it is approved for use only in patients with Tourette disorder.

    (2) Experimental agents include sulpiride, remoxipride, rimcazole, tiospirone, and a host of other drugs that show promise for helping treatment-resistant symptoms or for treating patients with severe side effects from other medications.

3. Barbiturates. Amobarbital and **pentobarbital** have been used in the past for acute sedation of patients resistant to sedation with neuroleptics. Because of the risks of respiratory depression and other side effects, these drugs are not recommended. Benzodiazepines can be used more safely.

4. **Propranolol and other β blockers.** These medications have been reported to be effective in treating acute psychotic episodes in conjunction with neuroleptics. Propranolol appears to increase neuroleptic levels in the blood and to treat akathisia effectively.

5. **Lithium** may be an effective treatment when there is an affective component to the patient's illness or when there is uncertainty about the diagnosis (i.e., whether it is schizophrenia or a schizoaffective disorder). In some cases, lithium may be combined with neuroleptics to improve treatment in resistant cases. Recent literature reports that lithium may be the most effective adjunctive pharmacologic treatment for schizophrenia. It may be effective in some cases where affective symptoms are not evident or may not be present.

6. **Anticonvulsants.** Early reports of the effectiveness of **carbamazepine** and **valproate** as either adjunctive treatments or stand-alone treatments for schizophrenia have not proved to be correct. These medications even as an adjunctive treatment have not been impressive, and they tend to lose intitial effectiveness over the first month.

7. **ECT** has a secondary role in the treatment of schizophrenia and other acutely psychotic conditions. It is perhaps most effective in patients with affective and catatonic symptoms. Some studies suggest that ECT is acutely more effective than neuroleptics for the treatment of psychotic symptoms, although the risks and public perceptions of this treatment render it clearly a secondary line of treatment.
   Indications for ECT include:
   a. When life-threatening circumstances, such as severe catatonia or extreme suicidal ideation, are present
   b. When massive doses of neuroleptics are required, and smaller doses can be given following ECT
   c. When the patient is refractory to standard treatment regimens

DIRECTIONS: Each of the numbered items or incomplete statements in this section is followed by answers or by completions of the statement. Select the ONE lettered answer or completion that is BEST in each case.

1. Which of the following symptoms of schizophrenia is most likely to be acutely responsive to treatment with medications, milieu therapy, and other inpatient treatment methods?

(A) Auditory hallucinations
(B) Apathy
(C) Poverty of thought content
(D) Anhedonia
(E) Social withdrawal

2. A patient who has been diagnosed as schizophrenic asks his psychiatrist about the chances of a younger sister developing the same illness. Leaving aside the question of whether this information should or should not be shared with the patient, the psychiatrist knows that the biologic sister's chances of developing schizophrenia are about

(A) 70%
(B) 40%
(C) 25%
(D) 12%
(E) 1%

3. A 21-year-old man is referred to the psychiatrist through a student health service. The psychiatrist notes that the young man seems suspicious, talks vaguely with strange word usage, and seems unable to come to the point or include information in his speech. On further questioning, the man denies hallucinations but does appear to have a number of magical beliefs, which are generally inconsistent with those of the counterculture but which he has elaborated in an unusual way. His psychosocial functioning seems mildly to moderately impaired, but it seems to have been that way throughout much of junior high school and high school. The most likely diagnosis for the young man at this point is

(A) a personality disorder
(B) undifferentiated schizophrenia
(C) pseudoneurotic schizophrenia
(D) paranoid schizophrenia
(E) organic delusional syndrome

4. Which one of the following is true about socioeconomic factors influencing schizophrenia?

(A) In India, schizophrenia is more common among upper castes, partially disproving the drift hypothesis of schizophrenia
(B) In general, work should be avoided in patients with schizophrenia because of the harmful effects of job stress
(C) In the United States, the higher socioeconomic classes have higher rates of new cases of schizophrenia than lower socioeconomic classes
(D) Schizophrenic patients generally do poorly in times of low unemployment
(E) Large cities appear to offer protective effects against the development of new cases of schizophrenia

5. A 50-year-old woman with a history of multiple hospital admissions for treatment of schizophrenia over the last 30 years is now a patient in a community mental health center. She has been stable over the last 2 years, except for one hospitalization when the landlord tried to evict her for playing her stereo too loudly. She has been maintained on 10 mg/day of trifluoperazine and 8 mg/day of trihexyphenidyl. Because of her stable course, her psychiatrist decides to see if she can manage with less neuroleptic and cuts her dose in half. Within 2 days, she begins to experience unusual movements, including thrusting her lips and chin out at odd times, odd writhing wiggles of her trunk and some difficulty talking. The most likely explanation is

(A) parkinsonian symptoms related to the change in neuroleptic dose
(B) partial complex seizures related to the reduction of the anticonvulsant effect of the neuroleptic
(C) she is responding to tactile hallucinations with her unusual behavior
(D) she has developed Parkinson disease, which is being unmasked by the withdrawal of her dopamine-blocking neuroleptic
(E) she is exhibiting a withdrawal-emergent dyskinesia

DIRECTIONS: Each of the numbered items or incomplete statements in this section is negatively phrased, as indicated by a capitalized word such as NOT, LEAST, or EXCEPT. Select the ONE lettered answer or completion that is BEST in each case.

6. Negative symptoms of schizophrenia include all of the following EXCEPT

(A) affective blunting and flattening
(B) hallucinations of voices speaking to the patient
(C) lack of motivation and initiative
(D) anhedonia
(E) poverty of thought content

7. A 25-year-old man who has carried a diagnosis of schizophrenia for the past 6 years lives with his parents and does not work. They complain that he is an extreme "couch potato." Most days, he sits watching television. Once or twice a week, he goes to the downtown area with encouragement from parents, but only sits in a diner drinking coffee and smoking. When interviewed, the patient appears hypoactive. Answers to questions are minimal and very concrete. He will perform tasks only if each step is carefully outlined. He moves slowly and stops moving when he seems to run out of ideas of what to do next. He is taking 30 mg/day of thiothixene, prescribed by the community mental health center and has tried three other neuroleptics in the past. He has hallucinations almost constantly and has a system of bizarre delusional beliefs involving Elvis and extraterrestrial visitations. Which of the following is the LEAST potentially productive strategy to help this patient and his family?

(A) Consider switching to clozapine or risperidone
(B) Consider prescribing methylphenidate or an antidepressant
(C) Consider a psychosocial rehabilitation program and vocational skills training
(D) Consider cognitive/behavioral therapy or cognitive remediation to increase activity and expressiveness
(E) Consider lowering the daily neuroleptic dose to see if some of the problems are related to parkinsonian bradykinesia, while being careful to watch for the emergence of increasing psychotic symptoms

8. Evidence used to support genetic transmission of schizophrenia includes all of the following EXCEPT

(A) risks of developing schizophrenia in relatives of schizophrenics range from 3.5%–6%, in contrast to the rates of 0.02%–1.7% in the general population
(B) monozygotic twins have a concordance rate between 33% and 60% for schizophrenia if one member of the pair has schizophrenia
(C) monozygotic and dizygotic twins of the same sex have roughly the same rates of concordance for schizophrenia
(D) adoption studies find no role for vertical cultural transmission of schizophrenia in families as evidenced by no increased rate of schizophrenia in nonbiologic relatives of schizophrenics
(E) increased rates of schizophrenia spectrum disorders are found in biologic relatives of schizophrenic adoptees

9. A patient with a second psychotic episode has been in the hospital for 5 days with neuroleptic treatment. As the psychotic symptoms begin to resolve, the patient appears to be decreasingly active, has limited range of emotional expression, and says that he is sad. Sleep is normal in amount because of the neuroleptic sedation. Reasonable theories of the patient's condition include all of the following EXCEPT

(A) the patient is experiencing increasing bradykinesia and reductions in facial motility from the parkinsonian effects of the neuroleptics
(B) the patient is experiencing deficit symptoms of schizophrenia, and the complaint of sadness is usual with the remission of hallucinations and delusions
(C) the patient is responding to the sedative effects of the neuroleptics
(D) the patient is experiencing a major depressive episode and may need antidepressant medications in addition to neuroleptics
(E) the patient is responding with fear to an overstimulating ward milieu as demands for participation in groups from staff increase

DIRECTIONS: Each set of matching questions in this section consists of a list of four to twenty-six lettered options (some of which may be in figures) followed by several items. For each numbered item, select the ONE lettered option that is most closely associated with it. To avoid spending too much time on matching sets with large numbers of options, it is generally advisable to begin each set by reading the list of options. Then, for each item in the set, try to generate the correct answer and locate it in the option list, rather than evaluating each option individually. Each lettered option may be selected once, more than once, or not at all.

Questions 10–13

Match each clinical presentation with the best pharmacotherapeutic agent.

(A) Phenothiazines
(B) Novel neuroleptics
(C) Depot neuroleptics
(D) β blockers
(E) Anticholinergics

10. A 35-year-old patient has been hospitalized 10 times in the past year for relapse of symptoms. With each hospitalization, the patient quickly recompensates with monitored medications and the ward milieu.

11. A young, male patient with acute psychotic relapse complains of stiffness in his neck and drools excessively.

12. A patient with chronic delusional and hallucinatory symptoms demonstrates a lack of spontaneity, a lack of creativity, and finds it difficult to motivate himself to do anything other than sit in his apartment.

13. A patient with a previous psychotic episode has been medication-free for 1 year when she is brought to the psychiatric hospital with acute hallucinations of the devil telling her to kill her mother, beliefs that her mother is putting thoughts in her head, and acute agitation.

Questions 14–18

For each enzyme listed below, select the response most likely to be associated with it.

(A) Associated at one time with theories that methyl donors exacerbate schizophrenia
(B) Synthetic enzyme in noradrenergic neuronal systems
(C) No known contribution to schizophrenia
(D) The "muscle" isoenzyme is increased in schizophrenics and relatives of schizophrenics
(E) The "B" isoenzyme of this group is associated with cerebral ventricular enlargement in schizophrenics

14. Creatine phosphokinase

15. Dopamine-β-hydroxylase

16. Monoamine oxidase

17. Catechol-O-methyltransferase

18. Lactate dehydrogenase

ANSWERS AND EXPLANATIONS

1. The answer is A *[I; VIII B, C, G].* Generally, the positive symptoms of schizophrenia, including alterations in thinking, perceptions, and behavior, such as hallucinations and delusions, are more responsive to acute treatment than the negative symptoms of schizophrenia. Negative symptoms include affective flattening, social withdrawal, apathy, anhedonia, and poverty of thought and content of speech. Negative symptoms of schizophrenia may be more responsive to rehabilitation programs and other psychosocial interventions than to acute inpatient treatments.

2. The answer is D *[III F].* Leaving aside the adjustment of the percentage of risk for the sister's age, the risk of a full sibling developing schizophrenia is 10%–12%, according to an average of most studies of this topic. The risk for the general population is 1%.

3. The answer is A *[VI A 3–4, B 3].* The key feature of the presentation of the 21-year-old man described in the question is the lack of a clear episode of psychosis without which he cannot be diagnosed as schizophrenic. Diagnostic systems, which include dated concepts, such as "process schizophrenia" are no longer considered valid. Although organic mental syndrome is possible, there is no evidence that would lead the clinician to suspect this over a personality disorder, such as schizotypal personality disorder.

4. The answer is A *[III E].* In worldwide studies, meaningful work and a place in society is a factor in better courses for schizophrenia, while urban environments and lower socioeconomic conditions appear to be a risk factor both for the development of and poorer courses of schizophrenia. It is thought that in India, upper castes experience higher levels of social stress, accounting for this unusual finding.

5. The answer is E *[VIII K 1 f (1) (e)].* The first clue should be the type of movement problem. The description, though minimal, fits the description of a choreoathetotic movement disorder pattern. In contrast, parkinsonian movement problems tend to include characteristic tremor, mask-like facial mobility, and bradykinesia. Most parkinsonian symptoms are worse early in the course of increasing or beginning new medication (except akathisia), and this woman was on a stable dose of drug for years, which was then decreased. Thus, the second clue is the time frame of the problem in relation to drug level. Neuroleptics tend to reduce seizure threshold, not to raise it. Tactile hallucinations are a possible cause of these symptoms but are less likely than the common cause of this dyskinesia-like movement pattern. Although it is possible that the dyskinesia appeared spontaneously on reduction of neuroleptic dose, it is more likely that there were earlier symptoms of the dyskinesia that would have been detected by tests like the Abnormal Involuntary Movement Scale (AIMS).

6. The answer is B *[I A 2].* Hallucinations and delusions are positive symptoms of schizophrenia. "Positive" symptoms are those that are additions to the patient's mental state, in contrast to absent, or "negative" symptoms. Negative symptoms are those subtracted from the patient's mental state, such as loss of affect and lack of motivation and initiative.

7. The answer is B *[VIII J, K 2 b (4) (b)].* Although there is no definitive solution to what are probably negative symptoms of schizophrenia, any of the strategies listed in this question, except prescribing methylphenidate or an antidepressant, is reasonable to try. There is no evidence that antidepressants improve negative symptoms, and the use of methylphenidate may increase psychotic symptoms. Despite the paucity of evidence for their use, antidepressants are often prescribed in the mental health system, under the assumption that patients are depressed. Cognitive remediation and cognitive/behavioral therapy for negative symptoms are experimental but might be attempted if local expertise in these fields is available.

8. The answer is C *[III F].* Monozygotic twins raised together have a concordance rate for schizophrenia of 91%; if raised apart, they are concordant at a rate of 78%, according to one study. Some studies show high rates of mental illness in relatives of schizophrenics, and adoption studies have shown that there is no increased rate of schizophrenia in nonbiologic relatives of schizophrenics. If there were equal rates of schizophrenia in monozygotic and dizygotic twins, there would be strong evidence for an environmental as opposed to a genetic mode of transmission of schizophrenia, but this has not been found to be true.

9. The answer is D *[VIII C, K 1–2]*. Depressive symptoms associated with acute psychotic episodes tend to resolve with the resolution of the psychotic symptoms, and no antidepressant treatment is necessary. Parkinsonian symptoms may indeed cause the patient to appear depressed, but all that may be needed is control of emerging parkinsonian symptoms. Sedation can produce a similar picture. Too-active demands for participation in ward milieu may produce withdrawal in a patient too ill for this activity.

10–13. The answers are: 10-C *[VIII K 1]*, **11-E** *[VIII K 1 f (1) (a)]*, **12-B** *[VIII K 2]*, **13-A** *[VIII K 1]*. A history of 10 hospitalizations in the past year provides clues that the patient is having difficulty taking the oral antipsychotic medications prescribed. The patient may be unable to afford the medication, or may be too disorganized to take it. Some patients become suspicious of oral medications because of a transient exacerbation of the illness. In all of these cases, depot neuroleptics, administered with an injection every 2 weeks, may be the most effective solution.

The acute dystonia and drooling described in the young, male patient are typically found shortly after starting neuroleptics. These are typical parkinsonian side effects of neuroleptics, and are usually easily reversed by administering an anticholinergic medication.

The patient with chronic delusions presents one set of commonly found negative symptoms. Older neuroleptics are of little value in treating these symptoms. Several of the newer, novel neuroleptics may offer significant benefits in reducing symptoms. They may also offer relief to patients with chronic positive symptoms unrelieved by older medications.

Early in the course of a psychotic episode, the standard practice is to try treatment with standard neuroleptic medications. In some cases, the potential side effects of the novel neuroleptics, and in all cases, the costs of these newer medications, make their use as a first-line treatment of acute psychotic symptoms a less than ideal choice. In the future, this situation may change as some of the new medications are released and prices are decreased.

14–18. The answers are: 14-D, 15-B, 16-E, 17-A, 18-C *[VII B 2 a–d]*. The muscle form (not brain as might be expected) of creatine phosphokinase has been found to be increased in schizophrenics and relatives of schizophrenics. This may reflect increased levels of muscle breakdown due to as yet unknown processes or simple increases in muscular activity in this group.

Dopamine-β-hydroxylase (DBH) catalyzes the transformation of dopamine to norepinephrine in noradrenergic neurons. It has been found to be reduced in schizophrenics with increased ventricular size, although its overall significance is yet unclear. Low levels of DBH appear to be correlated with better psychosocial functioning than high levels.

Recent research has focused on the role of monoamine oxidase, subtype B, which is found to be associated with changes in ventricular size in schizophrenia. It is likely to be a nonspecific indicator of pathology rather than being directly associated with schizophrenia.

Catechol-O-methyltransferase (COMT) is a major extracellular route for the metabolism of catecholamines. It was originally found that *l*-methionine exacerbated the symptoms of schizophrenics, and this finding was replicated with betaine. Attention was focused on the possible role of COMT in schizophrenia. However, other amino acids without a likely role in donating methyl groups were found to produce similar symptoms. Interest in this enzyme has waned to some extent.

To date there has been no indication that lactate dehydrogenase is involved in schizophrenia.

Chapter 3

Mood Disorders
Nancy A. Breslin

I. **DEFINITION.** The prominent feature of mood disorders is a **disturbance of mood** along the happy–sad axis. Disorders featuring anxious mood are described in Chapter 4. The *Diagnostic and Statistical Manual of Mental Disorders,* 4th edition (DSM-IV) classifies mood disorders to include **major depressive disorder, bipolar I disorder, bipolar II disorder, dysthymia, cyclothymia, mood disorder due to a general medical condition,** and **substance-induced mood disorder.**

II. **HISTORY.** Serious investigation into the etiology and classification of mood disorders began in the middle of the nineteenth century. As in other areas of psychiatry and medicine, prevailing theories have continually shifted, particularly regarding the tendency to view mood disorders as a problem with the brain (a biologically based illness) or a problem with the mind (a psychologically based illness).

A. **Nineteenth century.** In the **middle-to-late nineteenth century,** a number of clinicians began to see the possibility of differentiating forms of "insanity."

1. Rather than lumping all such patients together, **Emil Kraepelin** noted that some psychotic patients had a cyclical pattern and prominent mood symptoms (manic–depression) and others had a more chronic pattern that also featured cognitive impairment (i.e., **dementia praecox,** now called **schizophrenia**).

2. Because other mental disorders, such as Alzheimer disease and neurosyphilis, were found at the turn of the twentieth century to have neuropathologic correlates, it was assumed by many that schizophrenia and mood disorders were also due to brain diseases.

B. **Twentieth century**

1. In the **twentieth century,** particularly in the United States, psychoanalytic theorists believed that many mood disorders stemmed from the psychological response to loss. A differentiation was often made between **endogenous** (caused by biologic factors) and **exogenous** (caused by loss or other environmental stresses) depression. With the emphasis on psychological factors, less effort was put into the neurochemical and neuroanatomic research of mood disorders during the first half of the century.

2. In the **1950s,** appreciation of the biologic underpinnings of mood disorders was stimulated by the serendipitous observation that two drugs affect depression.
   a. **Iproniazid,** which was being studied as a treatment for tuberculosis, was found to elevate the mood of the (often depressed) patients. Knowledge that this drug acted as a **monoamine oxidase inhibitor (MAOI)** lead to speculation that low levels of monoamines [e.g., norepinephrine (NE), serotonin (5-HT), dopamine] might play a role in the etiology of depression.
   b. Similarly, the antihypertensive drug **reserpine** (which **depletes monoamines** presynaptically) was found to cause depression in some patients.

3. It is currently believed that the interaction of biologic and psychosocial factors determine which individuals will develop mood disorders. The exogenous–endogenous

dichotomy is no longer seen as a critical distinction because patients with and without obvious environmental causes of their depressions can have similar prognosis and treatment response.

III. DIAGNOSIS

A. **Identification of mood episodes.** The diagnosis of a mood disorder requires the identification of mood episodes. These are not diagnoses. Rather, they are the building blocks a clinician uses in making the diagnosis of a mood disorder (see III B). The DSM-IV defines **four types of mood episodes:** major depressive episode, manic episode, mixed episode, and hypomanic episode. The criteria for each require that the mood symptoms lead to serious distress or dysfunction and that they are not due to the effects of drugs, alcohol, or a medical condition.

1. **Major depressive episode (MDE).** The criteria for MDE are shown in Table 3-1. To be characterized as MDE, symptoms must represent a change from baseline and must persist for at least 2 weeks.
   a. A patient must exhibit **either depressed mood or a notable decrease in interest or pleasure**. Another name for the inability to experience pleasure is **anhedonia**. Loss of interest commonly extends to **loss of libido**.

TABLE 3-1. DSM-IV Diagnostic Criteria for Major Depressive Episode

A. At least five of the following symptoms have been present during the same 2-week period and represent a change from previous functioning; at least one of the symptoms is either (1) depressed mood or (2) loss of interest or pleasure.

   1. Depressed mood most of the day, nearly every day, as indicated by either subjective report (e.g., feels sad or empty) or observation made by others (e.g., appears tearful); in children and adolescents, can be irritable mood
   2. Markedly diminished interest or pleasure in all, or almost all, activities most of the day, nearly every day (as indicated either by subjective account or observation made by others)
   3. Significant weight loss or weight gain when not dieting (e.g., more than 5% of body weight in 1 month), or decrease or increase in appetite nearly every day; in children, consider failure to make expected weight gains
   4. Insomnia or hypersomnia nearly every day
   5. Psychomotor agitation or retardation nearly every day (observable by others, not merely subjective feelings of restlessness or being slowed down)
   6. Fatigue or loss of energy nearly every day
   7. Feelings of worthlessness or excessive or inappropriate guilt (which may be delusional) nearly every day (not merely self-reproach or guilt about being sick)
   8. Diminished ability to think or concentrate, or indecisiveness, nearly every day (either by subjective account or as observed by others)
   9. Recurrent thoughts of death (not just fear of dying); recurrent suicidal ideation without a specific plan; or a suicide attempt or a specific plan for committing suicide

B. The symptoms cause clinically significant distress or impairment in social, occupational, or other important areas of functioning.

C. The symptoms are not due to the direct effects of a substance (e.g., drugs of abuse, medication) or a general medical condition (e.g., hypothyroidism).

D. The symptoms are not better accounted for by bereavement (i.e., after the loss of a loved one, the symptoms persist for longer than 2 months or are characterized by marked functional impairment, morbid preoccupation with worthlessness, suicidal ideation, psychotic symptoms, or psychomotor retardation).

    b. Patients typically exhibit **neurovegetative symptoms** of depression, such as changes in sleep and appetite. Sleep impairment may involve initial insomnia (trouble falling asleep), middle insomnia (awakening during the night), or terminal insomnia (early morning awakening). Whereas sleep and appetite usually decrease in MDE, in atypical depression the patient notes oversleeping and increased appetite with weight gain.

    c. **Fatigue** and **impaired concentration** are common.

    d. **Psychomotor activity** may be increased (agitation: pacing, hand wringing) or decreased (retardation: including soft speech, lack of eye contact, immobility).

    e. Feelings of **worthlessness** and **guilt** are often present. The guilt may be **delusional** (i.e., a fixed, false belief, such as thinking that one has committed a great crime or caused a natural disaster).

    f. **Thoughts of death** or **suicidal ideation** are also common features of an MDE. Suicidal ideation can range from passive ideas (e.g., wishing one would develop cancer) to active plans.

2. **Manic episode.** This features a distinct period of elevated or irritable mood that lasts at least 1 week. DSM-IV criteria are given in Table 3-2. Features of mania include the following.

    a. **Grandiosity** involves an elevated opinion of one's features and accomplishments. A manic patient may feel extraordinarily attractive, engage in name dropping, exaggerate educational and career achievements, and feel superior to other people. **Grandiose delusions** may also be seen, such as a patient's belief that he has achieved world peace or owns a billion-dollar company.

    b. During a manic episode, **most patients need little sleep.** Whereas depressed individuals complain about their short nights, patients with mania feel well rested after only 2 or 3 hours of sleep.

    c. **Pressured speech,** as observed by the clinician, may reflect the **flight of ideas,** or **racing thoughts,** which the patient experiences.

TABLE 3-2. DSM-IV Diagnostic Criteria for a Manic Episode

A. A distinct period of abnormally and persistently elevated, expansive, or irritable mood lasts at least 1 week (or any duration if hospitalization is necessary).

B. During the period of mood disturbance, at least three of the following symptoms have persisted (four if the mood is only irritable) and have been present to a significant degree:

    1. Inflated self-esteem or grandiosity
    2. Decreased need for sleep (e.g., feels rested after only 3 hours of sleep)
    3. More talkative than usual or pressure to keep talking
    4. Flight of ideas or subjective experience that thoughts are racing
    5. Distractibility (i.e., attention too easily drawn to unimportant or irrelevant external stimuli)
    6. Increase in goal-directed activity (e.g., socially, at work or school, or sexually) or psychomotor agitation
    7. Excessive involvement in pleasurable activities that have a high potential for painful consequences (e.g., the person engages in unrestrained buying sprees, sexual indiscretions, or foolish business investments)

C. The mood disturbance is sufficiently severe to cause marked impairment in the occupational functioning or in usual social activities or relationships with others or to necessitate hospitalization to prevent harm to self or others, or there are psychotic features.

D. The symptoms are not due to the direct effects of a substance (e.g., drugs of abuse, medication) or a general medical condition (e.g., hyperthyroidism).

Note: Manic episodes that are clearly precipitated by somatic antidepressant treatment (e.g., medication, electroconvulsive therapy, light therapy) should not count toward a diagnosis of bipolar I disorder.

    d. Manic patients are **easily distracted** and will become interested in various environmental stimuli. This can lead to difficulty in engaging such a patient during an interview. During mental status testing, vigilance tests, such as the continuous performance task (CPT), will show evidence of this dysfunction.

    e. An **increase in goal-directed activities** is often seen, as well as participation in **potentially dangerous activities,** such as gambling, sexual promiscuity, or reckless driving.

3. Mixed episode. This describes a period during which a patient meets criteria for **both manic episode and MDE over a 1-week period**. Such a patient might exhibit pressured speech, irritability, and the need for little sleep, while feeling worthless and suicidal.

4. Hypomanic episode. This is similar in many ways to a manic episode but is less severe. Differences in the criteria include the following.

    a. The episode need only last 4 days.

    b. The episode must not lead to hospitalization, must not include psychotic features (e.g., delusions), and must not cause severe social or occupational impairment.

B. **Diagnosis of mood disorders.** Differentiation of the mood disorders listed below relies upon the presence or absence of the mood episodes discussed in III A 1–4. Table 3-3 may help to clarify the various diagnoses.

1. Major depressive disorder

    a. Diagnosis. This diagnosis requires the presence of one or more MDEs and the absence of any manic, hypomanic, or mixed episodes.

    b. Associated clinical features

        (1) Psychotic features are seen in some patients and are most often **mood congruent** (i.e., the content of the delusion or hallucination reflects depression). A mood-congruent delusion might be the belief that one has committed terrible crimes or sins. A mood-congruent hallucination might be a voice that tells one to die or says that one is a loser.

        (2) Melancholia refers to a more severe subtype of major depression and features more profound anhedonia and neurovegetative symptoms. Early morning awakening and significant weight loss are common.

        (3) Mortality and morbidity. In addition to the risk of suicide, patients with major depressive disorder have a higher risk of illness or death due to medical causes.

        (4) Psychiatric comorbidity. Patients with major depression are at risk for several other psychiatric conditions (e.g., alcohol or other substance abuse, anxiety disorders).

    c. Epidemiology

        (1) Risk and prevalence. The lifetime risk of developing major depressive disorder is about 15% overall; the prevalence in women is roughly twice the prevalence in men. The risk is similar in different countries and across races.

TABLE 3-3. Differentiation of Mood Disorders

Diagnosis	Major Depressive Episode	Milder Depression	Manic or Mixed Episode	Hypomania
Major depressive disorder	+	±	−	−
Dysthymic disorder	−*	+	−	−
Bipolar I disorder	±	±	+	±
Bipolar II disorder	+	±	−	+
Cyclothymia	−	+	−†	+

+ = This syndrome must be present to make the diagnosis; − = this syndrome must be absent to make the diagnosis; ± = this syndrome may be present or absent.
*A major depressive episode must not occur during the first 2 years of the illness.
†A manic episode must not occur during the first 2 years of the illness.

(2) Age of onset. The age of onset can range from childhood to old age; the mean age is approximately 40 years.

(3) Recurrence. Approximately 50% of people who have one episode of major depression will have one or more additional episodes.

d. Differential diagnosis. The symptoms seen in patients with major depressive disorder can overlap with symptoms of many other illnesses.

(1) Other psychiatric disorders that may have symptoms similar to major depressive disorder include dysthymia, adjustment disorder with depressed mood, schizoaffective disorder, dementia, anxiety disorders, and personality disorders.

(2) Substance-induced mood disorders may be caused by intoxication with depressant drugs (e.g., alcohol, opiates, barbiturates), withdrawal from stimulants (e.g., cocaine, amphetamines), or treatment with medications such as steroids, some antihypertensives (i.e., reserpine, propranolol), and cimetidine.

(3) Mood disorders due to a general medical condition. Depression has been associated with a number of medical illnesses, including hypothyroidism, left anterior stroke, pancreatic cancer, Parkinson disease, sleep apnea, and tuberculosis.

(4) Normal bereavement can feature many symptoms of a major depressive episode and may meet the criteria for it, as well. A diagnosis of major depressive disorder is not usually made unless the criteria are still met 2 months after the loss. There are some symptoms that are atypical for normal bereavement, such as hallucinations unrelated to the loss and prolonged functional impairment, which are more suggestive of major depression. One must recognize that the symptoms and duration of "normal" bereavement vary among cultures.

2. Dysthymic disorder

a. Diagnosis

(1) This diagnosis is made when a patient presents with a **chronic depression** (at least 2 years in duration) that has **not** been **severe enough to meet the criteria for MDE.** Rather than the five symptoms required of MDE, the patient must have two of the following: increased or decreased appetite, increased or decreased sleep, low energy, low self-esteem, poor concentration or decision-making ability, and hopelessness.

(2) If a patient experiences an MDE after 2 years of dysthymia, more than one diagnosis is made (dysthymic disorder and major depressive disorder).

(3) In addition, the patient must never have met criteria for manic episode, mixed episode, or hypomanic episode.

b. Associated clinical features. Dysthymic disorder is associated with social impairment, health problems, alcohol and other drug abuse, and major depressive disorder. Coexistence of dysthymic disorder and major depression is sometimes referred to as **double depression**.

c. Epidemiology. The lifetime risk of dysthymia is about 5% overall; the prevalence rate in women is about twice that in men. Patients who develop dysthymia before age 21 are more likely to develop major depressive disorder later.

d. Differential diagnosis is similar to that of major depressive disorder (see III B 1 d).

3. Bipolar I disorder. Bipolar is a misnomer for this illness, since a single manic episode is enough for the diagnosis (i.e., one only needs one "pole"). However, most patients experience manic and depressive symptoms, and the first episode may be manic, hypomanic, depressed, or mixed. Of course, if the first episode is hypomanic or depressed, the proper diagnosis will not be made until the later emergence of mania.

a. Diagnosis. The diagnosis of bipolar I disorder is made when a patient has experienced **at least one manic or mixed episode,** unless the symptoms were caused by a substance (including antidepressants) or a general medical condition. Major depressive episodes may or may not have ever been present.

b. Associated clinical features

(1) Psychotic features. Delusions, hallucinations, and disorganization can be seen during manic episodes, with severity similar in degree to that in schizophrenia. These are most often **mood congruent**. A mood-congruent delusion in mania might be the belief that one has found a cure for cancer or won an Academy Award. Mood-congruent hallucinations might include hearing the voice of God.

    (2) Morbidity and mortality. Attempted and completed suicide are both common in patients with bipolar I disorder. Comorbid medical problems can deteriorate because of poor compliance, which is caused by grandiosity or generally impaired judgment. Reckless behavior can increase the risk of sexually transmitted diseases and injuries.

    (3) Psychiatric comorbidity. Alcohol and other forms of drug abuse frequently complicate manic episodes and can carry into other phases of this disorder. Eating disorders, anxiety disorders, and attention deficit hyperactivity disorder are also associated with bipolar illness.

  c. Epidemiology. The lifetime risk of bipolar I disorder is about 1% and is similar in men and women and across racial groups. The mean age of onset is 21 years. More than 90% of people who have a manic episode will have additional episodes of mania or major depression.

  d. Differential diagnosis

    (1) Other psychiatric disorders. Similar symptoms are seen in bipolar II disorder and cyclothymia. When psychotic symptoms exist, it can be difficult to differentiate bipolar I disorder from schizophrenia or schizoaffective disorder. However, if a patient has ever had delusions or hallucinations for at least 2 weeks in the absence of mania or major depression, then a psychotic disorder (rather than a mood disorder with psychotic features) must be diagnosed. Narcissistic personality disorder also has overlapping features.

    (2) Substance-induced mood disorder. Intoxication with stimulants, such as cocaine or amphetamine, can mimic mania. Antidepressant drugs can occasionally cause a patient to "switch" from depression to mania. Other prescription medications (e.g., corticosteroids, dopamine agonists, anticholinergics, cimetidine) can also precipitate manic symptoms.

    (3) Mood disorder due to a general medical condition. Manic symptoms can be seen with infectious diseases, with acquired immune deficiency syndrome (AIDS), endocrinopathies (e.g., Cushing disease, hyperthyroidism), lupus, and a variety of neurologic disorders (e.g., epilepsy, multiple sclerosis, Wilson disease).

4. Bipolar II disorder. This disorder is officially recognized for the first time in the DSM-IV.

  a. Diagnosis. This diagnosis is made when a patient has had **at least one MDE and one hypomanic episode** in the absence of any manic or mixed episodes.

  b. Associated features. Suicide is a risk, particularly during depressive episodes. As with major depression and bipolar I disorder, comorbidity with substance abuse or anxiety disorders is common.

  c. Epidemiology. The lifetime risk is approximately 0.5% and is higher in women than in men. There do not appear to be racial differences.

  d. Differential diagnosis is similar to bipolar I disorder (see III B 3 d).

5. Cyclothymic disorder. This disorder could be described as dysthymia with intermittent hypomanic periods. Like dysthymia, it is a chronic rather than episodic illness.

  a. Diagnosis. A patient who, over at least 2 years, experiences **repeated episodes of hypomania and depression (not severe enough to meet criteria for major depressive disorder)** is diagnosed with cyclothymic disorder. During the first 2 years the patient may not have an MDE, manic, or mixed episode. If such episodes occur after 2 years, more than one diagnosis may be made (e.g., cyclothymia and bipolar I disorder).

  b. Associated features. Substance abuse and social and occupational dysfunction are commonly seen.

  c. Epidemiology. The lifetime risk of cyclothymia is about 1%; it is slightly higher in women than in men. The age of onset is usually in the teens or early adulthood, and the course tends to be chronic. Up to 50% of people with cyclothymic disorder may ultimately develop bipolar disorder.

    d. The **differential diagnosis** of cyclothymia is similar to that of bipolar I disorder (see III B 3 d). In addition, the features of cyclothymia must be differentiated from the mood swings seen in borderline personality disorder.

  6. **Mood disorder due to a general medical condition** and **substance-induced mood disorder** are two other mood disorder diagnoses in the DSM-IV. As noted previously, other mood disorder diagnoses (e.g., major depressive disorder) are not made if medical illness or drug use appears to be the cause of the symptoms. Clinical examples include the following.

    a. If a 69-year-old man who recently suffered a left anterior stroke now has the symptoms of an MDE, the appropriate diagnosis would be mood disorder due to cerebrovascular accident, with a major depressive-like episode.

    b. A 32-year-old woman who presents to an emergency department with manic behavior has traces of amphetamine in her urine. The symptoms clear over several days without pharmacologic treatment. The diagnosis would be amphetamine-induced mood disorder with manic features, with onset during intoxication.

IV. ETIOLOGY.

Over the years, mood disorders have been thought to represent brain disease, to reflect intrapsychic conflicts, and then back to represent a biologic process. The etiology is probably multifactorial.

A. **Genetic factors.** Both major depressive and bipolar disorders run in families, which does not necessarily indicate genetic transmission. However, a variety of research techniques have shown the etiology of mood disorders to be at least partly genetic.

  1. **Family studies**

    a. **Major depressive disorder.** Approximately 50% of people with major depressive disorder have a first-degree relative with a mood disorder, which is more often depression than bipolar disorder. Concordance for identical twins is approximately 50%, whereas siblings (including fraternal twins) have an approximate 15% risk. When one twin of a concordant pair has major depression, the other twin usually has depression rather than bipolar illness.

    b. **Bipolar disorder.** Approximately 90% of people with bipolar illness have a first-degree relative with a mood disorder, most frequently bipolar illness. Concordance has been estimated to range between 33% and 90% for monozygotic twins and between 5% and 25% for other siblings. If the twin of a bipolar patient becomes ill, the disorder may be either bipolar or depressive.

  2. **Adoption studies** in both major depression and bipolar disorder have supported a genetic etiology.

  3. **Linkage studies**

    a. Studies have suggested that bipolar disorder is inherited in some families in an **X-linked pattern** and that in other families the disorder is linked to **chromosome 11**. Further study with the Amish pedigree involved in the latter finding failed to confirm the linkage.

    b. **Chromosome 18** has also been implicated in some studies.

    c. Linkage studies are difficult because investigators are unsure whether to expect genetic patterns for particular mood disorders (e.g., pure major depression) or for a spectrum of diseases (e.g., major depression and dysthymia; major depression and bipolar disorder).

B. **Neurochemical factors.** A number of neurotransmitters have been implicated in mood disorders, particularly **NE** and **5-HT**.

  1. **NE** association with mood disorders is based upon a variety of findings.

    a. Many effective antidepressant medications (e.g., desipramine, nortriptyline) block NE reuptake immediately and **down-regulate β-receptors** after several weeks. Since the latter effect correlates with the onset of action, it has been speculated that **adrenergic function may be abnormal in depression**.

b. Measurements of NE or its metabolites in cerebrospinal fluid (CSF), plasma, and urine have shown variable results.
c. Increased NE activity has been speculated to be involved in mania.

2. **5-HT** has been of more interest since the introduction of primarily serotonergic antidepressants.
   a. The **selective serotonin reuptake inhibitors (SSRIs),** such as fluoxetine, have proved to be effective antidepressants.
   b. 5-HT and 5-hydroxyindoleacetic acid (5-HIAA; a serotonin metabolite) have been found in low levels in depressed patients in some studies, and 5-HT depletion (e.g., by a tryptophan-depleted diet) can worsen depression.

3. **Dopamine** is less solidly linked to depression, but there is some suggestive evidence.
   a. Bupropion is an effective antidepressant that is dopaminergic without directly affecting 5-HT or NE transmission.
   b. Parkinson disease, which involves dopaminergic dysfunction, often leads to depressive symptoms.

4. **Other neurotransmitters,** including γ-aminobutyric acid (GABA) and neuropeptides, have also been implicated in mood disorders.

C. **Other biologic factors**

1. **Neuroendocrine regulation** appears to be related to mood disorders.
   a. The hypothalamic-pituitary-adrenal (HPA) axis may be disrupted in depression, as the dexamethasone suppression test (DST) demonstrates. Normally, administration of dexamethasone (a synthetic corticosteroid) suppresses the HPA axis, and serum cortisol levels drop. Depressed patients, however, have been found to exhibit **nonsuppression** (cortisol remains elevated). The DST is not selective or specific enough to be used in routine clinical care, but it points to endocrine involvement.
   b. **Hypothyroidism** may mimic depression, and **hyperthyroidism** may mimic mania. In addition, a subset of depressed patients release a low amount of thyroid-stimulating hormone after being given thyrotropin-releasing hormone.

2. **Sleep and circadian rhythm**
   a. Problems with sleep are common in mood disorders. Depressed patients may experience insomnia or hypersomnia, and manic patients typically have a decreased need for sleep.
   b. **Polysomnography** shows that many depressed patients have **shortened rapid eye movement (REM) latency** (i.e., the time from falling asleep to the first REM period is about 60 minutes rather than 90 minutes). Other abnormalities of sleep architecture are also found.
   c. **Sleep deprivation** is an effective treatment for depression, although depression returns after the next night's sleep.

3. **Kindling** is a phenomenon observed when repeated, subthreshold stimulation of the brain eventually results in seizure activity. It has been postulated that bipolar illness follows a similar paradigm.
   a. **Anticonvulsant drugs,** such as carbamazepine and valproic acid, are effective treatments for bipolar disorder.
   b. The temporal pattern of mood disorders may be suggestive of kindling. For instance, some patients have a first episode of illness in response to stress (e.g., a loss), with subsequent episodes following lower-grade stress, and spontaneous episodes eventually occurring.

D. **Psychological and social factors**

1. **Stress** commonly precedes the first episode of both major depression and mania. It has been speculated that such stress can precipitate brain changes, which make an individual more vulnerable to future mood episodes.

2. **Loss of a parent** before the age of 11 years has been linked to depression in adulthood.

3. Some psychodynamic theorists have proposed that depression represents **anger turned inward;** that is, a person becomes angry at a loved one (often one who was lost) but, because such anger is intrapsychically unacceptable, the patient experiences depression and self-hatred.

4. Animal studies have lead to the model of depression as **learned helplessness**. An animal exposed to inescapable shock will, over time, fail to escape the shock even when given the opportunity. Antidepressant medications reverse this behavior.

5. Depressed individuals often express inaccurate, negative cognitions (e.g., "I've never done anything right"). **Cognitive therapy,** aimed at changing these cognitions, can improve depressive symptoms in many individuals.

V. TREATMENT

A. **Overall treatment planning.** Mood disorders vary in symptoms and severity, but some overall guidelines exist.

1. **Treatment setting**
   a. **Type of clinician.** Most patients with mood disorders are treated by clinicians other than mental health professionals.
      (1) **Primary care physicians** provide much of the care for disorders that respond well to medication, although this can present several problems, including:
         (a) Inadequate diagnosis
         (b) Limited time for supportive therapy (which improves compliance and treatment response)
         (c) A tendency to use lower-than-needed doses of medication (which is less of a problem now that SSRIs, which have a wider therapeutic index, have been introduced)
      (2) **Psychiatrists** are able to provide both medication and psychotherapy.
      (3) Psychologists, psychiatric social workers, and other mental health professionals often provide assessment and psychotherapy.
   b. **Location of treatment.** Patients with mood disorders are most often treated in **outpatient settings,** although dangerous or disorganized patients and those who have failed outpatient treatment may require **hospitalization.** An intermediate setting is the **psychiatric day hospital,** which provides daytime support, supervision, and therapy, and the patient returns home at night.

2. **Diagnostic evaluation.** The various mood disorders are treated quite differently. Therefore, it is important to establish, for instance, if a patient with a current MDE has a prior history of mania. Comorbid psychiatric and medical problems must also be identified or ruled out. Such an evaluation can be done in either an inpatient or outpatient setting.

3. **Assessment of safety.** All mood disorders carry a risk of suicide. All clinicians who deal with these patients must be familiar with assessment of suicidal risk, so that appropriate steps can be taken (e.g., **voluntary or involuntary hospitalization**) when needed to ensure the patient's safety. In addition, bipolar patients may engage in behavior which, while not suicidal, is dangerous to themselves or others. Evidence of such behavior requires similar steps to protect the patient.

B. **Treatment of major depressive disorder**

1. **Hospitalization.** Whereas most patients with major depression can safely be treated as outpatients, a subset of patients require hospitalization, which can serve several functions.

  a. Safety for a suicidal or severely psychotic patient can often be best ensured in a hospital.
  b. Treatment can, at times, be more rapidly instituted in the hospital setting.
     (1) Medication doses can be advanced more rapidly in a setting where side effects can be rapidly identified and alleviated.
     (2) Electroconvulsive therapy (ECT), at times an outpatient procedure, is more commonly done on inpatients.
  c. Support, in the form of individual and group therapies and general staff availability, is intensive in a hospital setting.

2. **Outpatient treatment.** Various levels and modalities of outpatient treatment are available.
  a. A **combination of psychotherapy and medication** is probably the most effective treatment for major depression. This may be provided by one clinician (e.g., a psychiatrist) or different clinicians (e.g., an internist and a social worker).
  b. Several **models of psychotherapy** for depression have been utilized.
     (1) Psychodynamic, or psychoanalytically oriented, psychotherapy is probably the most commonly used with depressed patients, although it is also the least well studied.
     (2) Two forms of time-limited therapy, **cognitive therapy** and **interpersonal therapy,** have been found in controlled studies to be effective treatments for depression.
  c. Since **support** appears to be an important variable both in treatment and safety, a number of supportive measures (in addition to individual therapy) are often utilized.
     (1) Family or friends are often involved in some phase of treatment.
     (2) Day hospitalization may be used instead of or as a transition from inpatient hospitalization.
     (3) Supportive living arrangements (group homes) may be recommended for patients with more refractory symptoms, more limited social supports, or comorbid factors.

3. **Somatic therapies (medication and ECT).** All of the somatic therapies listed have proved similarly effective in treating MDEs. Response to all of the antidepressant medications takes time, with full response usually seen within 4–6 weeks. When choosing a treatment for an individual patient, the clinician must consider prior treatment response in the patient or a family member, comorbid psychiatric or medical problems, and factors that might make side effects of a particular drug more or less problematic.
  a. Tricyclic antidepressants were the standard drug treatment for several decades, and they are still used for many patients. All tricyclic antidepressants are hepatically metabolized, renally excreted, and have a narrow therapeutic index. Relatively long half-lives allow once-daily dosing. Cardiotoxicity shared by these drugs leads to the lethality of overdose.
     (1) Tertiary tricyclics (e.g., imipramine, amitriptyline) are the oldest of this class. Their use is limited by a side-effect profile that includes prominent sedative and anticholinergic effects.
     (2) Secondary tricyclics (e.g., nortriptyline, desipramine) tend to be less anticholinergic, less sedating, and less likely to cause orthostatic hypotension.
  b. MAOIs were discovered in the 1950s, but have not been popular because of the **hypertensive crisis** that can be precipitated when these drugs interact with sympathomimetic agents (including a diet high in tyramine, which is found in ripe cheese, for example). Other side effects of these agents include orthostatic hypotension, weight gain, and insomnia. A new class of **reversible inhibitors of monoamine oxidase A (RIMAs),** which appear to be as effective as the standard MAOIs but much safer, may soon be available.
  c. SSRIs, which were introduced in the 1980s, have the advantages of once-daily dosing and a wide therapeutic index. **Fluoxetine, sertraline, paroxetine,** and **fluvoxamine** are currently available. Limitations include side effects (e.g., nausea, insomnia,

anxiety, sexual dysfunction) and drug interactions (fluoxetine and paroxetine significantly affect the hepatic P_{450} system; combination with other serotonergic drugs can
precipitate a potentially lethal **serotonin syndrome**).

d. **Triazolopyridines** include **trazodone** and **nefazodone**. Both of these agents have a
short half-life (necessitating multiple daily dosing) and a wide therapeutic index.
Trazodone is very sedating, whereas nefazodone is not; neither drug has prominent
anticholinergic effects. Male patients on trazodone run a risk of developing
priapism.

e. **Bupropion** is an aminoketone that blocks the reuptake of dopamine rather than
5-HT or NE. Whereas it is not highly lethal in overdose, it has a narrow therapeutic
index because of a dose-related tendency to cause **seizures**. Side effects include restlessness, tremors, and nausea. Multiple daily dosing is usually required.

f. **Venlafaxine** has been called a selective 5-HT–NE reuptake inhibitor. It has a wide
therapeutic index and requires twice-daily dosing. Side effects resemble those associated with SSRIs and are dose dependent.

g. **ECT.** When performed with present-day equipment and anesthetic procedures, ECT
is a safe and effective treatment for major depressive disorder.

(1) The use of ECT remains limited, however, because of bias remaining from the
years when it was a much cruder procedure. Use of ECT is often reserved for
patients with psychotic depressions and those who have failed or are unable to
tolerate trials of antidepressant medications.

(2) Common **complications** are confusion immediately after the procedure and
memory loss, which usually resolves within 6 months. There is no evidence that
ECT causes permanent brain damage.

C. Treatment of bipolar I and bipolar II disorders

1. **Hospitalization.** As is the case with major depressive disorder, a subset of patients with
bipolar disorder require hospitalization, usually because of the risks of suicide during
the depressed phase or out-of-control behavior during the manic phase.

a. **Containment of manic behavior** can prevent potentially disastrous consequences for
a patient, including financial loss, arrest, and destroyed relationships.

b. **Initial or reinstituted treatment** with antipsychotic medication and mood stabilizers
can be done rapidly in the hospital.

c. Since **compliance** is often an issue in the treatment of bipolar patients, intensive psy-
choeducation and the enlistment of family and friends can also be important goals of
hospitalization.

2. **Outpatient treatment**

a. A **combination of psychotherapy and medication** is also important in treating bipolar
disorder.

(1) **Compliance** is a large problem, particularly as many bipolar patients prefer
hypomania to euthymia and, once manic symptoms begin, they believe that
they know better than their physicians. A strong **treatment alliance** and frequent
visits aid compliance and enable early intervention, if signs of mania begin.

(2) During a depressed phase, psychotherapeutic approaches as noted for major
depression are appropriate.

b. Approximately one-third of patients with bipolar disorder develop a degree of
chronic functional impairment. These patients may benefit from programs such as
day hospitals, vocational rehabilitation, or **supportive living arrangements**.

3. **Somatic therapies.** Several drugs have been found to demonstrate **mood-stabilizing**
properties (i.e., they are effective in treating both mania and depression) in bipolar
patients. **ECT** is also effective for both phases of the illness.

a. **Lithium,** usually the first-line treatment for bipolar disorder, has been found effective
as an acute treatment for mania and depression and as a prophylactic agent.

(1) During **acute mania,** approximately 80% of patients respond to lithium, although such response may take 1–2 weeks. Antipsychotic drugs, such as haloperidol, are often coadministered during this initial period to control behavior and psychosis.

(2) During **acute bipolar depression,** approximately 80% of patients also respond to lithium, although it may take 6–8 weeks to see the full effect.

(3) Lithium is effective at preventing future episodes of depression and mania, with **relapse rates** reduced by approximately 50% compared with placebo.

(4) **Side effects** of lithium include tremor, sedation, nausea, polyuria, polydypsia, memory problems, and weight gain. Hypothyroidism occurs in some patients.

(5) Lithium is **renally excreted** (it is treated by the kidney like sodium), so impaired renal function can lead to toxicity.

(6) Lithium has a **narrow therapeutic index,** and high serum levels can lead to seizures, confusion, coma, and cardiac dysrhythmia. In the case of severe overdose, dialysis is effective.

b. Valproate. In recent years, valproate has been found in some studies to be as effective as lithium in treating bipolar illness.

(1) In patients with **acute mania,** some evidence suggests that valproate may be a more effective treatment than lithium for mixed episodes, whereas lithium may be more effective for traditional manic episodes.

(2) The role of valproate in **bipolar depression** is less clear.

(3) As a **prophylactic agent,** valproate appears to have a role, particularly in the case of **rapidly cycling patients**.

(4) **Side effects** include dose-related symptoms (e.g., nausea, tremor, sedation, hair loss, weight gain) and rare, idiosyncratic responses, including hepatic failure, pancreatitis, and agranulocytosis.

(5) Valproate is **hepatically metabolized,** so it is vulnerable to pharmacokinetic drug interactions.

(6) Valproate has a **wide therapeutic index,** although it can be fatal in overdose.

c. Carbamazepine

(1) Carbamazepine appears to be effective in patients with **acute mania** and **bipolar depression**.

(2) When used for **prophylaxis,** it appears to reduce the frequency and severity of manic and depressive episodes.

(3) Common, dose-related **side effects** include blurred vision, ataxia, nausea, fatigue, hyponatremia, and asymptomatic leukopenia. Rare, idiosyncratic effects include agranulocytosis, liver failure, Stevens-Johnson syndrome, and pancreatitis.

(4) Carbamazepine is **hepatically metabolized** and induces its own metabolism (so dosage adjustment may be needed over time). Pharmacokinetic drug interactions are seen with other hepatically metabolized drugs.

(5) Carbamazepine is **toxic at high doses** (serum levels must be monitored) and can be lethal in overdose.

d. Several other drugs, **without documented mood-stabilizing properties,** still have a role in the treatment of bipolar disorder.

(1) **Antipsychotic drugs** are commonly used during the acute phases of mania or psychotic depression because they provide symptomatic relief while mood stabilizers are taking effect. These agents are not usually used as maintenance treatment because of the risk of **tardive dyskinesia,** unless mood stabilizers alone have been unsuccessful or poorly tolerated.

(2) **Benzodiazepines,** particularly **clonazepam,** may be used to treat mania. Sedation and a full night's sleep can markedly improve symptoms in some patients.

(3) **Antidepressants** are frequently used in the depressed phase of bipolar illness, either alone or in combination with a drug such as lithium. However, this practice is not well studied. Clinicians must be cautious because most antidepressant agents have been reported to precipitate mania in some patients.

D. **Treatment of dysthymia and cyclothymia** is less well studied than treatment of mania and depression.

1. **Dysthymia** was traditionally treated with psychotherapy and was believed to be poorly responsive to antidepressant medication.
   a. It now appears that this disorder may respond to drug treatment, and that **SSRIs** and **MAOIs** are more effective than tricyclic antidepressants.
   b. Of the psychotherapies, **cognitive therapy** and **behavioral therapy** have the best data to support their use.

2. **Cyclothymia** can be treated with mood-stabilizing drugs. Antidepressants frequently precipitate manic symptoms in these patients. Supportive psychotherapy is also important.

DIRECTIONS: Each of the numbered items or incomplete statements in this section is followed by answers or by completions of the statement. Select the ONE lettered answer or completion that is BEST in each case.

1. The prevalence rate is similar in men and women for

(A) major depressive disorder
(B) dysthymic disorder
(C) bipolar I disorder
(D) bipolar II disorder
(E) cyclothymic disorder

2. Which one of the following individuals is most likely to have a first-degree relative with a mood disorder?

(A) A woman with major depressive disorder
(B) A man with major depressive disorder
(C) A man with dysthymia
(D) A woman with bipolar I disorder
(E) A woman with cyclothymia

3. The dexamethasone suppression test (DST) is best described by which one of the following statements?

(A) DST is a sensitive screening tool for major depressive disorder
(B) DST is a selective screening tool for major depressive disorder
(C) DST explains why hypothyroidism is associated with depressive symptoms
(D) DST differentiates nonpsychotic, depressed patients from those patients with psychotic features
(E) DST usually shows nonsuppression of cortisol in depressed patients

4. Of the following treatments, which one is probably the most effective treatment for major depressive disorder?

(A) A tricyclic antidepressant
(B) A selective serotonin reuptake inhibitor (SSRI)
(C) Cognitive therapy
(D) Hospitalization
(E) Combined treatment with medication and psychotherapy

5. Common side effects of selective serotonin reuptake inhibitors (SSRIs) include which one of the following?

(A) Dry mouth, constipation, and orthostatic hypotension
(B) Sedation and priapism
(C) Restlessness, tremors, and seizures
(D) Nausea, insomnia, and sexual dysfunction
(E) Confusion and memory loss

6. The diagnosis of cyclothymic disorder requires which one of the following criteria?

(A) Repeated episodes of hypomania and depression
(B) A minimum duration of 6 months
(C) At least one prior major depressive episode (MDE)
(D) At least one prior manic episode
(E) Comorbid substance abuse

7. The percentage of patients with cyclothymia who will ultimately develop bipolar disorder is approximately

(A) 5%
(B) 25%
(C) 50%
(D) 75%
(E) 90%

8. The noradrenergic effect of antidepressant drugs that is thought to best correlate with the onset of clinical efficacy is the

(A) acute blockade of norepinephrine (NE) reuptake
(B) acute increase of NE in the synapse
(C) blockade of α_1-receptors
(D) blockade of β-receptors
(E) down-regulation of β-receptors

DIRECTIONS: Each of the numbered items or incomplete statements in this section is negatively phrased, as indicated by a capitalized word such as NOT, LEAST, or EXCEPT. Select the ONE lettered answer or completion that is BEST in each case.

Questions 9–10

A 64-year-old male accountant presents to his internist with a 6-week history of worsening depression, insomnia, weight loss, poor concentration, fatigue, and suicidal ideation. He also believes that his evil thoughts caused the recent death of his mother.

9. This patient's current symptoms are consistent with all of the following diagnoses EXCEPT

(A) major depressive disorder
(B) bipolar I disorder
(C) bipolar II disorder
(D) mood disorder due to a general medical condition
(E) dysthymic disorder

10. The patient's belief about his mother would best be described as

(A) thought insertion
(B) thought broadcasting
(C) a mood-congruent delusion
(D) a mood-incongruent delusion
(E) a melancholic symptom

11. Evidence that monoamines are involved in the pathogenesis of mood disorders include all of the following EXCEPT

(A) reserpine induces depression in some patients
(B) valproate is an effective treatment for mania
(C) nortriptyline is an effective treatment for depression
(D) fluoxetine is an effective treatment for depression
(E) iproniazid improves mood in patients with tuberculosis

12. Common side effects of tricyclic antidepressants include all of the following EXCEPT

(A) orthostatic hypotension
(B) dry mouth
(C) diarrhea
(D) blurred vision
(E) sedation

13. Effective treatments for dysthymic disorder include all of the following EXCEPT

(A) selective serotonin reuptake inhibitors (SSRIs)
(B) monoamine oxidase inhibitors (MAOIs)
(C) electroconvulsive therapy (ECT)
(D) cognitive therapy
(E) behavioral therapy

DIRECTIONS: Each set of matching questions in this section consists of a list of four to twenty-six lettered options (some of which may be in figures) followed by several items. For each numbered item, select the ONE lettered option that is most closely associated with it. To avoid spending too much time on matching sets with large numbers of options, it is generally advisable to begin each set by reading the list of options. Then, for each item in the set, try to generate the correct answer and locate it in the option list, rather than evaluating each option individually. Each lettered option may be selected once, more than once, or not at all.

Questions 14–16

Match each clinical feature with the associated drug.

(A) Lithium
(B) Valproate
(C) Carbamazepine
(D) Clonazepam
(E) Haloperidol

14. This drug is associated with a significant risk of tardive dyskinesia

15. This agent may be particularly effective in bipolar patients who exhibit rapidly cycling illness

16. Side effects of this agent include tremor, nausea, polyuria, and weight gain

ANSWERS AND EXPLANATIONS

1. The answer is C *[III B 1 c, 2 c, 3 c, 4 c, 5 c].* Of the mood disorders listed, only bipolar I disorder has a similar prevalence in men and women. For cyclothymic disorder, there is only a slight increase in prevalence in women over men.

2. The answer is D *[IV A 1].* Family studies have shown that whereas approximately 50% of patients with major depressive disorder have a first-degree relative with a mood disorder, 90% of patients with bipolar disorder have a first-degree relative with a mood disorder. The gender of the patient is irrelevant to the answer.

3. The answer is E *[IV C 1 a].* The dexamethasone suppression test (DST) involves the administration of a synthetic corticosteroid, followed by measurement of serum cortisol levels. Whereas nondepressed individuals respond to the drug with decreased cortisol, many patients with major depressive disorder demonstrate nonsuppression and, thus, elevated cortisol levels. It is no longer used routinely because it lacks adequate specificity or selectivity for major depression. It does not differentiate psychotic patients and does not explain the association between thyroid disorders and mood symptoms.

4. The answer is E *[V B].* All of the medications available to treat major depression appear to be similarly effective, although they vary widely in other respects (e.g., therapeutic index, side-effect profile). While selective serotonin reuptake inhibitors (SSRIs) are, in many cases, safer and better tolerated than tricyclics, they do not appear to be more effective. Cognitive therapy has been shown to be effective as a treatment for major depression but not superior to medication. Combined psychotherapy and medication treatment appears to be the most successful option. Hospitalization is necessary for a subset of patients but is not a specific treatment.

5. The answer is D *[V B 3].* Common side effects of selective serotonin reuptake inhibitors (SSRIs), such as fluoxetine, include nausea, insomnia, anxiety, and sexual dysfunction. Dry mouth, constipation, and orthostatic hypotension are commonly seen with tricyclic agents. Sedation is commonly seen with trazodone, and priapism also can occur with this drug. Restlessness and tremors are associated with bupropion, which can lead to seizures at high dosage. Confusion and memory loss are associated with electroconvulsive therapy (ECT).

6. The answer is A *[III B 5].* The DSM-IV criteria for cyclothymic disorder require repeated episodes of hypomania and of depressive symptoms that are not severe enough to meet criteria for major depressive episode (MDE). The minimum duration for diagnosis is 2 years for adult patients (only 1 year is required when making the diagnosis in children and adolescents). Not only are prior major depressive or manic episodes not required, but their presence during the first 2 years of illness rules out a diagnosis of cyclothymia. Although substance abuse is commonly associated with cyclothymia, it is not required to make the diagnosis.

7. The answer is C *[III B 5 c].* The onset of cyclothymia is usually in adolescence or early adulthood, and the course tends to be chronic. Up to 50% of affected individuals will ultimately have a manic or mixed episode and thus be diagnosed with bipolar disorder.

8. The answer is E *[IV B 1 a].* Blockade of norepinephrine (NE) reuptake at the presynaptic membrane occurs shortly after noradrenergic antidepressants are administered, so NE increase in the synapse is similarly rapid. Likewise, α_1-blockade occurs shortly after dosing. The down-regulation of β-receptors, however, takes several weeks. This time course correlates well with the onset of antidepressant effect. These drugs are not β-blockers, or down-regulation at this receptor would not occur.

9–10. The answers are 9-E, 10-C *[III A 1, B 1 b (1)].* The patient's symptoms are consistent with a major depressive episode (MDE). MDE can be a feature of several mood disorders, including major depressive disorder, bipolar I and bipolar II disorders, mood disorder due to a general medical condition, and substance-induced mood disorder. To differentiate these, one would need a history of any prior mood episodes, concurrent medical problems, and drug and alcohol use. Whereas the patient could certainly have an underlying dysthymia, his current symptoms require that one of the above listed diagnoses be made. Dysthymia alone could not account for his current symptoms.

Believing that thoughts can cause someone to die is delusional. Because the patient's symptoms are those of an MDE, and the delusion has a depressing content (causing someone to die), the belief would be described as a mood-congruent delusion. Delusions can occur in melancholic patients, but they are not a specific symptom of melancholia. Thought insertion is the belief that thoughts have been placed into the patient's head, and thought broadcasting is the belief that others can hear the patient's thoughts. Neither is related to this case.

11. The answer is B *[IV B]*. The efficacy of drugs that enhance monoamine transmission and the tendency of some monoamine depleters to induce depression serve as evidence for the role of catecholamines and indoleamines in the etiology of depression. Reserpine depletes monoamines by inhibiting their accumulation in presynaptic vesicles. Nortriptyline blocks norepinephrine (NE) reuptake, and fluoxetine blocks serotonin (5-HT) reuptake. Iproniazid inhibits monoamine oxidase, so it also results in increased availability of NE, 5-HT, and dopamine at the synapse. Valproate, however, is an anticonvulsant that acts through the γ-aminobutyric acid (GABA) system; thus, it is not directly relevant to the monoamine hypothesis of mood disorders.

12. The answer is C *[V B 3 a]*. Tricyclic antidepressants have a variety of side effects, many of which are related to postsynaptic receptor-blocking effects. Blockade of muscarinic receptors cause anticholinergic symptoms such as dry mouth, constipation, blurred vision, and tachycardia. Blockade of histamine receptors produces sedation. Orthostatic hypotension is caused by adrenergic (α_1)-blockade. Diarrhea is not a common side effect of this drug class.

13. The answer is C *[V D 1]*. Although dysthymia was long thought to be refractory to pharmacotherapy, it is now thought that many patients may respond to medications, particularly selective serotonin reuptake inhibitors (SSRIs) and monoamine oxidase inhibitors (MAOIs). Of the psychotherapies, the best evidence exists for the effectiveness of cognitive and behavioral approaches. Dysthymia is not an indication for electroconvulsive therapy (ECT).

14–16. The answers are: 14-E *[V C 3 d]*, **15-B** *[V C 3 b]*, **16-A** *[V C 3 a]*. All of the agents listed are useful at times in the treatment of bipolar disorder. An antipsychotic drug such as haloperidol is commonly used in combination with a mood stabilizer during the first week or two of treatment for acute mania (because mood stabilizers have a more delayed onset of action). However, antipsychotic medications are not a first choice for prophylaxis because of the risk of tardive dyskinesia. Tardive dyskinesia is a late-onset movement disorder that features choreoathetotic movements of the face and extremities.

Valproate is a mood stabilizer that appears to be particularly effective in patients who have a pattern of rapid cycling illness (i.e., at least four episodes of mood disorder within a 12-month period).

Lithium, usually considered the first-line treatment for bipolar disorder, has side effects that include tremor, sedation, nausea, polyuria, polydypsia, memory problems, weight gain, and hypothyroidism.

Chapter 4

Anxiety Disorders
Steven L. Dubovsky

I. **OVERVIEW.** Anxiety is abnormal fear that is out of proportion to any external stimulus. Significant anxiety is experienced by 10%–15% of general medical outpatients and 10% of inpatients. Of the physically healthy population, 25% of individuals are anxious at some point in their lives. Approximately 7.5% of these people have a diagnosable anxiety disorder in any given month. Until recently, anxiety was viewed primarily as a psychological response to internal or external stress; however, some types of anxiety are independent of identifiable stress.

A. **Panic versus generalized anxiety**

1. **Panic anxiety** arises spontaneously and does not have particular content associated with it. Panic anxiety may evolve gradually in nine stages:
   a. Spontaneous subclinical (limited symptom) anxiety attacks
   b. Gradual progression to full-blown panic attacks
   c. Hypochondriacal fears of occult disease
   d. Development of **anticipatory anxiety** about panic attacks
   e. Phobic avoidance of situations in which panic attacks occur or from which escape might be difficult if panic did occur
   f. Generalized avoidance (agoraphobia)
   g. Abuse of drugs or alcohol to control anxiety
   h. Depression
   i. Social limitations

2. **Panic attacks** are unprovoked, sudden episodes of anxiety that usually reach their peak within a few minutes and subside in less than an hour. A sense of dread, which is the most prominent psychological symptom, may be masked by or seem to be in reaction to the physical symptoms that frequently accompany panic attacks:
   a. Palpitations or rapid heart beat
   b. Sweating
   c. Tremor or shaking
   d. Dyspnea or feelings of smothering
   e. Feeling of choking
   f. Chest pain
   g. Feeling dizzy or faint
   h. Derealization (feelings of unreality) or depersonalization (feelings of detachment from oneself)
   i. Feelings of losing control or going crazy
   j. Fear of dying
   k. Paresthesias
   l. Chills or hot flashes

3. **Generalized anxiety** involves excessive worry about actual circumstances, events, or conflicts.
   a. Panic anxiety and generalized anxiety often accompany each other. Subpanic anxiety may mimic generalized anxiety, whereas anticipatory anxiety is a type of generalized anxiety.

b. Whereas panic anxiety does not involve fear of any specific circumstance, general-ized anxiety involves worry about specific circumstances.

c. Symptoms of generalized anxiety fluctuate more than those of panic anxiety.

B. **Diagnostic categories of anxiety.** Information about symptoms and diagnostic categories is taken from the *Diagnostic and Statistical Manual of Mental Disorders*, 4th edition (DSM-IV). In addition to the specific symptoms listed with each category, all DSM-IV categories of anxiety include significant distress or interference with normal functioning or routines caused by the symptoms.

1. Panic disorder

a. Symptoms. Panic disorder consists of recurrent panic attacks characterized by sudden apprehension or fear (see I C 1–3) and usually accompanied by autonomic arousal that is not a reaction to physical exertion, a life-threatening situation, a sub-stance, a medical factor, or another disorder (e.g., panic evoked by a phobic stimu-lus). To meet criteria for panic disorder, at least one panic attack must be followed by 1 month or more of persistent concerns about having more panic attacks, worries about the consequences or implications of the panic attack (e.g., that the patient is losing control or having a heart attack), or a change in behavior caused by the panic attacks (e.g., not leaving the house).

b. Panic disorder may be accompanied by agoraphobia (see I B 2).

c. Treatment. Panic disorder is treated with antidepressants, benzodiazepines, and behavioral therapies.

2. Agoraphobia

a. Symptoms include anxiety about being in situations from which escape might be difficult or embarrassing or for which help may not be available in the event of panic or other forms of discomfort or distress. Agoraphobic situations may include being away from home, sitting in the middle of a row of seats in a theater, being on a bridge, or traveling in a car or airplane. Such situations are either avoided or endured only by having a companion nearby. Otherwise, remaining in the situation causes marked distress or panic.

b. If agoraphobia complicates panic disorder, the diagnosis is **panic disorder with agoraphobia**. If agoraphobia occurs in the absence of panic disorder, the diagnosis is **agoraphobia without a history of panic disorder**.

3. Generalized anxiety disorder

a. Symptoms include at least 6 months of unrealistic worry about a number of life cir-cumstances accompanied by at least three of six additional symptoms of anxiety, including restlessness or feeling keyed up, easy fatigability, difficulty concentrating or mind going blank, irritability, muscle tension, and insomnia.

b. Treatment. Benzodiazepines, buspirone, and antidepressants are the drugs used to treat generalized anxiety disorder. Relaxation training, hypnosis, biofeedback, and related treatments are also useful.

4. Obsessive-compulsive disorder

a. Symptoms include persistent intrusive, recurrent ideas, thoughts, feelings, images, or impulses (**obsessions**), which are experienced as senseless or repugnant and which the patient tries to ignore or resist. Repetitive stereotyped physical or mental actions (**compulsions**), which the patient recognizes as senseless and tries to resist, may also occur. Compulsions are performed with a subjective sense of necessity to prevent some future event or in response to an obsession or some rigid rule.

b. Treatment of obsessive-compulsive disorder is with the tricyclic antidepressant clomipramine and selective serotonin reuptake inhibitors (SSRIs) such as fluoxetine, paroxetine, sertraline, and fluvoxamine. Behavioral therapies may be as effective as medications in some cases and are usually combined with these treatments.

5. Specific phobias

a. Symptoms. Excessive or irrational fear in response to the presence or anticipation of a specific object or situation (e.g., height, spiders, blood). Although the anxiety is recognized as inappropriate, the phobic stimulus is avoided or endured only with intense distress.

b. Subtypes

(1) Animal type. Fear of animals or insects usually begins in childhood.

(2) Natural environmental type. This subtype, which also usually begins in childhood, is characterized by fear of storms, height, and other events in the environment.

(3) Blood-injection-injury type. This phobia subtype, which is characterized by anxiety in response to seeing blood or injury or getting an injection, is often familial and is associated with fainting.

(4) Situational type. This subtype is characterized by fear cued by specific situations such as elevators, bridges, and enclosed places but without panic disorder or other agoraphobic symptoms. However, situational phobia is similar to panic disorder with agoraphobia in its age of onset, familial aggregation, and sex ratios.

(5) Other type. This category includes irrational fears of other stimuli, such as illness, or fears of falling if not near a wall or other means of physical support (**space phobia**).

c. Treatment. Specific phobias are usually treated with behavioral therapies.

6. Social phobia

a. Symptoms include a marked and persistent fear of humiliating oneself, sometimes accompanied by panic attacks in social or performance situations that involve social scrutiny. Panic attacks may occur in social situations.

b. Treatment. Social phobia is treated with monoamine oxidase (MAO) inhibitors, group therapy, behavior therapy, and occasionally with β-adrenergic blocking agents.

7. Posttraumatic stress disorder describes a syndrome of distress, re-experiencing, avoidance, and arousal that develops after exposure to events or circumstances that involved actual death or injury or a threat to the physical integrity of oneself or others and that evoked intense fear, helplessness, or horror.

a. Symptoms of posttraumatic stress disorder may appear immediately after the trauma, or they may be delayed for 6 months or more (**posttraumatic stress disorder with delayed onset**). Symptoms include:

(1) Re-experiencing the initial trauma occurs via intrusive memories of the event, dreams about the trauma, feeling as if the trauma were continuing to occur, and intense distress on exposure to cues that recall the event.

(2) Avoidance of stimuli associated with the trauma and numbing of overall responsiveness occurs.

(3) Symptoms of **excessive arousal** include insomnia, angry outbursts, hypervigilance, exaggerated startle response, and difficulty concentrating.

b. Treatment of posttraumatic stress disorder involves discussion of the trauma as a means of achieving retroactive mastery. At times, confrontations with perpetrators can be helpful. Group therapy is often very helpful. Adjunctive techniques (e.g., biofeedback) and medication (especially SSRIs and carbamazepine) may be useful.

8. Acute stress disorder is a diagnosis new to DSM-IV. A traumatic event defined exactly as for posttraumatic stress disorder produces anxiety or arousal, avoidance, re-experiencing, and acute or delayed dissociative symptoms. Acute stress disorder begins within 1 month of the event and lasts 2 days to 4 weeks. A traumatic event (see I B 7) is followed by posttraumatic stress disorder that is accompanied by detachment or absence of emotional responsiveness, decreased awareness of surroundings, derealization, depersonalization, or dissociative amnesia. Three or more of these symptoms (including emotional numbing) must be present to make the diagnosis.

9. **Anxiety disorder due to a general medical condition.** This diagnosis, which replaces the DSM-III-R diagnosis of organic anxiety disorder, refers to anxiety caused by medical and surgical disorders (see I D 1–6).

10. **Substance-induced anxiety disorder.** This diagnosis is made when a psychoactive substance is responsible for anxiety symptoms (see I D 7). In the DSM-III-R this diagnosis would have been included with organic anxiety disorder.

11. **Other primary psychiatric disorders** may be associated with anxiety, which may be prominent or may be the presenting complaint.
   a. **Depression.** Approximately 70% of depressed patients also feel anxious, and 20%–30% of apparent cases of anxiety are caused by an underlying depression. Approximately 40%–90% of patients with panic disorder become depressed, and 20%–50% of depressed patients have panic attacks. Depressed patients with blood relatives who are anxious are more likely to experience anxiety plus depression than those with a family history of depression only.
   b. **Psychosis.** As control of mental processes is lost, a patient experiencing psychotic disorganization due to mania, schizophrenia, or brief reactive psychosis often displays considerable anxiety, which initially may obscure the underlying severe disturbance of thinking, affect, or behavior.
   c. **Mania.** Especially in younger patients, bursts of overstimulation, excess energy, and racing thoughts may be experienced as panic attacks.
   d. **Delirium and dementia.** Anxiety is the most common emotion experienced by patients with acute organic mental syndromes (delirium), who are frightened by a sudden disruption of cognitive abilities, and by demented patients, whose mental syndromes are made worse by an intercurrent illness or by a sudden change in the environment (e.g., a change in the roommate of a hospitalized demented patient).
   e. **Adjustment disorder with anxiety.** Patients experience anxiety or impairment in excess of those that would normally be expected within 3 months of exposure to an obvious stress. In contrast to posttraumatic stress disorder, anxiety and other symptoms appear soon after the onset of the traumatic event and are expected to resolve within 6 months of the stress abating or the patient achieving a new level of functioning.
   f. **Factitious disorder.** Rarely, patients consciously simulate a mental disorder, including anxiety, for the sole purpose of becoming a patient. The patient often relates an improbable history and has been hospitalized numerous times, often under different names. In contrast, **malingering** refers to the conscious simulation of a condition for some obvious gain (e.g., obtaining benzodiazepines). Malingering is more common in a patient with a history of lying, drug abuse, and antisocial behavior.

C. **Signs and symptoms.** A subjective state of anxiety may be obvious, or it may be masked by physical or other psychological complaints.

1. **Psychological symptoms**
   a. Apprehension, worry, fear, and anticipation of misfortune
   b. Sense of doom or panic
   c. Hypervigilance
   d. Irritability
   e. Fatigue
   f. Insomnia
   g. Predisposition to accidents
   h. Derealization (the world seems strange or unreal) and depersonalization (the patient feels unreal or changed)
   i. Difficulty concentrating

2. **Somatic complaints**
   a. Headache
   b. Dizziness and light-headedness
   c. Palpitations and chest pain

    d. Upset stomach and diarrhea
    e. Frequent urination
    f. Lump in the throat
    g. Motor tension or restlessness
    h. Shortness of breath
    i. Paresthesias
    j. Dry mouth

3. Physical signs
    a. Diaphoresis
    b. Cool, clammy skin
    c. Tachycardia and arrhythmias
    d. Flushing and pallor
    e. Hyperreflexia
    f. Trembling, easy startling, and fidgeting

D. **Illnesses that cause anxiety.** Before investigating psychological causes of anxiety, it is important to exclude the possibility of physical disorders in which anxiety may be a presenting complaint even before other signs of disease become evident.

1. Cardiovascular disorders
    a. Arteriosclerotic heart disease
    b. Paroxysmal tachycardias
    c. Mitral valve prolapse
    d. Hyperdynamic β-adrenergic circulatory state

2. Pulmonary disorders
    a. Pulmonary embolism
    b. Hypoxemia
    c. Asthma
    d. Chronic obstructive lung disease

3. Disorders of the endocrine system and metabolism
    a. Hypoglycemia
    b. Hyperthyroidism or hypothyroidism
    c. Hypocalcemia
    d. Cushing syndrome
    e. Porphyria

4. Tumors
    a. Insulinoma
    b. Carcinoid tumor
    c. Pheochromocytoma

5. Neurologic disorders
    a. Multiple sclerosis
    b. Temporal lobe epilepsy
    c. Organic mental syndrome of any etiology
    d. Ménière disease

6. Infections
    a. Tuberculosis
    b. Brucellosis

7. Drug-related disorders
    a. Abstinence syndromes [i.e., withdrawal from central nervous system (CNS) depressants such as alcohol, tranquilizers, sleeping pills]
    b. Intoxication with sympathomimetics
    c. Akathisia
    d. Caffeinism
    e. Chinese restaurant syndrome, resulting from the ingestion of monosodium glutamate (MSG)

E. **Anxiety that mimics disease states.** Anxiety may also mimic physical disease. For example, patients with **hyperventilation syndrome** complain of shortness of breath, weakness, paresthesias, headache, and carpopedal spasm. These patients are often unaware of the psychological stresses that lead to hyperventilation and may either deny feelings of anxiety or feel that any anxiety that is experienced is secondary to not being able to breathe. Symptoms abate when the patient is calmed and respiratory rate decreases. Treatment consists of instructing the patient to breathe into a paper bag, which is held over the nose and mouth. Carbon dioxide accumulates and reverses the respiratory alkalosis caused by hyperventilation.

II. **PSYCHOLOGICAL COMPONENTS OF ANXIETY.** A significant number of patients display anxiety symptoms that do not meet criteria for any specific DSM-IV diagnosis but are still a cause of significant distress or disability. These forms of anxiety often reflect the meaning of the illness.

A. **Situational anxiety.** Severe stress may temporarily overwhelm any person's ability to cope. Even minor stress can have important symbolic meaning.

1. **Symptoms.** Even a relatively minor situation may feel overwhelming because it recalls other situations in which the patient was unable to cope or that aroused unresolved conflict. The intensity and nature of anxiety that evolves from a stressful situation depend on the meaning of the illness and the patient's previous level of adjustment. A relatively well-adjusted patient may experience only transient symptoms, whereas an underlying psychosis may be precipitated in a more marginally compensated patient.

2. **Treatment.** When patients must contend with acute, ongoing stress, antianxiety medication (when appropriate) and support should be offered. In addition, patients should be encouraged to talk about what the stress means to them. A greater sense of mastery, which is incompatible with the helplessness of anxiety, is facilitated by having the patient put the situation into words and use relaxation techniques and related therapies (see III B).

B. **Anxiety about death.** Even nonfatal illnesses may remind patients of their mortality.

1. **Symptoms.** Persistent fear of death, even in terminally ill patients, symbolizes concern about loss of control, pain, isolation, helplessness, and the prospect of losing important relationships.

2. **Treatment.** Reassurance that the patient will not be left alone and in pain often decreases the apparent fear of death.

C. **Anxiety about mutilation, loss of prowess, and loss of attractiveness** is especially common in patients who feel that love, approval, and self-esteem are dependent on their strength or beauty.

1. **Symptoms.** Patients become frightened if an illness threatens their appearance or prowess. They express excessive fear of side effects and after effects of the illness, complain continuously, or fail to improve as expected. Patients may also attempt self-reassurance by demonstrating attractiveness (e.g., by behaving seductively) or strength (e.g., by exercising conspicuously) in inappropriate or even dangerous ways.

2. **Treatment.** Patients should be reassured that they still possess valued traits. The reaction of their families to the illness or surgery should be evaluated.

D. **Anxiety about loss of self-esteem.** Patients whose self-esteem is fragile are especially vulnerable to experiencing illness as an imperfection, weakness, or failure, which can lead to attempts to bolster a sense of self-worth by boasting about importance and superiority.

1. **Symptoms.** Patients may adopt a self-important air, insisting on being treated only by the most senior or well-known physician and treating others as worthless inferiors.

Attempts to convince these patients that they are not as important as they think only increases their insecurity, which is covered up with greater protestations of their own importance and, by comparison, the unimportance of others.

2. **Treatment.** Patients should be approached with appropriate deference and should be reassured that they are still important. Reasonable requests for special consideration should be granted during an acute illness.

E. | **Separation anxiety.** Regressed adults (i.e., those who function psychologically more as children than as adults) may become frightened when they are separated from important caretakers. This state commonly is encountered in physically ill people, as well as in overly dependent individuals and some patients with psychotic and personality disorders.

1. **Symptoms.** Separation distress may be expressed directly as anxiety, or indirectly with complaints of pain or by ringing for the nurse whenever the patient is left alone.

2. **Treatment.** Family and close friends should be encouraged to be with the patient as much as possible, and unrestricted visiting should be allowed. The nursing staff should be encouraged to visit the patient frequently for brief periods of time, and a roommate should be provided. The patient's room should be close to the nurse's station to facilitate frequent, brief visits.

F. | **Stranger anxiety**

1. **Symptoms.** Patients who suffer from separation anxiety also may react adversely to unfamiliar people, including new physicians, nurses, and visitors. In a hospitalized adult, this can lead to distress at changes of shift or in other situations in which there are new caretakers.

2. **Treatment.** As much continuity in personnel as possible should be provided (e.g., the same nurse should be assigned to the patient each day). Unrestricted visiting by those familiar to the patient should be allowed, and unfamiliar visitors should be limited. Changes in roommates should be minimized.

G. | **Anxiety about loss of control**

1. **Symptoms.** Illness and hospitalization may be threatening to an individual with a strong need to feel in complete control of his life and his environment, especially when others must make decisions about the patient's life. The patient may attempt to gain a sense of control by refusing to comply with the physician's advice, by becoming excessively demanding, by making the physician feel helpless, or by otherwise asserting control over those who are in a caretaking role or who are healthy.

2. **Treatment.** The patient should be allowed as much control as possible over his own care. For example, the patient's opinion about therapeutic decisions should be solicited, and the patient should be consulted about which treatment schedules would make the most sense to him.

H. | **Anxiety about dependency.** Patients who fear loss of control also commonly have anxiety about being dependent on others, which is precipitated by being ill. Fear of dependency is common in people whose normal dependency needs were not met in childhood (e.g., because of parental illness or unavailability).

1. **Symptoms.** Extremely strong dependency wishes, which have been unchanged since childhood, threaten to break through when the patients are put in a dependent position (e.g., becoming ill). Because patients are afraid that they will not be able to control dependency needs, they reject attempts of others to be helpful and become hostile toward potential caretakers. They may also assert their independence by being noncompliant, failing to keep appointments, or ignoring signs of increasing illness.

2. **Treatment.** When possible, patients should be reassured that the illness and the dependency required by it are temporary. They should be helped to maintain as much independent function as possible.

I. Anxiety about intimacy

1. **Symptoms.** Patients with concerns about dependency may be afraid of becoming too close emotionally to caretakers or loved ones, which leads to the maintenance of a greater-than-normal emotional distance, to attempts to ward off (e.g., through hostility) people who are nice or express concern, and to distress at expressions of friendliness or intimacy.

2. **Treatment.** Intimacy should not be forced. The patient's sense of formality should be respected.

J. Anxiety about being punished

1. **Symptoms.** Patients with an underlying sense of guilt about real or imagined transgressions may have a conscious or unconscious expectation of punishment. They may attempt to relieve guilt or avoid worry about when they will be punished by means of self-inflicted punishment (e.g., through an unhappy marriage, repeated accidents, not recovering from an illness, or alcoholism).

2. **Treatment.** The suffering of patients should be acknowledged, and attempts should be made to uncover the source of their guilt. Patients with a desire for insight may benefit from expressive psychotherapy.

K. Signal anxiety

1. **Symptoms.** When awareness of a previously unconscious, unresolved psychological conflict is stimulated by some external occurrence (e.g., the patient had mixed feelings about a parent and the patient's age is the same as that of the parent at the time of death), anxiety may signal the emergence of the conflict. This anxiety may call forth **psychological defenses (ego defenses),** which are unconscious mechanisms that avoid anxiety by keeping the conflict out of the patient's awareness.
   a. **Repression** (forgetting) is an automatic process by which memories, thoughts, and feelings are excluded from awareness.
   b. **Rationalization** is the act of explaining away psychologically meaningful data (e.g., "I'm anxious only because my blood sugar seems low").
   c. **Reaction formation** is feeling the opposite of one's true emotions in order not to be aware of it (e.g., experiencing excessive affection toward someone who actually elicits hostility).
   d. **Isolation of affect** is experiencing the content of a thought without its associated emotions.
   e. **Denial** is remaining unaware of some aspect of reality (e.g., feeling that one does not have to be afraid of the consequences of an illness because one is not really sick).
   f. **Projection** is attributing one's own motives to someone else.
   g. **Projective identification** is incompletely projecting an intense emotional state, usually anger, onto another individual while inducing the emotion in the object of the projection through provoking behavior. Patients also experience the original emotion but feel that this is only because they are attempting to protect themselves from the other individual's affect.

2. **Treatment.** When it is possible and practical, an attempt to resolve the underlying conflict should be undertaken. When patients cannot tolerate an awareness of their motives, they should be helped to develop less disabling defenses against them (e.g., isolation of the affect rather than denial of it, or denial of anxiety rather than denial of the situation that causes it). Behavioral and adjunctive measures (e.g., relaxation training), which are useful for control of situational anxiety, may help to lessen signal anxiety.

III. TREATMENT OF ANXIETY

A. **Psychotherapy** is effective for situational anxiety and anxiety related to identifiable intrapsychic conflict. It is not effective for panic attacks and phobias. Psychotherapy may be facilitated by medication and behavioral techniques.

1. **Supportive therapy.** Psychotherapy that is primarily supportive is useful for acutely ill patients, patients under severe stress, and patients with limited emotional and psychosocial resources (e.g., because of dementia or personality disorders).
   a. **Support of defenses.** The principal therapeutic approach involves encouraging defenses that are as adaptive as possible, for example:
      (1) Patients with acute myocardial infarction should be helped to minimize the immediate danger because intense fear may contribute to the onset of lethal arrhythmias. However, when symptoms first appear, denial may lead to a fatal delay in seeking medical attention. Later in the course of the illness, denial of the need for treatment may cause noncompliance.
      (2) Marginally compensated schizophrenic patients might be encouraged not to pay too much attention to psychotic thoughts that cannot be dealt with constructively by directing their attention to problems in everyday living that can be solved.
      (3) People who are anxious because they feel out of control may gain a sense of mastery through intellectualization.
   b. **Reality testing.** Patients who tend to distort reality can be helped to assess the situation more objectively by the physician offering her own observations and tactfully pointing out lapses in reality testing.
   c. **Advice** should be given, especially when the patient attempts to avoid anxiety through destructive or self-destructive behavior. For example, the patient might be advised to stop attempting to relieve anxiety by arguing with a spouse and to go for a walk instead.
   d. **Adaptive behavior** by the patient should be reinforced (encouraged).

2. **Expressive psychotherapy.** Patients whose anxiety reflects intrapsychic conflicts and who are able to understand and are interested in understanding themselves may gain more control of their symptoms by uncovering the psychological meaning of the anxiety and resolving conflict more effectively. Before applying expressive psychotherapy, it is important to assess a patient's ability to be aware of emotions without acting on or being overwhelmed by them. Components of expressive psychotherapy include:
   a. **Clarification** of the patient's statements in order to make them more comprehensible
   b. **Confrontation** of aspects of reality or the patient's emotions that the patient is ignoring (e.g., "You say that you are not anxious, but you look very nervous.")
   c. **Interpretation** of unconscious thoughts and feelings to bring them into the patient's awareness (e.g., "Do you think that you are anxious around your boss because he is so much like your father?")

B. **Behavior therapy** is effective for phobias, anticipatory anxiety, some forms of panic anxiety, generalized anxiety, situational anxiety, and obsessive-compulsive disorder.

1. **In systematic desensitization,** patients are taught deep muscle relaxation, which is incompatible with the tension of anxiety. The patient is then taught to visualize a scene involving thoughts that are the opposite of anxious thinking, such as feeling safe, relaxed, and in control. Next, the patient imagines anxiety-provoking situations.
   a. As soon as anxiety begins to emerge, the scene that induces relaxation is re-evoked until the anxiety ceases. Anxiety-provoking and comforting scenes are repeatedly paired until the thought of the former no longer causes anxiety.
   b. Beginning with the situation that provokes the least anxiety, the patient gradually moves up a hierarchy of situations to the ones that are most feared. Hypnosis may be used to facilitate the process.

    c. When the patient can visualize the most anxiety-provoking scene while still feeling relaxed, less anxiety will be experienced in the corresponding real-life situation.

    d. However, to consolidate this gain, "in vitro" densensitization in the doctor's office must usually be followed by "in vivo" desensitization in actual situations by using a combination of relaxation and exposure while again progressing from the least to the most anxiety-provoking situation.

2. Graduated in vivo exposure places phobic patients (who are usually accompanied by a family member, friend, or physician for reassurance) in situations that evoke anxiety. Systematic desensitization may be necessary first if the patient becomes overwhelmingly anxious in the phobic situation. Relaxation techniques and hypnosis are used to change the association between phobic situations and anxiety to an association of those situations with relaxation and control.

3. Panic control therapy is a modification of cognitive behavioral therapy, which is an established treatment for depression. Panic control therapy involves reassessing expectations (cognitions) that the patient will have a panic attack. The patient is also taught to stop interpreting minor physical sensations (e.g., dizziness, shortness of breath from hyperventilation) as a sign of impending catastrophe. This prevents these perceptions from precipitating panic attacks.

4. Response prevention is a technique for treating compulsions. The patient refrains from engaging in a compulsive behavior (e.g., hand washing) for increasing lengths of time while using adjunctive techniques to control the resulting anxiety. Response prevention is less effective in the absence of specific compulsions.

5. Stop thinking is a mental variant of response prevention in which a patient repeats an obsessive thought until it seems overwhelming and then terminates the thought while saying "stop" out loud.

6. Adjunctive behavioral techniques may be useful for patients who suffer from any type of anxiety.

    a. Relaxation techniques. Because an individual cannot feel tense and relaxed at the same time, any method that decreases tension tends to relieve anxiety.

    b. Hypnosis is an altered state of consciousness that permits heightened concentration and attention. Hypnosis helps the patient to concentrate on thoughts that are calming and therefore incompatible with anxiety. Patients who have excessive fear of loss of control or who have organic brain disease often cannot be hypnotized.

    c. Biofeedback is a technique that is useful for patients who prefer to learn to relax with a machine or without anyone else present. It also has been used to treat migraine and tension headaches and mild essential hypertension. The level of muscular tension, usually in the forearm or frontalis muscles, is "fed back" through a visual or auditory stimulus to help patients learn to decrease motor tension and, with it, anxiety.

C. **Psychopharmacology.** Medication is indicated for the treatment of panic anxiety, acute situational anxiety, generalized anxiety disorder, agoraphobia, obsessive-compulsive disorder, posttraumatic stress disorder, and other anxiety disorders when these conditions are not responses to specific trauma or conflict. It is also indicated if a 3-month trial of psychotherapy and behavior therapy for treatment of exogenous anxiety is unsuccessful. Adjunctive use of antianxiety medication may facilitate psychotherapy and behavior therapy. Approximately 30% of chronically anxious patients do not recover with appropriate pharmacotherapy. If complete recovery does not follow appropriate drug therapy, the diagnosis may be incorrect (e.g., the patient may have anxiety secondary to a personality disorder or psychosis) or anxiety may be caused by a medical or substance-related disorder.

1. Benzodiazepines are the most effective antianxiety drugs. They are most useful for acute situational anxiety, anticipatory anxiety associated with panic attacks, generalized anxiety disorder, and panic disorder.

a. Uses

   (1) Panic anxiety. The most widely used benzodiazepines for treating panic disorder are alprazolam (Xanax), which is a triazolobenzodiazepine, and clonazepam, which is a benzodiazepine anticonvulsant.

     (a) Recovery should be apparent after 4 weeks of treatment with a dosage of 2–10 mg/day of alprazolam or 1–5 mg/day of clonazepam.

     (b) If improvement has not occurred within 4 to 6 weeks, another medication should be tried (see III C 2).

     (c) Equivalently high doses of other benzodiazepines (e.g., 20–100 mg of diazepam) appear to be equally effective for panic disorder, but are difficult to tolerate and require taking too many pills.

   (2) Generalized and situational anxiety. Benzodiazepines are effective for generalized and situational anxiety. The benzodiazepine antianxiety drugs differ mainly in their elimination half-lives, potency, and lipid solubility. These properties vary for different preparations. For example, alprazolam has a short half-life, high potency, and high lipid solubility; diazepam has a long half-life, intermediate potency, and high lipid solubility; and chlordiazepoxide has a long half-life, low potency, and low lipid solubility.

     (a) Long-acting benzodiazepines include diazepam (Valium), chlordiazepoxide (Librium), chlorazepate (Tranxene), prazepam (Centrax), and clonazepam (Klonopin). Long-acting preparations can be given less frequently during the day, although they are usually administered at least twice daily to minimize peaks in blood level. Discontinuation syndromes appear more gradually, last longer, and are often more attenuated than after discontinuation of shorter-acting benzodiazepines.

     (b) Short-acting benzodiazepines include midazolam (Versed), lorazepam (Ativan), oxazepam (Serax), alprazolam (Xanax), and halazepam (Paxipam). Short-acting drugs must be given more frequently (i.e., as often as every 2 to 3 hours for some patients taking alprazolam). Discontinuation syndromes are more severe and abrupt than with longer-acting benzodiazepines, but the syndromes last a shorter period of time.

   (3) Insomnia. Benzodiazepines, such as flurazepam (Dalmane), temazepam (Restoril), triazolam (Halcion), and estazolam (ProSom) are used to treat acute insomnia associated with stress, jet lag, or a change in sleep phase. Zolpidem (Ambien) is a nonbenzodiazepine hypnotic that is selective for a subtype of the benzodiazepine receptor (type 1 receptor), which results in fewer side effects and withdrawal syndromes. Quazepam (Doral) also is selective for the type 1 receptor; however, with chronic treatment a metabolite accumulates that is a nonselective long-acting benzodiazepine. Any benzodiazepine can be used to treat insomnia as well as anxiety.

b. Administration. The best results of benzodiazepines are obtained when treating time-limited anxiety that occurs in response to clear-cut stress and when treatment lasts less than 8 weeks. Chronically anxious patients or patients with limited intrapsychic or external resources may need long-term therapy. Because generalized anxiety disorder follows a relapsing course, repeated treatment episodes are often necessary.

c. Addiction to benzodiazepines is rare in medical patients. However, individuals with a history of alcohol or drug abuse, physician shopping, and antisocial behavior are at risk of abusing benzodiazepines. The most frequently abused benzodiazepines are diazepam, alprazolam, and lorazepam.

d. Abstinence syndromes (withdrawal symptoms) may appear up to 10 days after abrupt discontinuation of moderate doses of benzodiazepines that have been taken for more than 1 month. Signs and symptoms of withdrawal include anxiety, insomnia, irritability, and, at times, psychosis, delirium, and seizures. Some patients may experience prolonged attenuated withdrawal symptoms lasting up to 1 year. Withdrawal is more abrupt and severe after discontinuation of short-acting benzodiazepines.

e. **Common side effects** include sedation, memory problems, and impaired psycho-motor performance. Tolerance develops to the sedative effects but not to the anxi-olytic effects or impaired performance. Alcohol and benzodiazepines have additive effects in impairing driving. Benzodiazepines may cause or aggravate depression. Because of drug accumulation, use of longer-acting benzodiazepines is a common cause of falls in the elderly.

2. **Heterocyclic antidepressants**
   a. **Uses**
      (1) **Panic disorder.** All antidepressants except bupropion have been found effective for panic disorder.
      (2) **Generalized anxiety disorder.** The tricyclic antidepressants have been noted to be as effective as the benzodiazepines in the treatment of generalized anxiety disor-der, even if the antidepressant is not sedating and the patient is not also depressed.
      (3) **Obsessive-compulsive disorder.** In high doses, clomipramine and the SSRIs are effective for treating patients with obsessive-compulsive disorder. In most cases, these medications reduce symptoms but do not cure them.
      (4) **Posttraumatic stress disorder.** Intrusive recall, depression, anxiety, and arousal may respond to SSRIs. Arousal and recurrence of symptoms may respond to carbamazepine. Arousal may improve with antidepressants or a benzodiazepine. However, high comorbidity with substance-related disorders necessitates caution with this class of medication.
      (5) **Insomnia.** Sedating antidepressants (e.g., trazodone, amitriptyline, doxepin) often are effective as treatments for chronic insomnia. Tolerance to the hypnotic effect usually does not develop.
   b. **Administration.** Standard antidepressant dosages (e.g., 150–300 mg/day of imipra-mine or its equivalent) are often necessary to treat anxiety, but lower dosages often suffice for insomnia. High dosages (e.g., 80 mg/day of fluoxetine) are usually needed to improve patients with obsessive-compulsive disorder. It is often recommended that antidepressants be discontinued after 6 to 12 months of having no symptoms, but chronic treatment is often required to prevent relapse.

3. **MAO inhibitors**
   a. **Uses.** MAO inhibitors are used to treat atypical depression or depression with "reverse" vegetative symptoms, such as eating and sleeping too much and having no energy. MAO inhibitors are also useful for panic disorder, social phobia, and depres-sion accompanied by mood reactivity (i.e., being temporarily cheered up by positive interactions), prominent anxiety, and treatment resistance.
   b. **Administration.** Phenelzine (45–90 mg/day) and tranylcypromine (20–80 mg/day) are used most frequently in the United States. Because of a high prevalence of rapid metabolism, higher doses may be necessary.
   c. **Side effects.** MAO inhibitors may produce hypertensive crises when administered with foods that are high in tyramine content (e.g., cheese) and by sympathomimetic substances. Fatal serotonin syndrome can occur when MAO inhibitors are combined with SSRIs, fenfluramine, and other serotoninergic compounds.

4. **Buspirone (BuSpar)**
   a. **Uses.** Buspirone is an azaspirone antianxiety drug that is used for the same indica-tions as the benzodiazepines. In contrast to the benzodiazepines, buspirone is a par-tial agonist of the serotonin 5-HT$_{1A}$ receptor.
   b. **Administration.** Buspirone must be given in a divided dose (10–40 mg/day) for 1 month before it is effective.
   c. **Side effects.** Buspirone does not cause sedation, physical dependence, psychomotor impairment, or abstinence syndromes, and it does not raise the seizure threshold. It has few clinically important interactions other than serotonin syndrome when co-administered with MAO inhibitors. Since higher doses cause dysphoria, patients do not escalate the dose (as may occur with benzodiazepines). Because buspirone is not a CNS depressant, it will not suppress withdrawal from benzodiazepines and cannot be directly substituted for them.

5. **Barbiturates**
   a. **Uses.** Barbiturates should not be prescribed for anxiety or insomnia except for the very rare patient who has been taking them for years and cannot be withdrawn.
   b. **Side effects.** Barbiturates (e.g., phenobarbital, secobarbital), propanediols (e.g., meprobamate), and related compounds (e.g., glutethimide) cause addiction and severe abstinence syndromes. They are extremely dangerous if taken in overdose.

6. **Antihistamines** (e.g., hydroxyzine, diphenhydramine) are frequently used as antianxiety drugs and hypnotics for elderly patients and for those in whom addiction may be a problem. However, they are not as predictably effective as other antianxiety drugs, and their anticholinergic and sedating side effects can aggravate memory loss and loss of coordination.

7. **Neuroleptics (antipsychotic drugs)**
   a. **Uses**
      (1) Neuroleptics are indicated for anxiety associated with psychoses such as schizophrenia, mania, and psychotic depression.
      (2) Low doses of neuroleptics may temporarily reduce self-destructive behavior in some patients with borderline personality disorder; however, continued benefit has not been demonstrated.
   b. **Side effects.** The danger of long-term side effects, especially that of tardive dyskinesia, precludes continued administration of neuroleptic medications to nonpsychotic patients.

8. **β-blocking agents** (e.g., propranolol) are indicated for patients whose anxiety is accompanied by signs of adrenergic stimulation and for patients with performance anxiety. They are not as predictably effective as the benzodiazepines or the antidepressants in relieving generalized anxiety. High doses can diminish the possibility of brain-injured patients assaulting other people. One dose may be useful in relieving stage fright. Atenolol may reduce social phobia in some patients, but findings have been inconclusive.

BIBLIOGRAPHY

American Psychiatric Association: *Diagnostic and Statistical Manual of Mental Disorders,* 4th ed. Washington, DC, American Psychiatric Association, 1994.

DIRECTIONS: Each of the numbered items or incomplete statements in this section is followed by answers or by completions of the statement. Select the ONE lettered answer or completion that is BEST in each case.

1. A patient with panic anxiety can become agoraphobic if

(A) phobic and anxious traits are inherited together
(B) the patient becomes frightened of situations in which anxiety attacks were experienced
(C) a stressful experience occurs
(D) the patient has deep-seated conflicts
(E) medication side effects predominate

2. In contrast to generalized anxiety, panic anxiety is best described as

(A) unrealistic
(B) excessive
(C) concerned with everyday events
(D) spontaneous
(E) accompanied by hyperventilation

3. An example of a specific phobia is fear of

(A) horses
(B) public transportation
(C) bridges
(D) social situations
(E) crowds

4. Posttraumatic stress disorder differs from adjustment disorder in that

(A) it occurs in veterans
(B) impairment of social functioning occurs
(C) it persists long after the stress has abated
(D) it is characterized by preoccupation with the stress
(E) it can be accompanied by depression

5. A 25-year-old woman who recently had an extramarital affair feels that her physician disapproves strongly of her behavior, which is not really objectionable. This is an example of the defense of

(A) denial
(B) repression
(C) reaction formation
(D) isolation
(E) projection

6. Soon after admission to the coronary care unit for his first myocardial infarction, a 45-year-old businessman refuses to be examined by the house officers and demands to see the most senior cardiologist in the hospital. He tells this individual that his secretary must be permitted unrestricted visiting privileges because he has many important business deals that require prompt attention. He adopts a condescending attitude toward the physicians and nurses. A reasonable management plan while the patient is acutely ill would include which one of the following?

(A) Telling the patient that he must do what the doctors say or risk serious consequences
(B) Restricting visits by the secretary until the patient is well
(C) Discussing fears of dependency, loss of control, and damage to self-esteem
(D) Agreeing that the patient is an important person
(E) Referring the patient to a psychiatrist

7. A 30-year-old man complains of panic attacks and anticipatory anxiety. Which one of the following drugs would be effective for his treatment?

(A) Haloperidol
(B) Fluoxetine
(C) Meprobamate
(D) Pentobarbital
(E) Carbamazepine

8. A 25-year-old man has had long-standing fears of humiliating himself in social interactions. As a result, he has become increasingly isolated. Recently, he has been waking up early in the morning and has found himself wishing he were dead. An appropriate treatment might include which one of the following medications?

(A) Chlordiazepoxide
(B) Buspirone
(C) Hydroxyzine
(D) Phenelzine
(E) Chlorpromazine

DIRECTIONS: Each of the numbered items or incomplete statements in this section is negatively phrased, as indicated by a capitalized word such as NOT, LEAST, or EXCEPT. Select the ONE lettered answer or completion that is BEST in each case.

9. Correct statements about diazepam include all of the following EXCEPT

(A) addiction is rare in medical practice
(B) doses for generalized anxiety are effective for panic disorder
(C) use should not exceed 8 weeks
(D) it can be used as a hypnotic
(E) antipsychotic properties may accompany the anxiolytic effect

10. Correct statements about buspirone include all of the following EXCEPT

(A) it is not addicting
(B) it has the same indications as the benzodiazepines
(C) it suppresses benzodiazepine withdrawal
(D) it has a delayed onset of action
(E) it is prescribed in divided dose

11. Treatment modalities that are usually helpful for posttraumatic stress disorder include all of the following EXCEPT

(A) discussion of the precipitating event
(B) relaxation techniques
(C) biofeedback
(D) systematic desensitization
(E) administration of selective serotonin reuptake inhibitors (SSRIs)

DIRECTIONS: Each set of matching questions in this section consists of a list of lettered options followed by several numbered items. For each numbered item, select the ONE lettered option that is most closely associated with it. Each lettered option may be selected once, more than once, or not at all.

Questions 12–16

Match each clinical situation listed below with the medication most likely to be associated with it.

(A) Diazepam
(B) Trazodone
(C) Pentobarbital
(D) Fluoxetine
(E) Phenelzine

12. Too dangerous for routine use as a hypnotic

13. Effective for obsessive-compulsive disorder

14. Helpful for social phobia

15. Risks of addiction overrated

16. Used as a hypnotic for patients who do not wish to be sedated during the day

Questions 17–21

Match the subtype of phobia with its defining fear.

(A) Agoraphobia
(B) Social phobia
(C) Blood-injection-injury phobia
(D) Natural environmental phobia
(E) Space phobia

17. Humiliation

18. Elevators

19. Venipuncture

20. Falling down

21. Thunderstorms

1. The answer is B *[I A 1 e].* Patients with panic anxiety become progressively more phobic of situations in which they experienced spontaneous anxiety attacks. Although biologic factors are implicated in panic disorder and agoraphobia, these conditions do not seem to be inherited together. Phobias that develop after exposure to a frightening situation are called specific phobias, and they are only associated with panic when the patient is actually in the phobic situation. Patients may become phobic of benign situations that stimulate unconscious conflicts; however, the symbolism of the phobia is usually apparent, and spontaneous panic attacks do not occur. Antidepressants often initially increase anxiety, but they do not cause phobias.

2. The answer is D *[I A 1, 3].* By definition, all anxiety is unrealistic or excessive. Hyperventilation occurs with all types of anxiety. Whereas generalized anxiety involves excessive worry about everyday events, panic attacks arise spontaneously and are not associated with any specific event or concern.

3. The answer is A *[I B 5].* Agoraphobia is fear of situations in which help might not be available or escape might not be possible, such as being in crowds or on public transportation. Fear of humiliating oneself in social or performance situations indicates social phobia. Specific phobias include fears of specific circumscribed objects or situations, such as horses (animal phobia), that are not primarily associated with being alone, in public places, or in social or performance situations.

4. The answer is C *[I B 7].* Posttraumatic stress disorder may persist for years after the stress has abated. This condition may develop after any traumatic event involving a threat to life or physical integrity that evokes intense fear, helplessness, or horror. A soldier, or anyone else under stress, may develop the more acute adjustment disorder, which resolves when the stressful situation ceases. Preoccupation with a stressful event is characteristic of many kinds of anxiety as an attempt to master the stress retroactively. Either disorder impairs social or other aspects of functioning. Patients with acute stress disorder and posttraumatic stress disorder frequently have depressive symptoms.

5. The answer is E *[II K 1].* Projection is attributing to others one's own unacceptable feelings, thoughts, or impulses. Denial involves ignoring elements of external reality, whereas repression involves forgetting memories, thoughts, and feelings that cause internal conflict. Reaction formation, which involves adopting attitudes or interests that are the opposite of the underlying mental state, and isolation, which involves repressing the affect associated with the mental state, are defenses that help to support repression.

6. The answer is D *[II D].* Although a few acutely ill patients may benefit at some point from discussions of fears of dependency, loss of control, or damage to their self-esteem, confronting this issue during the acute phase of the illness tends to increase anxiety. Attempts to assert the physician's control over the situation are likely to make the patient feel more threatened and increase attempts to reassure himself by becoming more demanding. A referral at this point will make the patient feel rejected or insulted. Supporting the patient's self-esteem and allowing him some control will decrease the patient's need to keep demonstrating his importance.

7. The answer is B *[I B 7 b; III C 1, 2].* Antidepressants, including the selective serotonin reuptake inhibitors (SSRIs) such as fluoxetine but not bupropion, are effective treatments for panic disorder. Neuroleptics should be reserved for psychotic anxiety. Carbamazepine is not effective against panic attacks unless they are a symptom of partial seizures. The dangers of addiction and withdrawal preclude the use of meprobamate as an anxiolytic.

8. The answer is D *[I B 6; III C 3].* The diagnosis in this case is probably social phobia complicated by depression. Benzodiazepines, such as chlordiazepoxide, may help the patient to tolerate a social situation acutely, but they are not specific treatments for social phobia, and they may aggravate depression. Buspirone is useful for generalized anxiety disorder, and possibly depression, but not for social phobia. Antihistamines, such as hydroxyzine, are occasionally helpful for anxiety in patients at risk of abusing benzodiazepines, but they have no effect on social phobia. Monoamine oxidase (MAO) inhibitors, such as phenelzine, can treat both depression and social phobia.

9. The answer is B *[III C 1]*. High doses of diazepam are often necessary to treat panic attacks. Diazepam, like any other benzodiazepine, can be used as a hypnotic, although daytime sedation may occur. Benzodiazepines should usually be prescribed for limited periods of time, although recurrent treatment is often necessary for generalized anxiety disorder. Diazepam does not have antipsychotic properties.

10. The answer is C *[III C 4]*. Buspirone has the same indications as the benzodiazepines. It is not habituating or sedating and has no major interactions other than that with the monoamine oxidase (MAO) inhibitors. Buspirone is given in divided doses. Its onset of action may be delayed up to 1 month. If it is directly substituted for a benzodiazepine, a central nervous system (CNS) depressant withdrawal syndrome may occur.

11. The answer is D *[I B 7 b]*. Discussion of the patient's feelings about the traumatic event is a cornerstone of treatment of posttraumatic states. Biofeedback, meditation, and related relaxation techniques are useful adjuncts in the treatment of any anxiety disorder. However, systematic desensitization is a treatment for agoraphobia and specific phobias. SSRIs may reduce arousal, depression, and intrusive recall.

12–16. The answers are: 12-C, 13-D, 14-E, 15-A, 16-B *[III C]*. Barbiturates, such as pentobarbital, carry risks of addiction, withdrawal, and death from overdose that make them too dangerous for routine use for insomnia or anxiety. Selective serotonin reuptake inhibitors (SSRIs), such as fluoxetine, and clomipramine are the only medications shown to be effective for obsessive-compulsive disorder. Monoamine oxidase (MAO) inhibitors, such as phenelzine, have been found effective for social phobia. Dependence on benzodiazepines is rare in medical practice. A combination of sedation and a short elimination half-life make trazodone an effective hypnotic.

17–21. The answers are: 17-B, 18-A, 19-C, 20-E, 21-D *[I B 2, 5, 6]*. Agoraphobia, which may occur with or without panic disorder, is characterized by fear of being trapped in situations from which escape would be difficult or embarrassing (e.g., elevators, crowded theaters). Social phobia involves fear of humiliating oneself in social or performance situations. Blood-injection-injury phobia is a familial form of specific phobia that produces fainting at the sight of blood. Natural environmental phobia is a type of specific phobia involving fears of natural events (e.g., thunderstorms). Space phobia is the fear of falling down if a source of physical support (e.g., a wall) is unavailable.

Chapter 5

Cognitive and Mental Disorders Due to General Medical Conditions

Roderick Shaner

I. **INTRODUCTION.** The term "organic mental disorders" has been used to denote disorders that are caused by general medical conditions or by substances (e.g., abused drugs, medications, and toxins). This classification can erroneously imply that other (primary) mental disorders are nonorganic. In the *Diagnostic and Statistical Manual of Mental Disorders,* 4th edition (DSM-IV), psychopathology formerly attributed to organic mental disorders is classified in three new groups:

A. **Delirium, dementia, and other cognitive disorders** is a newly named group of mental disorders that are characterized by cognitive disturbances.

B. **Mental disorders due to general medical conditions.** Specific mental disorders due to general medical conditions are now described with other disorders that present with similar syndromes. For example, what was formerly called an organic mood disorder and described in the DSM-III-R organic mental disorders section is now called mood disorder due to a general medical condition and is described in the DSM-IV mood disorder section.

   1. **Diagnosis.** A mental disturbance is due to a general medical condition when evidence suggests that the disturbance results from the direct physiologic effect of the medical condition.

   2. **Etiology.** The proposed general medical etiology should be known to cause the particular mental disturbance, and a temporal relationship should exist between the course of the general medical condition and the mental disturbance.

   3. **Differentiation.** The disturbance should not be better explained by a primary mental disorder or one that is substance-induced.

C. **Substance-induced mental disorders.** Specific substance-induced mental disorders are now described with other disorders that present with similar syndromes. For example, what was formerly called a cocaine delusional disorder and described in the DSM-III-R organic mental disorders section is now called cocaine-induced psychotic disorder and is described in the DSM-IV section on schizophrenia and other psychotic disorders.

   1. **Diagnosis.** A mental disturbance is substance-induced if evidence suggests that the disturbance developed in association with substance use.

   2. **Etiology.** The proposed substance should be known to cause the particular mental disturbance.

   3. **Differentiation.** The disturbance should not be better explained by a primary mental disorder or one that is due to a general medical condition.

II. **COGNITIVE DISORDERS** are characterized by the syndromes of delirium, dementia, and amnesia. All are caused by general medical conditions, substances, or a combination of these factors. Disturbances of cognition involve symptoms such as confusion, memory impairment, speech and language difficulties, and impairment of ability to plan or engage in complex tasks.

A. **Delirium** (Table 5-1)

1. **Diagnostic features**
   a. **Clouding of consciousness.** Individuals with clouding of consciousness have reduced clarity of awareness of the environment. Ability to focus, sustain, or shift attention is impaired. Affected individuals may appear confused, perplexed, or alarmed; and they may have difficulty in responding to reassurance or in following directions.
   b. **Impaired cognition.** Individuals with delirium often have a marked disturbance of recent memory and may be unable to give a meaningful history. They may be disoriented to time and place. Speech may be rambling, incoherent, or sparse. The affected individual may have trouble in finding words or in identifying objects or people. Perceptual disturbances may include illusions and hallucinations. Often, actual perceptions are misinterpreted, and ordinary noises or objects are perceived as dangerous or disturbing. Hallucinations are often visual, but other senses can be involved. Persecutory delusions based on sensory misperceptions are common.
   c. **Short and fluctuating course.** Delirium develops over a course of hours or days and fluctuates in severity. The individual may have relatively lucid intervals of minutes or hours. Often, delirium worsens at night or during isolation.
   d. **Not better explained for by dementia.** When delirium is superimposed on a preexisting dementia, it is considered an associated feature of the dementia, not a separate diagnosis.
   e. **Caused by a general medical condition or by a substance.** A comprehensive medical assessment should be undertaken to establish the relationship of the delirium to a general medical condition or to a substance. The disturbance should not be better explained by a primary mental disorder, such as a manic episode occurring during the course of bipolar disorder. A general medical condition is more likely to be responsible for a delirium if its onset or exacerbation corresponds in time period to the course of the delirium and if it has previously been reported to cause delirium. Similarly, it is more likely that a substance is responsible for a delirium if history or laboratory results indicate that use of the substance corresponds in time period to the delirium and if the substance is known to cause delirium.

TABLE 5-1. DSM-IV Classifications for Cognitive Disorders

Amnesia
   Amnestic disorder due to a general medical condition
   Substance-induced persisting amnestic disorder
   Amnestic disorder not otherwise specified

Delirium
   Delirium due to a general medical condition
   Substance-induced delirium
   Delirium due to multiple etiologies
   Delirium not otherwise specified

Dementia
   Dementia of the Alzheimer type
   Vascular dementia
   Dementia due to human immunodeficiency virus (HIV) disease
   Dementia due to head trauma
   Dementia due to Parkinson disease
   Dementia due to Huntington disease
   Dementia due to Pick disease
   Dementia due to Creutzfeldt-Jakob disease
   Dementia due to other general medical conditions
   Substance-induced persisting dementia

2. **Associated features and diagnoses**
   a. **Disturbance in the sleep–wake cycle.** Individuals with delirium are often somnolent during daytime periods or awake and agitated at night. They may have difficulty falling asleep and marked confusion upon arousal.
   b. **Disturbance in psychomotor behavior.** Psychomotor behavior may be disorganized, with purposeless movements, psychomotor agitation, or decreased psychomotor activity.
   c. **Emotional disturbances.** Individuals with delirium are often emotionally labile. They may be extremely agitated and frightened, or withdrawn and apathetic. Periods of irritability, belligerence, or euphoria can occur. Symptoms of delirium can cause affected individuals to strike out, struggle, or attempt to flee, sometimes resulting in patient injuries.
   d. **Abnormal electroencephalogram (EEG).** EEG abnormalities are common in delirious patients, usually showing either generalized slowing or fast wave activity.
   e. **Evidence of general medical conditions or substance use**
      (1) Individuals with delirium often have signs and symptoms of the underlying general medical condition. Metabolic disturbances are especially common.
      (2) Individuals with substance-induced delirium may have toxic levels of the responsible substance and other physical problems associated with the substance. In many cases, delirium results from multiple concurrent etiologies.

3. **Epidemiology.** Children and the elderly are most susceptible to delirium. Studies indicate that up to 25% of elderly hospitalized patients have delirium.

4. **Differential diagnosis.** Delirium should be distinguished from other mental disorders that present with confusion, disorientation, and perceptual disturbances. Intoxication or withdrawal from many drugs of abuse can cause these symptoms, but the diagnosis of substance-induced delirium should not be made unless the symptoms exceed those that would be expected during typical intoxication or withdrawal.

5. **Etiologies.** Delirium most often results from a variety of general medical conditions and from substances that interfere with brain function. Some research findings suggest that the reticular-activating system and cholinergic neurotransmission are specifically affected in delirium.
   a. **General medical conditions** most often associated with delirium include systemic infections, metabolic disturbances, hepatic and renal diseases, seizures, and head trauma.
   b. **Substance-induced delirium** is associated with high, sustained, or rapidly decreasing levels of many drugs, especially in predisposed individuals (e.g., the elderly, the severely ill).

6. **Treatment.** Delirium is treated by correction of the underlying physiologic problems. A quiet, well-lighted room and frequent orientation can decrease agitation. The protective use of restraint or antipsychotic medications to control or decrease severe agitation is sometimes indicated to prevent injury.

B. **Dementia** (see Table 5-1)

1. **Diagnostic features.** The essential feature of dementia is deterioration of memory and cognition that is due to general medical conditions or is substance-induced. Dementia is diagnosed only if the cognitive deficits are present for at least several months and are not merely manifestations of a fluctuating course of delirium. In dementia, cognitive deficits should be apparent even with clarity of consciousness. A disturbance of both memory and at least one of the following aspects of cognition is necessary for diagnosis of dementia.
   a. **Memory impairment** is the hallmark of dementia, and often develops insidiously as the condition progresses. Early on, the individual may appear more absentminded and distracted, misplacing personal objects and becoming disoriented in unfamiliar surroundings. This person may often lose keys or become lost. As dementia progresses, learning deficits become more prominent, and recent memories are lost.

Older memories are the most resistant to loss in dementia, but individuals with progressive dementia ultimately forget even their own names. In addition to social and occupational compromise, memory impairment can lead to physical dangers, such as fires from forgotten cooking or exposure from wandering away while in a disoriented state.

b. Aphasia is an impairment or loss of language function. The affected individual may have difficulty constructing sentences, finding words, naming objects, or comprehending instructions. Speech may become halting, and aphasic individuals may become frustrated and attempt to substitute more general words, such as "it," "that," or "thing," rather than the correct noun. Communication becomes increasingly more difficult, sometimes resulting in mutism.

c. Apraxia is an inability to execute complex motor behaviors, such as bathing, dressing, driving, or drawing. The difficulty is not due to impaired sensory or motor function.

d. Agnosia is a failure to recognize or identify previously known objects, and is not due to impaired sensory function. An affected individual may be unable to recognize common objects or utensils and may not recognize familiar persons.

e. Disturbance in executive function refers to impaired ability to think abstractly and plan, initiate, sequence, monitor, and stop complex behavior. Individuals with dementia may have difficulty conceptualizing or solving problems, such as creating a report, making a grocery list, or adjusting the thermostat in a house.

2. Cortical and subcortical dementias. Some clinicians distinguish between cortical and subcortical dementias, but the relationship of neuroanatomic lesions to symptoms is not entirely clear.

a. Cortical dementia is characterized by the early appearance of aphasia memory loss, and difficulties with calculation. Disturbances of speech and psychomotor behavior are less predominant. These cortical signs usually are not present in subcortical dementia.

b. Subcortical dementia is characterized by the early appearance of problems with executive functioning and recall, dysarthria, motor skill impairment, and personality changes.

3. Associated features and diagnoses

a. Emotional changes. Individuals with dementia often become emotionally uninhibited and labile. They may have outbursts of anger, anxiety, or despair. Depressive symptoms are common and may exacerbate cognitive deficits.

b. Personality disturbances. Even with relatively mild dementia, individuals may undergo marked changes in personality, becoming uninhibited, socially inappropriate, or moody. Irritability and argumentativeness may increase. Expansiveness and euphoria are sometimes present.

c. Psychotic symptoms. Delusions, especially of a persecutory nature, may be present in individuals with dementia. Hallucinations can also occur.

d. Neuroimaging. Abnormal findings on computed axial tomography (CAT) and magnetic resonance imaging (MRI) are common and reflect the pathophysiology of the underlying general medical condition. Neurodegenerative diseases often cause generalized or focal cerebral atrophy, with enlarged cerebral ventricles and cortical sulci. Vascular disease, neoplasms, and traumatic injuries may cause focal lesions. Functional neuroimaging with positron emission tomography (PET) or single photon emission computed tomography (SPECT) may show evidence of focal hypometabolic activity before structural changes are visible.

e. Evidence of general medical conditions or substance use. Individuals with dementia may have signs and symptoms of the underlying general medical condition. Some neurodegenerative diseases are associated with motor and sensory deficits. Cerebrovascular lesions may be associated with focal motor and sensory deficits as well as with evidence of systemic vascular disease. Other dementing generalized medical conditions have characteristic physical findings, such as evidence of infection, endocrine disturbance, or head trauma. Substance-induced persisting dementia may be associated with physical signs of prolonged substance abuse, such as alcohol-related liver disease.

4. **Epidemiology.** The prevalence of dementia varies by age: 5% of the population older than age 65; 20% of the population older than age 85. More than 75% of dementia is caused by Alzheimer disease or cerebrovascular disease.

5. **Course.** Depending on the underlying cause, the onset of dementia may be sudden or gradual. Function may stabilize or deteriorate further, with intensification of social, occupational, and psychological problems. In children, dementia may result in developmental delays rather than deterioration of function.

6. **Familial pattern.** Some types of neurodegenerative dementias are heritable [see dementia of the Alzheimer type (DAT)].

7. **Differential diagnosis**
   a. **Transient substance-induced impairments** may present with cognitive deficits, but they resolve relatively quickly.
   b. **Mental retardation** is distinguished from dementia by evidence of characteristic developmental abnormalities in social, emotional, and language skills. If childhood-onset dementia is responsible for the mental retardation, both conditions are diagnosed.
   c. **Major depressive disorder** can present as difficulties with mental concentration that mimic cognitive deficits, but neuropsychologic tests usually reveal intact cognitive function.
   d. Dementia should be distinguished from less severe, **age-related cognitive decline** in the elderly.
   e. Substance-induced cognitive impairment can be seen during some **intoxications or withdrawals,** but the deficits do not persist beyond the usual course of the intoxication or withdrawal.

8. **Etiologies.** Many medical conditions that involve diffuse or focal cerebral damage can cause dementia.
   a. **Neurodegenerative diseases** associated with dementia include Alzheimer disease, Parkinson disease, amyotrophic lateral sclerosis (ALS)–dementia complex, Huntington disease, and Pick disease.
   b. **Infectious causes** include human immunodeficiency virus (HIV) disease, Creutzfeldt-Jakob disease, viral and bacterial encephalitis and meningitis, and parasitic illnesses.
   c. **Cerebrovascular disease, epilepsy, traumatic brain injuries, and other intracranial processes (e.g., radiation, tumor), normal-pressure hydrocephalus, hypothyroidism, metabolic disorders (e.g., Wilson disease, storage diseases), and vitamin deficiencies (e.g., thiamine, niacin, pyridoxine, cobalamin)** are also causes.
   d. **Substance-induced persisting dementias** are most commonly caused by alcohol, inhalants, sedative–hypnotics, anxiolytics, anticonvulsants, heavy metals, insecticides, and solvents.

9. **Treatment**
   a. **Stabilization or correction of underlying general medical conditions** is the definitive treatment for dementia. When this treatment is effective, cognitive deficits may diminish with time.
   b. Severe agitation and psychotic symptoms may respond to **antipsychotic medications,** but care should be taken to avoid exacerbation of underlying medical conditions. The use of substances such as alcohol, anxiolytics, sedatives and hypnotics, and opioid analgesics may further impair cognition and should be avoided.
   c. **Familiar surroundings, reassurance, and support** decrease confusion and agitation and improve functional capacity.

  d. Family counseling is important for patients with both reversible and irreversible dementias.

C. **Amnestic disorders** (see Table 5-1)

1. **Diagnostic features.** The essential feature of amnestic disorders is impairment in memory, which does not occur solely during the course of delirium or dementia.
   a. **Memory impairment.** As with delirium and dementia, the memory impairment in patients with amnestic disorders is manifested by difficulty in learning new information and, less often, by inability to recall previously learned information. Immediate memory is usually relatively intact, but recent memory is severely affected. The individual may not be able to recount recent events and may be disoriented in terms of time and place.
   b. The memory impairment **does not occur exclusively during the course of a delirium or a dementia**. In amnestic disorders, other aspects of cognition are relatively intact. Clarity of awareness is preserved.

2. **Associated features and diagnoses**
   a. **Confusion.** Individuals with amnesia are often confused and disoriented as a result of recent memory impairment, and they may appear to be suffering from delirium.
   b. **Confabulation.** Individuals with memory impairment may imagine events to account for periods of time that they are unable to recall. They may adamantly defend their ideas.
   c. **Emotional changes.** Individuals with amnesia often have other subtle emotional changes. They sometimes appear inappropriately unconcerned and amotivated. Emotional lability is sometimes present.

3. **Epidemiology.** Although precise numbers are not available, amnestic disorders are more common in populations with a higher prevalence of alcohol abuse and head trauma. Young adult men and individuals with antisocial personality disorder are at greater risk.

4. **Course.** The onset of amnesia may be rapid when it results from trauma or acute biochemical injury (e.g., anoxia). More insidious onset is seen with neurodegenerative conditions or with chronic exposure to toxic substances. The clinical course depends on the underlying cause, and the symptoms may be transient or chronic.

5. **Differential diagnosis**
   a. **Delirium and dementia** are both characterized by prominent memory disturbances but are accompanied by other cognitive deficits.
   b. **Dissociative disorders** also involve disturbances of memory, but are often associated with emotional stress and unusual patterns of memory impairment.
   c. Substance **intoxication and withdrawal** often cause memory impairment, which does not persist.
   d. **Age-related cognitive decline** is associated with decreased acuity of memory, but not to a degree that causes significant functional impairment.

6. **Etiologies.** Bilateral damage (transient or chronic) to diencephalic and mediotemporal structures (e.g., mamillary bodies, fornix, hippocampus) may produce memory dysfunction in the absence of other cognitive symptoms. Such damage can be caused by thiamine deficiency associated with alcohol dependence, head trauma, cerebrovascular disease, hypoxia, local infection (herpes encephalitis), ablative surgical procedures, and seizures. Acute and chronic use of alcohol, anxiolytics, sedatives, and hypnotics can produce amnesia.

7. **Treatment.** As with delirium and dementia, stabilization or correction of the underlying general medical condition is the definitive treatment for amnestic disorders. Further physical or biochemical cerebral insults should be avoided. Familiar surroundings as well as reassurance and support are also helpful as the patient gradually becomes reoriented.

D. **Cognitive disorder not otherwise specified.** A variety of cerebral insults can lead to patterns of cognitive deficits, which are not better explained by delirium, dementia, or amnesia.

1. **Mild neurocognitive impairment.** Early in the course of neurodegenerative illness or after mild cerebral damage from various causes, symptoms of cognitive impairment are sometimes evident in the absence of dementia. In addition, subtle changes in personality are often present in such conditions.

2. **Postconcussion syndrome.** Chronic physical discomfort and disturbances in cognition sometimes follow significant closed head trauma with transient loss of consciousness and amnesia. In such cases, sleep disturbances, headaches, and dizziness are often present. Automobile accidents are a common cause of concussion injury.

III. MENTAL DISORDERS DUE TO GENERAL MEDICAL CONDITIONS

A. **Catatonic disorder due to a general medical condition**

1. Catatonia is a syndrome characterized by **abnormalities of psychomotor activity,** which include any of the following:
   a. **Motoric immobility** (e.g., catatonic rigidity, waxy flexibility)
   b. **Excessive motor activity** (e.g., catatonic excitement)
   c. Extreme **negativism or mutism** (e.g., passive resistance to instructions, failure to speak)
   d. **Peculiarities of voluntary movement** (e.g., purposeless repeated movements, bizarre posturing)
   e. **Echolalia** (e.g., immediate purposeless repetition of words)
   f. **Echopraxia** (e.g., purposeless imitation of movements)

2. Individuals with catatonia often appear bizarre and disturbed; this combination makes comprehensive medical assessment particularly difficult. The onset and course of catatonia depend entirely on the underlying general medical condition.

3. **Etiologies.** General medical conditions that cause catatonia include both generalized and focal cerebral insults and systemic illnesses. It is not known whether specific central nervous system (CNS) structures must be affected to produce catatonia.
   a. Neurologic conditions that can produce catatonia include **neoplasms, head trauma, cerebrovascular disease, and encephalitis**.
   b. Other general medical conditions associated with catatonia include **hypercalcemia, hepatic encephalopathy, homocystinuria, and diabetic ketoacidosis**.

4. **Differential diagnosis**
   a. **Delirium.** If catatonic behavior occurs exclusively during the course of delirium, it is not diagnosed separately.
   b. **Movement disorders** can mimic catatonia.
   c. **Schizophrenia, catatonic type,** presents with catatonia but is accompanied by other signs of schizophrenia and is not due to a general medical condition.
   d. **Mood disorders** can present with catatonia but are accompanied by a mood disturbance, such as depression or mania.

5. **Treatment.** Stabilization or correction of the underlying general medical condition is the definitive treatment for catatonia due to a general medical condition. Antipsychotic medications or restraints are sometimes indicated to prevent patient injury from disorganized behavior.

B. **Personality change due to a general medical condition.** The alteration of personality can include emotional lability, poor impulse control, aggressive or angry outbursts, apathy, or suspiciousness. Affected individuals may become reclusive, querulous, or combative. DSM-IV subtypes of personality change due to a general medical condition are designated as labile, uninhibited, aggressive, apathetic, paranoid, and combined and unspecified types.

1. The **pattern of personality changes** depends in part on the locus of the responsible lesion. Frontal lobe damage is characterized by disinhibition, shallow emotions, and occasionally euphoria (so-called frontal lobe syndrome).

2. **Etiologies.** Many of the same general medical conditions that cause dementia can cause personality change when the lesion is not severe or the clinical course is in its early stages. Head trauma is a major cause of personality change that does not progress to dementia.

3. **Differential diagnosis**
   a. Personality change due to a general medical condition must be distinguished from other mental disorders due to general medical conditions and from substance-induced mental disorders. Dementia and other cognitive disorders are characterized by memory impairment or other cognitive problems.
   b. Other mental disorders, whether they are primary or are due to a general medical condition, can secondarily result in personality change, such as those that result from depressed mood, delusional beliefs, or immersion in a substance-abusing subculture.

4. **Treatment.** Stabilization or correction of the underlying general medical condition is the definitive treatment for personality disorder due to a general medical condition. Unfortunately, full recovery after traumatic damage does not always occur. Social and occupational rehabilitation plays an important role in treatment, as do counseling and support for patients' families.

IV. GENERAL MEDICAL CONDITIONS THAT CAUSE MENTAL DISTURBANCES

A. Overview

1. **Examination of patients with mental disturbances.** The current availability of sensitive and specific diagnostic examinations makes it reasonable to screen for general medical conditions in almost all patients who have cognitive or behavioral changes.

2. **Pathophysiology.** General medical conditions and substances can adversely affect cerebral functioning through a number of mechanisms. Effects may be reversible or irreversible, depending on the nature of the lesion.
   a. **Disruption of metabolic homeostasis.** Levels of electrolytes, pH, hydration, and osmolarity can be altered by many metabolic and endocrine disorders and neoplasms.
   b. **Disruption of molecular synthesis.** Synthesis of neurotransmitters, neuroreceptors, cellular structures, and supporting elements can be disrupted by neurodegenerative disease, endocrine diseases, and nutritional deficiencies.
   c. **Deficiency of substrates.** Oxygen or metabolic substrates for oxidative metabolism may be deficient in pulmonary disease, cerebrovascular disease, nutritional disease, and metabolic diseases.
   d. **Electrophysiologic disruption.** Synaptic transmission can be altered biochemically or by seizures.
   e. **Tissue damage.** Brain tissue can be destroyed by trauma, infection, or neoplasms.

B. Neurodegenerative diseases

1. **Alzheimer disease** is a progressive neurodegenerative illness of unknown cause that produces characteristic brain lesions and dementia.
   a. **Etiology.** No definite cause for Alzheimer disease has been identified, but several of its abnormalities have been suggested as causes. Because none are absolutely pathognomonic for Alzheimer disease, a multifactorial etiology is plausible.
      (1) **Genetic lesions.** Several genetic lesions may produce Alzheimer disease. Chromosome 21 is the locus most commonly implicated. It is the site of the genes for amyloid precursor protein, and Alzheimer disease is very common in patients with Down syndrome (trisomy 21). Chromosomes 14 and 19 have also been implicated.

(2) Abnormal amyloid precursor protein metabolism. A product of amyloid precursor protein, beta/A4 (amyloid), is a major component of neuritic plaques.

(3) Tau protein. This substance, which is associated with cellular microtubules, is found in neurofibrillary tangles.

(4) Cholinergic neuronal dysfunction. Cholinergic neurons in the hippocampus are affected early in the course of Alzheimer disease, and cholinergic agonists (e.g., physostigmine and tacrine) may at least transiently improve some symptoms.

(5) Other abnormalities. Aluminum has been implicated, as it is a component of neuritic plaques. **Abnormal neuronal membrane phospholipid metabolism** has also been suggested as a cause of Alzheimer disease.

b. Histopathology. The classic histopathologic findings of Alzheimer disease are neuronal loss, neurofibrillary tangles, neuritic (i.e., amyloid, senile) plaques, granulovacuolar degeneration, and amyloid angiopathy. Mediotemporal lobes are most severely affected.

(1) Neuronal loss. Cholinergic neurons in the basal forebrain (including the nucleus basalis of Meynert) are affected early, but general neuronal loss ultimately occurs.

(2) Neurofibrillary tangles. Intraneuronal deposits of abnormal microtubular elements and phosphorylated tau protein are common.

(3) Neuritic plaques. Extraneuronal deposits of amyloid, aluminosilicates, dystrophic neuronal elements, and microglia are most prominent in the hippocampus and neocortex. They are also present in vascular tissue (amyloid angiopathy) throughout the body of individuals with Alzheimer disease.

(4) Granulovacuolar degeneration. Intracytoplasmic vacuoles are present in hippocampal neurons.

c. Gross pathology. Diffuse frontotemporal cerebral atrophy, widened cortical sulci, and enlarged cerebral ventricles are characteristic.

d. Epidemiology. Dementia of the Alzheimer type (DAT) is responsible for approximately 55% of cases of dementia. It is seldom evident before age 50 and is slightly more common in women. It affects 4% of the population older than age 65 and 20% of the population older than age 85. Incidence of Alzheimer disease is three to four times higher in relatives of patients, and concordance rate is 40% in monozygotic twins. Early-onset DAT is extremely common in individuals with Down syndrome.

e. Course

(1) The onset of Alzheimer disease is usually insidious, and the course usually progresses slowly.

(2) Early deficits commonly involve recent memory disturbances, mood disturbances, emotional lability, and impulsivity.

(3) DAT becomes clinically evident as the disease progresses. DSM-IV subtypes include DAT with delirium, delusions, depressed mood, and behavioral disturbances. .

(4) Late in the disease, motor disturbances supervene, especially gait disturbances, pathologic reflexes, and incontinence. Seizures occur in approximately 10% of cases.

(5) The duration from the onset of dementia to death is usually 8–10 years.

f. Differential diagnosis. Dementias due to other causes are the major differential diagnoses for DAT. The clinical diagnosis of DAT is one of exclusion and is usually confirmed at autopsy. Major depressive disorder can present with difficulties in mental concentration and apathy that can mimic dementia.

g. Treatment. The goals of treatment are to reduce behavioral disturbances and psychosis, improve mood, maintain adequate nutrition, and help caregivers cope with the burden of illness. Tacrine, a reversible acetylcholinesterase (AChE) inhibitor, is effective in transiently reversing or slowing cognitive decline in a small percentage of cases. Antipsychotic agents may be used to reduce agitation and psychosis. Caregivers should try to maintain adequate food intake and good hygiene; they should also encourage exercise as much as possible.

2. **Dementia due to Parkinson disease.** This common, progressive neurodegenerative disease involves loss of dopaminergic neurons in the substantia nigra. It is manifested by resting tremor, rigidity, bradykinesia, and gait disturbances.

   a. **Etiology.** The cause of Parkinson disease is unknown in the majority of patients. It has been associated with infection or exposure to toxins in some cases, but does not appear to have any genetic basis.

   b. **Histopathology.** A progressive loss of dopaminergic neurons occurs in the substantia nigra. Lewy bodies are found in the neuronal cytoplasm of the remaining dopaminergic neurons.

   c. **Epidemiology.** The prevalence of Parkinson disease is 1 in 1000. Dementia occurs in at least 20%–40% of cases.

   d. **Symptoms and course**

      (1) The onset of Parkinson disease is usually between age 50 and 65.

      (2) Motor symptoms include progressive tremor, rigidity, bradykinesia, and postural instability.

      (3) Dementia due to Parkinson disease is usually more evident in advanced disease, and it must be distinguished from the depressive symptoms that are also commonly present. The dementia is characterized by "subcortical" features, such as psychomotor slowing and disturbances of executive function.

      (4) Cognitive problems may be compounded by coexisting depression and by DAT and other age-associated cognitive impairments.

      (5) The course is progressive, but the rate is extremely variable.

   e. **Differential diagnosis.** Other diseases that cause movement disorders and dementia must be considered, including vascular dementia, progressive supranuclear palsy, Shy-Drager syndrome, amyotrophic lateral sclerosis (ALS)-dementia-Parkinson disease complex, and olivopontocerebellar degeneration. Antipsychotic medications can also produce parkinsonian symptoms. A diagnosis of Parkinson disease is usually confirmed at autopsy by the presence of Lewy bodies.

   f. **Treatment** of Parkinson disease involves use of dopamine precursors (e.g., levodopa, carbidopa), dopamine agonists (e.g., bromocriptine, pergolide), anticholinergic medications (e.g., benztropine, trihexyphenidyl), amantadine, and selegiline, a selective monoamine oxidase (MAO)-B inhibitor. Antiparkinsonian medications can produce personality changes, cognitive changes, and psychotic symptoms.

3. **Dementia due to Huntington disease.** This progressive neurodegenerative disease involves γ-aminobutyric acid (GABA)-ergic neurons of the basal ganglia, and is manifested by choreoathetosis and dementia.

   a. **Etiology.** Huntington disease is caused by a defect in an autosomal dominant gene located on chromosome 4.

   b. **Histopathology.** A loss of GABA-ergic neurons occurs in the striatum.

   c. **Gross morphology.** Functional neuroimaging reveals caudate hypometabolism at an early stage. Atrophy of the caudate nucleus, with resultant ventricular enlargement (boxcar ventricles), is common.

   d. **Epidemiology.** The prevalence is about 5 in 100,000. Fifty percent of offspring of patients with Huntington disease will acquire the illness.

   e. **Symptoms and course**

      (1) The **onset** of clinically evident Huntington disease usually occurs at approximately age 40, but the variation is wide.

      (2) **Early symptoms** include personality changes and subtle movement disturbances.

      (3) **Later symptoms.** As the disease progresses, choreoathetosis and dementia become evident. The dementia is characterized by "subcortical" features that include cognitive slowing and disturbances of executive function. Behavioral disorganization and psychotic features are fairly common.

      (4) Death usually occurs approximately 15 years after onset.

   f. **Differential diagnosis.** Other causes of dementia should be considered. Schizophrenia (especially with catatonic symptoms), schizoaffective disorders, mood disorders with psychotic and catatonic symptoms, and other psychotic disorders can resemble

Huntington disease. Other causes of choreoathetosis, including tardive dyskinesia from antipsychotic medications, are also in the differential diagnosis.

g. Treatment. Antipsychotic medications can ameliorate both choreoathetosis and psychotic symptoms. Family counseling, including genetic counseling, is essential.

4. Dementia due to Pick disease. Pick disease is a progressive neurodegenerative disease of the frontal and temporal lobes, and is manifested by personality and language changes followed by other symptoms of dementia.

    a. Etiology is unknown.

    b. Histopathology. Pick bodies (intraneuronal argentophilic inclusions) and Pick cells (swollen neurons) are found in affected areas of the brain.

    c. Gross morphology. Functional neuroimaging (PET or SPECT) reveals frontal and temporal hypometabolism before frontal and temporal atrophy become apparent by MRI.

    d. Epidemiology. Prevalence is unknown, but it may be relatively more common than previously believed.

    e. Symptoms and course

        (1) The **age of onset** of clinical symptoms is usually between age 50 and 60.

        (2) Early behavioral signs often include personality changes suggestive of frontal lobe disturbance, including disinhibition and emotional lability or apathy.

        (3) Dementia due to Pick disease usually follows several years later, with subcortical features including impairment in language and executive functioning.

    f. Differential diagnosis. Pick disease must be distinguished from other causes of dementia, especially a group of other diseases characterized by frontotemporal atrophy. Pick bodies are found only in patients with Pick disease.

    g. Treatment. There is no specific treatment for Pick disease.

C. **Cerebrovascular disease**

1. Etiology. The most common etiologies for cerebrovascular disease are systemic arterial hypertensive disease, valvular heart disease, and extracranial vascular disease.

2. Gross morphology. Cerebral angiography may reveal flow abnormalities or abnormal vasculature (e.g., aneurysms). Neuroimaging by computed tomography (CT) scan or MRI reveals lesions in brain structures, including hyperintensities and focal atrophy suggestive of old infarctions. Functional neuroimaging may reveal both global and focal reductions in cerebral metabolism, with asymmetric distribution.

3. Epidemiology. Vascular dementia is the second most common cause of dementia; DAT is the most common. It is responsible for perhaps 20% of cases of dementia and is more common in men than women.

4. Symptoms and course

    a. The **onset** of cerebrovascular disease may be preceded by evidence of systemic hypertensive illness or other vascular pathology. In addition, the patient may have a history of transient ischemic attacks. Depending on etiology, the onset of cerebrovascular disease may be sudden or insidious.

        (1) Large thrombotic or embolic strokes are associated with the sudden onset or exacerbation of symptoms.

        (2) Symptoms from smaller serial infarcts or damage from cerebral insufficiency may be more gradual, with personality changes and increasing disturbance of cognitive function.

        (3) Single strokes may be associated with specific motor, sensory, and cognitive deficits, but rarely result in dementia.

    b. Neurologic findings include abnormal reflexes, focal motor weakness, and gait disturbances.

    c. With extensive cerebrovascular disease, **vascular dementia** becomes apparent. Symptoms depend on the location of the lesions. Some common patterns include:

        (1) Binswanger disease. Multiple small infarctions of deep hemispheric structures produce subcortical dementia, pseudobulbar palsy, spasticity, and weakness.

      (2) Left hemispheric disease involves cortical dementia, with prominent aphasia and apraxia. Depressive symptoms are more common with left than with right hemispheric disease.

      (3) Right hemispheric disease is characterized by cortical dementia, with prominent anomia and visuospatial deficits.

    d. The **course** of the illness is often characterized by stepwise exacerbations, which correspond to progressive cerebrovascular compromise. The developing patterns of cognitive and motor deficits are highly variable, depending on the location of lesions. Symptoms may fluctuate as brain tissue surrounding new lesions recovers from embolic or thrombotic insults. The overall course reflects the nature of the underlying vascular pathology, the location of lesions, and the effectiveness of treatment.

  5. Differential diagnosis. Dementia due to neurodegenerative disease usually has a more insidious onset and gradual progression, with less scattered motor findings. Dementia due to other general medical conditions is usually accompanied by other suggestive physical findings.

  6. Treatment of cerebrovascular disease is directed at the underlying cause. Depending on the cause, control of hypertension, endarterectomy, correction of sources of emboli, and anticoagulant therapy may be indicated. Successful treatment may arrest or slow the course of dementia.

D. | **Infectious diseases**

  1. Mechanisms. Infectious agents can cause mental disorders through a variety of mechanisms:

    a. Physical destruction of brain tissue

    b. Inflammation of brain tissue, meninges, or cerebral vasculature

    c. Mass effects from infectious lesions

    d. Toxins

    e. Systemic metabolic alterations such as fever, renal failure, hepatic failure, or electrolyte disturbance

  2. Viral encephalitis can result in delirium, sometimes accompanied by headache, fever, and photophobia. Focal CNS herpesvirus lesions, usually in frontal or temporal lobes, can produce anosmia, personality changes, bizarre behavior, and complex partial seizures. Rabies encephalitis rapidly produces delirium. Subacute sclerosing panencephalitis (SSPE) can occur following measles infection in childhood and progresses from delirium with myoclonus, ataxia, and seizures to chronic dementia.

  3. Chronic viral infections can produce progressive destruction of CNS tissue resulting in dementia. The DSM-IV describes both dementia due to HIV disease and dementia due to Creutzfeldt-Jakob disease.

    a. Dementia due to HIV disease. HIV directly destroys brain parenchyma, and the course of the dementia is progressive. It becomes clinically apparent in at least 30% of individuals with acquired immune deficiency syndrome (AIDS). Diffuse multifocal destruction of brain structures occurs, and cognitive impairment may be accompanied by signs of delirium. Motor findings include gait disturbance, hypertonia and hyperreflexia, pathologic reflexes (e.g., frontal release signs), and oculomotor deficits. The differential diagnosis for dementia due to HIV disease includes other HIV-associated general medical conditions that cause dementia, including CNS tumors and opportunistic CNS infections. Mood disturbances in individuals with HIV infection may mimic cognitive impairment.

    b. Dementia due to Creutzfeldt-Jakob disease. This rare spongiform encephalopathy is caused by a slow virus (prion) and presents with dementia, myoclonus, and EEG abnormalities (e.g., sharp, triphasic, synchronous discharges). Over a course of several months, symptoms progress from vague malaise and personality changes to dementia. Other findings include visual and gait disturbances, choreoathetosis or other abnormal movements, and myoclonus. Atypical presentations and slower courses have been described in some patients. Kuru is a slow virus that causes dementia and motor disturbances found in New Guinea.

   c. Progressive multifocal leukoencephalopathy (PML). This demyelinating condition is caused by papovavirus JC (JCV) infection and usually occurs in immunocompromised hosts. Over several months, increasing multiple motor deficits and cognitive deficits lead to death. HIV infection has increased the incidence of PML.

4. Neurosyphilis (general paresis), which is a parenchymal form of CNS tertiary syphilis, typically occurs 5 to 30 years after incompletely treated primary syphilis. Personality changes are usually noted before the onset of dementia. Prominent psychotic symptoms are sometimes present. Physical findings include papilledema, optic atrophy, Argyll Robertson pupils [i.e., constriction reaction to near objects (accommodation reflexes present) but not to light (pupillary reflexes absent)], gait disturbances, and spasticity.

5. Acute bacterial meningitis usually has a rapid onset and presents with systemic signs of infection (e.g., high fever), accompanied by headache, stiff neck, and delirium.

6. Chronic meningitis has a more gradual onset of cognitive impairment, progressing in some cases to delirium. The most common infections are tuberculosis and cryptococcal and coccidioidal mycoses. **Syphilitic meningitis** is a form of tertiary syphilis that usually occurs 1 to 3 years after incompletely treated primary syphilis and presents with delirium. Chronic basilar meningitis is accompanied by pupillary abnormalities, ptosis, hearing impairment, and facial paralysis. Chronic hemispheric meningitis is accompanied by marked cognitive impairments and seizures.

7. Mass lesions resulting from granulomatous infections or abscesses can cause a variety of cognitive disturbances depending on the site of the lesions. Infections that most commonly produce mass lesions include tuberculosis, parasitic disease (cysticercosis, schistosomiasis), and mycoses.

E. **Myelin diseases.** Several diseases involve myelin, the white matter that sheaths neuronal axons, associated with motor and sensory disturbances. Depending on the nature of the disorder and sites affected, cognitive symptoms, personality changes, and mood disturbances can occur.

   1. Acute disseminated encephalomyelitis. This demyelinating illness of abrupt onset presents with delirium followed by sensory and motor deficits, seizures, and coma. The mortality rate is 50%, and marked residual neurologic and cognitive impairments are present. It sometimes follows viral illnesses or vaccinations and may have an immune origin.

   2. Multiple sclerosis (MS) is a multifocal demyelinating disease of unclear viral or immune origin with a waxing and waning clinical course. Episodes of focal disturbances occur and remit, sometimes with increasing residual motor and sensory deficits. It has an overall prevalence of about 50 in 100,000 and is slightly more common in women, with a peak incidence between age 20 and 40. It is more common in temperate climates.

     a. Sensory symptoms include transient visual impairment (initial presentation in 40% of patients) and impaired vibratory and position sense.

     b. Transient motor symptoms include nystagmus, dysarthria, tremor, ataxia, bladder dysfunction, and focal motor weakness.

     c. Personality changes depend on the loci of lesions but can include emotional lability, shallow emotions, depression, suspiciousness, apathy, and impulsiveness.

     d. Cognitive symptoms occur, and persisting dementia occasionally develops late in the course of the illness. The transient and patchy distribution of lesions often leads to somatic preoccupation in affected individuals and suggests a somatoform disorder.

   3. Other diseases of myelin. A number of other leukodystrophies caused by genetic lesions of myelin metabolism cause progressive neurologic impairment and dementia in children and adults. These diseases include metachromatic leukodystrophy (cerebroside sulfatase deficiency), globoid cell (Krabbe) leukodystrophy (galactocerebrosidase deficiency), and adrenoleukodystrophy.

F. **Epilepsy** is characterized by recurrent seizures and is associated with a variety of mental disturbances that occur both intra- and interictally.

1. **Definition.** Seizures, also referred to as convulsions or ictal episodes, are characterized by transient bursts of abnormal CNS electrical activity that cause disturbances of movement, autonomic activity, and consciousness. Seizure symptoms depend on the location of the seizure focus and the electrophysiologic state of the CNS.

2. **Etiologies** of seizures include focal brain lesions resulting from trauma, infections, and neoplasms. Metabolic disturbances, neurodegenerative diseases, and various substances may also precipitate seizures. Autism and mental retardation are associated with a higher incidence of seizures.

3. **Pathophysiology.** Seizures result from disturbances of the electrophysiologic activity of brain cells, leading to paroxysmal discharges, which spread to large groups of neurons and produce characteristic EEG findings.

4. **Types of seizures**
   a. **Generalized seizures** involve the entire brain.
      (1) **Tonic–clonic seizures** present with loss of consciousness and postural control, followed by generalized muscular rigidity (tonic phase). This is followed by rhythmic contractions (clonic phase) of the upper and lower extremities. Incontinence may occur. EEG tracings show a wide range of abnormalities.
      (2) **Absences** are characterized by brief disruptions of consciousness during which affected individuals may seem inattentive or unresponsive. There may be subtle motor findings, such as loss of muscle tone, chewing, or lip-smacking movements. EEG tracings show characteristic bilaterally synchronous 3-Hz spikes and slow wave activity. Absence epilepsy is more common in childhood.
      (3) **Atonic seizures** (drop attacks) are characterized by brief loss of consciousness and postural tone. Episodes can resemble the cataplexy symptom of narcolepsy.
      (4) **Myoclonic seizures** involve muscle contractions without loss of consciousness, and are seen in a variety of neurodegenerative diseases.
   b. **Partial seizures** involve specific brain foci.
      (1) **Simple partial seizures** present with motor, sensory, or autonomic disturbances, depending on the location of the seizure focus.
      (2) **Complex partial seizures** cause disturbances of consciousness, including decreased awareness and alterations of cognition, emotion, and sensory experience. Recurrent complex partial seizure is the most common form of adult epilepsy, sometimes called psychomotor epilepsy or temporal lobe epilepsy. During seizure episodes, affected individuals may have dreamlike sensations, and may exhibit poorly organized behavior that can appear inappropriate, bizarre, or violent. Complex partial seizures can resemble symptoms seen with dissociative fugue and depersonalization disorder.

5. **Symptoms**
   a. **Preictal symptoms** are often referred to as an **aura,** and can include motor, sensory, emotional, and cognitive experiences. Motor twitching, olfactory hallucinations (e.g., burning rubber), autonomic sensations (e.g., a feeling of epigastric discomfort), peculiar emotion states or reveries, and intrusive thoughts or memories have been described as components of auras.
   b. **Postictal mental symptoms** due to generalized seizures and complex partial seizures are characteristic of resolving delirium. The duration of confusion varies from minutes to hours. Amnesia is usually complete for intraictal events during generalized seizures. Varying degrees of amnesia for events occur during complex partial seizures. After tonic–clonic seizures, focal motor paralysis may be present for minutes, hours, or days (Todd paralysis).

    c. Interictal symptoms are absent in many patients with epilepsy. Some affected individuals, especially those with complex partial seizure disorders, may develop a variety of personality changes or cognitive deficits. Psychotic symptoms may also occur. Some of these symptoms may be due to subclinical seizure episodes. With long-standing and poorly controlled seizure disorders, cognitive deficits become more common.

6. **Other psychopathology associated with epilepsy.** Individuals with epilepsy have a higher incidence of mental disorders.

    a. Some mental disorders, such as mental retardation and autism, may stem from the same cause as the comorbid seizure disorder.

    b. In cognitive disorders and other mental disorders due to general medical conditions, seizures may be the physiologic cause of the comorbid mental disturbance.

    c. Individuals with epilepsy may develop mood, anxiety, or somatoform disorders as a result of the psychological stress associated with the illness. The incidence of suicide is relatively high in individuals with epilepsy.

7. **Differential diagnosis**

    a. Seizure-like episodes can occur in **conversion disorder** and **factitious disorder,** but there is rarely incontinence or physical harm (e.g., tongue biting) from tonic–clonic motor activity. Patients with factitious seizures are more likely to suffer from actual seizures as well.

    b. Dissociative disorders can present with alterations of consciousness and cognition that are suggestive of complex partial seizures. Distinguishing between these conditions is sometimes difficult, and may require repeated EEGs, or 24-hour EEG recordings. Nasopharyngeal EEG leads are sometimes used.

8. **Treatment.** Definitive treatment of epilepsy requires amelioration of the underlying cause through management of systemic illness or surgical removal of seizure foci in the brain. Control of epilepsy can often be accomplished with anticonvulsant medications. However, these medications actually may cause mental disturbances.

G. **Neoplasms.** Neoplastic disease can cause mental disturbances through a variety of physiologic mechanisms, including intracranial mass effects, destruction of brain tissue, seizures, metabolic alterations, production of neuropeptides and toxins, and autoimmune reactions.

1. The **type of mental disturbance produced** by neoplasia depends on the nature of the neoplasm, the location of the tumor, the size of the tumor, and the rate of tumor growth.

2. **Rapidly growing intracranial neoplasms** in any location can produce **delirium** accompanied by other signs of increased intracranial pressure, including headache, papilledema, and vomiting. Slowly growing intracranial neoplasms can produce more insidious changes in cognition and personality.

3. The **location of intracranial neoplasms** influences the nature of the mental disturbances and physical findings.

    a. Frontal lobe tumors may be associated with personality changes, including disinhibition, emotional lability, or apathy.

    b. Parietal lobe tumors may be associated with sensory deficits, agnosia, and visual neglect.

    c. Temporal lobe tumors may be associated with complex motor, perceptual, and behavioral symptoms that resemble complex partial seizures.

    d. Occipital lobe tumors may be associated with visual hallucinations.

    e. Brain stem tumors may lead to an alert yet immobile and mute state (akinetic mutism or vigilant coma).

4. **Neuropeptide- and hormone-secreting tumors** in any location can produce mental changes through direct effects on CNS activity or by alteration of systemic metabolism.

5. Paraneoplastic syndromes are distant effects of neoplasms mediated by tumor-induced autoimmune reactions, tumor-produced neurotoxic substances, and perhaps other mechanisms. Paraneoplastic syndromes can produce mental disturbances. Small-cell lung carcinoma can produce encephalitis and delirium. When limited to limbic structures (limbic encephalitis), the condition can produce memory impairment and personality changes.

6. Adjustment disorders arising from the psychosocial effects of neoplastic disease must be considered in the differential diagnosis of mental disorders due to neoplasms.

H. **Head trauma** leading to traumatic brain injury can produce subtle or profound cognitive symptoms and personality changes that may be transient or chronic. Head trauma can cause **brain injury** by direct destruction of brain tissue, by shearing of neuronal axons, by increased intracranial pressure, and by resultant vascular hemorrhage. The symptoms and course of resultant mental disturbances depend on the nature, location, and extent of damage.

1. Acute head trauma may result in immediate delirium or delirium that follows recovery of consciousness. The delirium is of variable duration, from a few seconds to days or weeks of confusion. Duration may reflect the extent of overall damage. Recovery is often gradual over several weeks, and often involves amnesia for events surrounding the trauma.

2. Subdural hematomas arising from head injury (present in 10% of individuals with serious head injury) may present with headache, cognitive or personality changes, and focal neurologic deficits reflecting the location of the lesion. Individuals with alcoholism are predisposed to development of posttraumatic subdural hematomas.

3. Postconcussion syndrome (diagnosed in the DSM-IV as cognitive disorder not otherwise specified) is a disturbance of at least 3 months' duration that sometimes follows significant head trauma. It is characterized by cognitive, somatic, and behavioral symptoms that include headaches, fatigue, sleep disturbances, dizziness, and personality changes.

4. Personality change sometimes results from head trauma, even in the absence of obvious cognitive changes.

5. Chronic amnestic disorder can result from damage to diencephalic and mediotemporal lobe structures (e.g., mamillary bodies, hippocampus, fornix).

6. Dementia due to head trauma is usually nonprogressive and may persist indefinitely, or may gradually ameliorate over many months or years. It is often accompanied by emotional lability and impulsivity. A history of head trauma is a risk factor for development of dementias due to neurodegenerative disorders.

7. In **children,** head trauma may lead to either loss of developmental competencies or a slowing of mental development. When either occurs, diagnoses of both mental retardation and dementia may be appropriate.

I. **Nutritional deficiencies.** Mental disturbances resulting from nutritional deficiencies are characterized by development of cognitive deficits and personality changes with occasional psychotic symptoms, and progression to dementia if untreated.

1. Etiologies. A number of nutritional substances are essential for the structural integrity of the CNS. Deficiencies can be due to inadequate intake, impaired absorption, and abnormal metabolism. Deficiency diseases are more common in areas of severe food shortage and in individuals with limited or unusual diets or alcoholism. Often, multiple deficiencies and general malnutrition are present in a single individual.

2. Thiamine (vitamin B_1) is required as a coenzyme for oxidative decarboxylation and for neural conduction.
   a. Beriberi results from thiamine deficiency caused by malnutrition. Individuals can present with high-output cardiac failure (wet beriberi), peripheral neuropathy with bilateral distal impairment of motor and sensory skills and reflexes (dry beriberi), and CNS damage with motor and cognitive impairments (cerebral beriberi).

b. **Wernicke encephalopathy and Korsakoff psychosis** describe forms of cerebral beriberi most commonly found in alcohol-dependent individuals.

   (1) Wernicke encephalopathy is characterized by the rapid onset of ataxia, oculomotor abnormalities (ophthalmoplegia and nystagmus), and delirium. Histopathologic changes occur in the mamillary bodies and walls of the third ventricle. Symptoms usually quickly resolve if thiamine is administered early.

   (2) Inadequately treated encephalopathy may result in alcohol-induced persisting amnestic disorder (Korsakoff psychosis), which is not responsive to treatment with thiamine. Associated symptoms include confabulation, personality changes, and motor deficits. Dementia may supervene.

3. **Nicotinic acid (niacin)** deficiency (pellagra) usually results from a dietary deficiency of tryptophan as a consequence of alcohol dependence, from some vegetarian diets, or from starvation. Symptoms include dermatitis, diarrhea, peripheral neuropathies, cognitive deficits, and personality changes that progress to delirium. Irreversible dementia can result if the deficiency is not treated.

4. **Pyridoxine (vitamin B$_6$)** deficiency leads to dermatitis, neuropathies, and cognitive changes. It is usually found only in association with use of medications (e.g., isoniazid) that act as pyridoxine antagonists.

5. **Cobalamin (vitamin B$_{12}$)** deficiency usually occurs when gastric mucosal cells fail to produce intrinsic factor necessary for ileal absorption of vitamin B$_{12}$. Symptoms include megaloblastic anemia (**pernicious anemia**), paresthesias and other sensory and motor peripheral neuropathies, gait disturbance, and cognitive disturbances. Delirium may occur and, if the deficiency is inadequately treated, irreversible dementia may supervene.

J. **Metabolic disorders** can cause mental disturbances through systemic metabolic alterations or by direct toxic effects on the CNS.

1. **Genetic metabolic diseases of childhood.** Disorders of lipid, carbohydrate, and protein metabolism can produce progressive mental retardation and other neurologic conditions in childhood. Some childhood disorders can be ameliorated by dietary control.

2. **Wilson disease (hepatolenticular degeneration)** is an autosomal recessive genetic illness characterized by abnormal copper metabolism that results in copper deposition and damage in the liver, renal tubules, and brain structures (e.g., corpus callosum, putamen). Personality changes may become apparent in early adulthood and progress to dementia if untreated. Gait disturbances, incoordination, and chorea also develop. Treatment often includes a copper-restricted diet and administration of chelating agents (e.g., D-penicillamine, zinc).

3. **Acute intermittent porphyria (AIP)** is an autosomal dominant genetic disorder characterized by abnormal heme biosynthesis and excessive accumulation of porphyrins. The disease leads to episodes of abdominal pain, motor neuropathies, and mental disturbances that range from personality changes to psychotic symptoms and delirium. AIP is more common in women and is often first apparent in young adulthood. Episodes are sometimes precipitated by barbiturates, estrogens, and sulfonamides. Treatment is symptomatic, involving analgesic and antipsychotic medications. Two other porphyrias, hereditary coproporphyria and variegated porphyria, have similar psychiatric symptoms.

4. **Hepatic encephalopathy** results from acute or chronic liver failure and presents with delirium accompanied by a characteristic flapping tremor (asterixis). Other symptoms include jaundice, hyperventilation, and EEG abnormalities. Treatment requires a nitrogen-restricted diet.

5. **Uremic encephalopathy** results from acute or chronic renal failure and presents with delirium accompanied by diffuse polyneuropathy, twitching, and hiccups. Untreated uremic encephalopathy may result in irreversible dementia. Treatment involves renal dialysis, which can also produce delirium.

6. **Disorders of glucose metabolism**
   a. **Hypoglycemic encephalopathy** results from the presence of excessive endogenous or exogenous insulin or the unavailability of glucose. Early symptoms include hunger, sweating, tremulousness, and anxiety. When untreated by administration of sugar, symptoms progress to delirium, coma, and seizures. Repeated hypoglycemic episodes can result in irreversible cognitive deficits.
   b. **Diabetic ketoacidosis** results from inadequately treated diabetes mellitus and presents with weakness, polyuria, polydipsia, nausea, vomiting, headache, and fatigue. Delirium may supervene. Dementia may result from repeated episodes.

7. **Fluid and electrolyte disturbances** cause mental disturbances that range from personality change to delirium.

8. **Hypoxia** can result from pulmonary, cardiovascular, and hematologic diseases, and toxins (e.g., carbon monoxide). Acute cognitive changes and delirium can result. Chronic amnestic disorder or dementia can be sequelae.

K. **Endocrine disorders** often cause changes in personality, mood, and cognitive function.

1. **Pituitary disorders.** Pituitary tumors may impair cognitive functions by causing pressure to hypothalamic and temporal lobe structures. Compression of the optic chiasm can cause bitemporal hemianopia. Endocrine disturbances reflect the area of the pituitary that is affected. Postpartum infarction and hemorrhage into the pituitary result in Sheehan syndrome, which is characterized by thyroid and adrenal failure with associated mental disturbances.

2. **Hypothalamic disorders.** Tumors of the hypothalamus may cause appetite and sleep disturbances accompanied by personality changes. Resultant metabolic disturbances from dysregulation of antidiuretic hormone can result in delirium from fluid and electrolyte disturbances.

3. **Thyroid disorders.** Disorders of thyroid metabolism can be caused by genetic lesions; by neoplasms of the thyroid gland, pituitary gland, or hypothalamus; by autoimmune diseases of the thyroid gland; by surgical or radiochemical ablation of the thyroid gland; by exogenous thyroxine; and by iodine deficiencies.
   a. **Hyperthyroid disorders** present with weakness and fatigue, insomnia, weight loss, tremulousness, palpitations, and sweating. Exophthalmos and lid lag are sometimes present. Anxiety and restlessness are early mental symptoms. Cognitive impairment and personality changes may emerge. In severe cases, manic and psychotic symptoms can develop. Cognitive deficits in the absence of anxiety can occur in the elderly. Treatment of the hyperthyroidism results in resolution of the associated mental disturbances.
   b. **Hypothyroid disorders.** Hypothyroidism (myxedema) presents with fatigue, somnolence, weakness, dry skin, brittle hair, cold intolerance, and hoarse speech. Depression and irritability are common. Cognitive slowing may progress to dementia. Occasionally, persecutory delusions and hallucinosis occur. Without timely treatment (i.e., exogenous thyroxine, iodine), residual dementia occurs. Untreated hypothyroidism in childhood results in mental retardation.

4. **Parathyroid disorders.** Disorders of parathyroid metabolism can be caused by genetic lesions, neoplasms of the parathyroid gland and other tissues, and surgical or radiochemical ablation of the parathyroid gland. In addition to parathyroid pathology, abnormal calcium metabolism can also result from diseases with bone lesions, such as Paget disease, multiple myeloma, and metastatic disease.
   a. **Hyperparathyroidism,** with resultant hypercalcemia, can cause muscular weakness, anxiety, and personality changes. Delirium, seizures, and death can occur in parathyroid storm.
   b. **Hypoparathyroidism,** with resultant hypocalcemia, leads to neuromuscular signs and symptoms, including increased excitability, transient paresthesias, cramping, twitching, tetany, and seizures. Delirium may occur even in the absence of tetany.

5. **Abnormalities of adrenal cortical functioning** can be caused by adrenal and pituitary neoplasms, excessive use of exogenous corticosteroids, or sudden cessation of corticosteroid use.

   a. **Adrenocortical hyperactivity (Cushing syndrome)** or excessive levels of exogenous corticosteroids produce a variety of mental disturbances. Restlessness, sleep disturbances, and mood symptoms are common. Mood changes can include agitated depression or manic symptoms. Psychotic symptoms are sometimes seen. Suicide can occur. Treatment of the underlying pathology or gradual taper of exogenous corticosteroids causes resolution of associated mental disturbances.

   b. **Chronic adrenal insufficiency (Addison disease)** produces apathy, fatigability, irritability, and depression. Occasionally, psychotic symptoms or delirium occurs. Treatment with corticosteroids eliminates the mental disturbances.

6. **Pheochromocytoma** is a catecholamine-secreting neoplasm of the adrenal medulla that can produce panic attacks, hypertension, excessive perspiration, palpitations, tremulousness, light-headedness, headaches, and pallor.

L. **Autoimmune disorders** can produce cognitive deficits and personality changes resulting from direct damage to brain tissue, damage to cerebral vasculature, and metabolic disturbances due to damage to other organ systems. Treatment of autoimmune disorders with steroids and other immunosuppressants can also produce mental disturbances.

1. **Systemic lupus erythematosus (SLE)** is characterized by damage to multiple organ systems resulting from deposition of antinuclear antibody–antigen complexes in renal glomeruli and systemic vascular beds. Arthralgias, cutaneous rashes, adenopathy, pericarditis, pleurisy, and renal failure are common manifestations. Mental disturbances are occasionally the initial presentation, and ultimately occur in at least 50% of SLE patients. Mental symptoms commonly involve personality changes. Mood symptoms and psychotic symptoms are sometimes present. Occasionally, delirium and dementia occur. Treatment of SLE with corticosteroids often produces mental disturbances, including psychosis and mood symptoms. The disease is much more common in women.

2. **Vasculitides.** Other autoimmune vasculitides may present with psychiatric symptoms when cerebral vasculature is involved. Such vasculitides may be associated with infection, transplant rejection, or other systemic autoimmune disease. Isolated vasculitis of the CNS sometimes occurs without identified associated illness and presents with headache, focal neurologic deficits, and altered mental status.

DIRECTIONS: Each of the numbered items or incomplete statements in this section is followed by answers or by completions of the statement. Select the ONE lettered answer or completion that is BEST in each case.

1. When examined in the emergency room, a 32-year-old man is noted to have an unsteady gait, a sixth cranial nerve palsy, and spider angiomas. He is confused and agitated. Which one of the following is the best immediate treatment?

(A) Anticoagulants
(B) Haloperidol
(C) Pentobarbital
(D) Salicylates
(E) Thiamine

2. Which one of the following is the most accurate statement about dementia?

(A) Dementia is always the result of substances or general medical conditions
(B) Demented individuals rarely have a depressed mood
(C) Individuals with dementia rarely develop delusions
(D) The ability to plan and carry out complex activities remains unimpaired until dementia is severe
(E) The ability to recall long-term memories is lost before the ability to recall more recent memories

3. A 46-year-old woman has been found unconscious in her garage. Her car was running, and all the doors to the garage were closed. On examination, the woman is confused. Which one of the following is the most likely cause of her confusion?

(A) Dissociative fugue
(B) Gasoline inhalation
(C) Hypoglycemia
(D) Hypoxia
(E) Lead poisoning

4. A 58-year-old man has gradually become more apathetic and moody. At times he is confused and forgetful. His gait is unsteady, and deep-tendon reflexes are diminished. He complains of tingling in his legs. Which one of the following is the most likely diagnosis?

(A) Cerebellar neoplasm
(B) Cobalamin (vitamin B_{12}) deficiency
(C) Hypothyroidism
(D) Manganese intoxication
(E) Multiple sclerosis (MS)

5. A 26-year-old woman presents with a history of episodic anxiety, emotional lability, confusion, and abdominal pain. She takes birth control pills but uses no other substances. Which one of the following is the most likely diagnosis?

(A) Absence (petit mal) seizures
(B) Acute intermittent porphyria (AIP)
(C) Exposure to organophosphates
(D) Premenstrual syndrome
(E) Wilson disease (hepatolenticular degeneration)

6. A 29-year-old man presents with a history of three distinct episodes of emotional lability. During the first episode, he experienced a right visual field deficit. During another episode, he experienced mild ataxia. Which one of the following is the most likely diagnosis?

(A) Cobalamin (vitamin B_{12}) deficiency
(B) Herpes encephalitis
(C) Multiple sclerosis (MS)
(D) Neurosyphilis
(E) Systemic lupus erythematosus (SLE)

7. Which one of the following is the most common cause of dementia?

(A) Alzheimer disease
(B) Cerebrovascular disease
(C) Head trauma
(D) Human immunodeficiency virus (HIV)
(E) Thiamine deficiency

8. A 23-year-old woman without a history of alcohol abuse reports that she has been troubled by morning episodes of tremulousness, anxiety, tachycardia, and sweating. Which one of the following test results is most likely to be abnormal?

(A) Serum ammonia measurement
(B) Serum glucose measurement
(C) Serum sodium measurement
(D) Thyroid function test
(E) Toxicologic screen

9. A 28-year-old woman presents with complaints of irritability and moodiness. She gives a history of brief episodes of auditory hallucinosis and suspiciousness. Her speech is slightly slurred. Which one of the following is the most likely diagnosis?

(A) Folate deficiency
(B) Hyperparathyroidism
(C) Pick disease
(D) Sydenham chorea
(E) Wilson disease

DIRECTIONS: Each set of matching questions in this section consists of a list of four to twenty-six lettered options (some of which may be in figures) followed by several items. For each numbered item, select the ONE lettered option that is most closely associated with it. To avoid spending too much time on matching sets with large numbers of options, it is generally advisable to begin each set by reading the list of options. Then, for each item in the set, try to generate the correct answer and locate it in the option list, rather than evaluating each option individually. Each lettered option may be selected once, more than once, or not at all.

Questions 10–13

For each of the following symptoms, select the most commonly associated neoplasm.

(A) Frontal lobe neoplasm
(B) Parietal lobe neoplasm
(C) Pituitary neoplasm
(D) Occipital lobe neoplasm
(E) Temporal lobe neoplasm

10. Trance-like states

11. Apathy

12. Uninhibited behavior

13. Visual hallucinations

Questions 14–17

For each of the following conditions, select the associated symptom.

(A) Anxiety attacks
(B) Depressive episodes
(C) Insidious personality changes
(D) Psychotic symptoms
(E) Reduced clarity of awareness

14. Pheochromocytoma

15. Adrenocortical hyperactivity (Cushing syndrome)

16. Pick disease

17. Delirium due to hyponatremia

1. The answer is E *[IV I 2 b]*. This case is most suggestive of Wernicke encephalopathy, which is a delirium characterized by gait disturbance, oculomotor abnormalities, and cognitive impairment. This delirium is due to acute thiamine deficiency, usually resulting from alcohol abuse. Treatment involves rapid administration of thiamine.

2. The answer is A *[II B]*. By definition, dementia is the result of physiologic disturbances. Dementia is classified as due to a general medical condition, substance-induced, or due to multiple causes.

3. The answer is D *[IV J 8]*. The circumstances of this case strongly suggest that the woman has been exposed to levels of carbon monoxide that would be sufficient to interfere with the oxygen-carrying capacity of her hemoglobin and result in cerebral anoxia and delirium. The other choices can cause cognitive disturbances, but are less likely causes in this case.

4. The answer is B *[IV I 5]*. The evidence of gradual cognitive, motor, and sensory impairments is most suggestive of cobalamin deficiency. Megaloblastic anemia is likely to be present. Multiple sclerosis (MS) might also cause such impairments, but the course would most likely be stuttering.

5. The answer is B *[IV J 3]*. The history is characterized by episodes of cognitive impairment, personality changes, mood disturbance, and abdominal pain. The episodes started when the patient began using estrogen. This history is most suggestive of acute intermittent porphyria (AIP), a disorder of heme synthesis that includes wine-colored urine. It is most common in women; often, it is first evident in the third decade of life and can be precipitated by estrogens and barbiturates.

6. The answer is C *[IV E 2]*. The patient has experienced relapsing and remitting symptoms involving a variety of central nervous system (CNS) sites, a course that is characteristic of multiple sclerosis (MS). The visual deficit is suggestive of optic nerve involvement, which is often an early symptom of this illness and is uncommon in any of the other choices. The peak incidence of MS is approximately age 30.

7. The answer is A *[IV B 1 d]*. Alzheimer disease causes 55% of cases of dementia. Vascular disease is the second most common cause (approximately 20%). Cerebrovascular disease, head trauma, human immunodeficiency virus (HIV), and thiamine deficiency cause dementia less frequently.

8. The answer is B *[IV J 6 a]*. The patient describes an episodic disturbance that occurs in the morning. This episode is most suggestive of hypoglycemia, which most often occurs after nighttime fasting or after vigorous exercise. Symptoms are strongly reminiscent of anxiety attacks. Hyperthyroidism might also present with anxiety and tremulousness, but it would not be limited to the morning.

9. The answer is E *[IV J 2]*. Wilson disease (hepatolenticular degeneration) usually becomes symptomatic in the second or third decade of life. The initial signs often include personality and mood changes. Transient episodes of psychosis may occur. The disease process involves the putamen and the corpus callosum, resulting in movement or muscular signs, such as the dysarthria manifested here.

10–13. The answers are: 10-E, 11-A, 12-A, 13-D *[IV G 2, 3]*. Temporal lobe neoplasms are most commonly associated with trance-like states and disturbances of complex behavior. Mood symptoms can be prominent. Frontal lobe neoplasms are most associated with insidious personality changes. These changes can include apathy or loss of inhibitions. Occipital lobe neoplasms are most often associated with visual symptoms, which can include misperceptions and hallucinations.

14–17. The answers are: 14-A *[IV K 6]*, **15-B** *[IV K 5 a]*, **16-C** *[IV B 4]*, **17-E** *[II A 1 a]*. Pheochromocytoma is a catecholamine-secreting neoplasm of the adrenal medulla, which can produce attacks of severe anxiety as well as hypertension and headaches. Adrenocortical hyperactivity produces excessive levels of corticosteroids that lead to restlessness, sleep disturbances, and mood symptoms. Psychotic symptoms occasionally occur, but are less likely. Pick disease is a neurodegenerative condition that results in personality disturbances and supervening dementia. Delirium due to hyponatremia or any other cause is distinguished by a reduced clarity of consciousness.

Chapter 6

Substance-Related Disorders
Steven L. Dubovsky

I. | **INTRODUCTION.** The *Diagnostic and Statistical Manual of Mental Disorders,* 4th edition (DSM-IV) recognizes two broad categories of disorders related to the use of psychoactive substances. Substance-use disorders are syndromes of pathologic use of a substance; substance-induced disorders are disturbances of thinking, emotion, or behavior caused by intoxication with or withdrawal from a psychoactive substance.

A. | **Substance use disorders** are subdivided into substance dependence and substance abuse.

1. **Substance dependence** is defined as a pathologic pattern of substance use that results in impairment or distress. Substance dependence is diagnosed when three or more of the following consequences of substance use occur together at any time in the same year:
   a. **Tolerance,** which is defined as:
      (1) A requirement for increased amounts of the substance to achieve the same effect, or
      (2) Decreased effect with continued use of the same amount of the substance
   b. **Withdrawal,** which is defined as:
      (1) Typical withdrawal syndrome for the substance (see I B), or
      (2) The substance or a related compound is taken to relieve or avoid withdrawal symptoms
   c. Use of the substance in greater amounts or for a longer time than was originally intended
   d. Unsuccessful attempts or wishes to cut down on or control substance use
   e. Significant amounts of time spent in activities necessary to obtain or use the substance or recover from its effects
   f. Giving up important social, occupational, or recreational activities because of substance use
   g. Continued use of the substance despite knowledge that it is causing or aggravating physical or mental problems

2. **Physiologic dependence** is defined in DSM-IV as the presence of either tolerance or withdrawal (I A 1 a, b).

3. **Substance abuse** in DSM-IV is a maladaptive pattern of abuse with fewer and different consequences than substance dependence. Substance abuse is diagnosed if one of the following four problems has occurred over a 12-month period, and if the patient does not meet criteria for substance dependence:
   a. Failure to fulfill major role obligations
   b. Recurrent use of a substance in situations in which it is hazardous (e.g., while driving)
   c. Recurrent legal problems resulting from substance use
   d. Continued use of a substance despite social or interpersonal problems caused by the substance (e.g., arguments with a spouse about substance use, getting into fights)

B. | **Substance-induced disorders** comprise a diverse group of physical and mental syndromes caused by psychoactive substances or their withdrawal:

1. **Substance intoxication** is a reversible, substance-specific syndrome (see II).

2. **Substance withdrawal** is a substance-specific syndrome that appears when a substance is withdrawn.

3. **Substance-induced delirium** is caused by taking a psychoactive substance. Of the substances in DSM-IV considered to be psychoactive, only nicotine is not thought to cause delirium.

4. **Substance-withdrawal delirium** is caused by withdrawal of alcohol, sedatives, hypnotics, anxiolytics, and some other substances.

5. **Substance-induced persisting dementia,** which is caused by intoxication with or withdrawal from substances (e.g., alcohol, inhalants, sedatives), is characterized by memory impairment plus one or more of four cognitive dysfunctions. These dysfunctions include aphasia, apraxia, agnosia, and disrupted executive function. The symptoms persist after intoxication or withdrawal has cleared.

6. **Substance-induced, persisting amnestic disorder** consists of impairment of recall of previously learned material or of the ability to learn new information. It is associated with the use of alcohol, sedatives, hypnotics, anxiolytics, and some other substances. The disorder persists after intoxication or withdrawal has resolved.

7. **Substance-induced psychotic disorder** is characterized by prominent hallucinations or delusions caused by substances such as alcohol, amphetamines, cannabis, cocaine, hallucinogens, inhalants, opioids, phencyclidine, and sedatives. According to the DSM-IV, the diagnosis cannot be based on hallucinations if the patient realizes that they are caused by the substance. If transient psychotic symptoms are associated only with delirium due to substance intoxication or withdrawal, the diagnosis is substance-induced delirium or substance-induced withdrawal delirium.

8. **Substance-induced mood disorder** refers to depressed or manic mood that either is clearly caused by substances such as alcohol, amphetamines, cocaine, hallucinogens, inhalants, opioids, phencyclidine, sedatives, and anxiolytics, or develops within a month of using these substances.

9. **Substance-induced anxiety disorder,** which is discussed in Chapter 4, consists of anxiety, panic attacks, obsessions, or compulsions that either are clearly caused by a substance or develop within a month of substance use or withdrawal.

10. **Substance-induced sexual dysfunction** either develops within 1 month of substance intoxication or is clearly caused by substances such as alcohol, amphetamines, cocaine, opioids, and a number of medications (e.g., reserpine, serotonin reuptake inhibitors).

11. **Substance-induced sleep disorder** either is obviously caused by a psychoactive substance or appears within 1 month of substance use or withdrawal. Typical offending agents include alcohol, amphetamines, caffeine, cocaine, opioids, sedatives, hypnotics, and anxiolytics.

12. **Hallucinogen-persisting perception disorder (flashbacks)** refers to the reexperiencing of perceptual symptoms that were caused by intoxication with a hallucinogen, but occur after the drug is no longer being taken.

C. **Addiction** is a term used by some clinicians to refer to overwhelming involvement with seeking and using drugs or alcohol and a high tendency to relapse after substance withdrawal. It is, therefore, a quantitative description of the degree to which drug use pervades an individual's life. Addiction may be described as a form of substance dependence as defined in I A.

1. It is possible for an individual to develop tolerance and undergo withdrawal without being addicted; that is, the individual's life is not organized around finding and using the drug. This is common in patients who become physically dependent on narcotics, tranquilizers, or sedatives during treatment of prolonged illness or insomnia but who do not experience intrusion of drug use into many aspects of their lives.

2. It may be possible to be addicted, in the sense that drug-seeking behavior is paramount in an individual's life, without being physically dependent.

D. **Substances subject to dependence and abuse.** DSM-IV categorizes substance-related disorders according to which 1 of 13 types of substances is used. All of these substances are felt to be associated with dependence and abuse, except caffeine (which in the DSM-IV is said to produce neither syndrome but has recently been shown to produce physical dependence) and nicotine (which causes dependence only). Any of these substances may produce the other syndromes listed in I B. The specific substance categories include:

1. Alcohol
2. Amphetamines
3. Caffeine
4. Cannabis
5. Cocaine
6. Hallucinogens
7. Inhalants
8. Nicotine
9. Opioids
10. Phencyclidine
11. Sedatives, hypnotics, and anxiolytics
12. Polysubstance
13. Other (e.g., digitalis, amyl nitrite)

II. **INTOXICATION SYNDROMES.** Because the manifestations and treatment of intoxication with different drugs vary drastically, it is crucial to be able to differentiate common intoxication syndromes.

A. **Alcohol** is frequently combined with other substances. The odor on the patient's breath that is characteristically associated with alcohol intoxication is caused by impurities in the preparation and is unreliable in diagnosing intoxication. In addition, head injuries and metabolic encephalopathies (e.g., ketoacidosis) are frequently mistaken for alcohol intoxication. Blood and urine screens may help to make the diagnosis. Central nervous system (CNS) concentration of alcohol parallels the concentration in the blood.

1. **Alcohol intoxication** is diagnosed in DSM-IV when the following signs appear in association with drinking:
   a. Slurred speech
   b. Loss of coordination
   c. Unsteady gait
   d. Nystagmus
   e. Impaired attention or memory
   f. Stupor or coma

2. **Mild intoxication** is characterized by disorganization of cognitive and motor processes. The first functions to be disrupted are those that depend on training and previous experience. As intoxication becomes more noticeable, the following changes occur:
   a. **Overconfidence.** If performance is initially impaired by psychological inhibitions, an individual may transiently function better after ingestion of small amounts of alcohol. However, although the intoxicated individual tends to feel more efficient, all aspects of physical and mental performance are decreased by alcohol.

      b. **Mood swings, emotional outbursts,** and **euphoria** may occur.

      c. **Initial enhancement of spinal reflexes** may develop as they are released from higher inhibiting circuits, followed by progressive general anesthesia of CNS functions.

      d. **An increased pain threshold** may be evident, whereas other sensory modalities are unaffected.

      e. **Nausea, vomiting, restlessness,** and **hyperactivity** may be present.

3. **Severe intoxication** is characterized by:

      a. Stupor or coma

      b. Hypothermia

      c. Slow, noisy respiration

      d. Tachycardia

      e. Dilated pupils (may be normal in some intoxicated individuals)

      f. Increased intracranial pressure

      g. Death (rare in the absence of ingestion of additional substances, trauma, infection, or unconsciousness lasting longer than 12 hours)

4. **Treatment** depends on whether or not the patient is conscious.

      a. **The conscious patient** needs little treatment except waiting for the alcohol to be metabolized.

        (1) Stimulants and caffeine do not hasten sobriety.

        (2) Restraint for severe agitation is safer than administration of tranquilizers or sedatives, which may potentiate the CNS depressant effects of alcohol.

        (3) In low doses, high-potency antipsychotic drugs (e.g., haloperidol) may decrease hyperactivity without increasing sedation.

      b. **The stuporous or unconscious patient** should be kept warm. It may also be necessary to:

        (1) Prevent aspiration, especially if gastric lavage is performed

        (2) Treat increased intracranial pressure with mannitol or by other measures (e.g., corticosteroids), in addition to the normal management of overdoses of CNS depressants

        (3) Remove alcohol by hemodialysis in extreme situations

B. **Sedatives, hypnotics, and anxiolytics**

1. **Specific substances**

      a. Benzodiazepine tranquilizers (e.g., diazepam, oxazepam, chlordiazepoxide, lorazepam, prazepam, chlorazepate, alprazolam, clonazepam)

      b. Benzodiazepine hypnotics or sleeping pills (e.g., flurazepam, temazepam, triazolam, estazolam)

      c. Barbiturates (e.g., phenobarbital, amobarbital, pentobarbital, and secobarbital)

      d. Drugs related to barbiturates [e.g., ethchlorvynol, glutethimide, propanediols (e.g., meprobamate), methyprylon, and paraldehyde]

      e. Chloral compounds (e.g., chloral hydrate)

2. **Mild-to-moderate intoxication** with benzodiazepines, barbiturates, and related compounds causes:

      a. Euphoria

      b. Hypalgesia (increased pain threshold)

      c. Increased seizure threshold

      d. Sedation

      e. Paradoxical excitement in:

        (1) Susceptible individuals

        (2) The elderly

        (3) Children

        (4) The presence of organic brain disease

      f. Nystagmus, dysarthria, ataxia, impaired attention and memory

      g. Psychomotor impairment

      h. Postural hypotension

3. **Severe intoxication** is usually due to purposeful overdoses in suicide attempts and accidental overdoses by addicts. A few patients, especially those with preexisting brain disease, may take too much medication because of drug automatism or continuing to ingest the drug in an altered state of consciousness. That is, the patient forgets that the drug has already been taken and continues to take more pills, usually in an effort to get to sleep. Severe intoxication can cause:
   a. Stupor and coma
   b. Respiratory depression
   c. Depressed reflexes
   d. Hypotension
   e. Decreased cardiac output
   f. Hypoxemia
   g. Bullous skin lesions and necrosis of sweat glands
   h. Hypothermia
   i. Coma
   j. Death
      (1) Death from barbiturate intoxication is usually caused by pneumonia or renal failure.
      (2) Short-acting preparations (e.g., amobarbital) are more lethal at lower doses than are long-acting compounds (e.g., phenobarbital).
      (3) Death from an overdose of benzodiazepines alone is rare.

4. **Treatment** of CNS depressant intoxication involves emesis if the ingestion has occurred within 1 half hour of initiation of treatment and the gag reflex is intact. Gastric lavage should be performed if these conditions have not been fulfilled. A cathartic agent should then be given to decrease intestinal absorption of the drug. For severe poisoning, the following steps are taken:
   a. Protection of the airway
   b. Oxygen administration
   c. Ventilation when necessary
   d. Prevention of further loss of body heat
   e. Correction of hypovolemia and maintenance of blood pressure with dopamine
   f. Forced diuresis with maximal alkalinization of the urine
   g. Hemodialysis

C. CNS stimulants

1. **Specific substances**
   a. **Amphetamines** and related compounds include dextroamphetamine, methylphenidate, and pemoline sodium. Medical indications for amphetamines include:
      (1) Attention deficit disorder in children
      (2) Depression in the elderly
      (3) Depression in medically ill patients who cannot tolerate antidepressants
      (4) Augmentation of antidepressants in treatment-resistant depression
      (5) Adult (residual) attention deficit disorder
      (6) Narcolepsy
   b. **Cocaine** is used to treat nosebleeds and is sometimes used as a local anesthetic in the ears, nose, and throat.
   c. **Phenmetrazine**
   d. **Phenylpropanolamine**
   e. **Antiobesity drugs.** Long-term treatment of obesity with stimulants is almost always unsuccessful because of tolerance.
   f. **Methamphetamine** (methedrine) is a synthetic amphetamine used only illicitly.

2. **Mild-to-moderate intoxication** produces:
   a. Elevated mood
   b. Increased energy and alertness

    c. Increased ability to perform repetitive tasks when the individual is tired or bored
    d. Decreased appetite
    e. Talkativeness
    f. Anxiety and irritability
    g. Insomnia
    h. Hypertension or hypotension
    i. Increased or decreased heart rate
    j. Hyperthermia
    k. Nausea or vomiting
    l. Loss of appetite and weight

3. Severe intoxication may produce a toxic psychosis. Although tolerance develops to many of the effects of stimulants, there is no tolerance to the tendency to develop psychotic symptoms, which may be indistinguishable from those of schizophrenia. **Signs and symptoms** include:
    a. Visual, auditory, and tactile hallucinations
    b. Delusions, especially of being infested with parasites
    c. Paranoia and loose associations in a clear sensorium
    d. Mania
    e. Fighting
    f. Hypervigilance
    g. Dilated pupils
    h. Elevated blood pressure and pulse (may be normal in some chronic abusers)
    i. Arrhythmias
    j. Seizures
    k. Exhaustion
    l. Coma
    m. Intracranial hemorrhage

4. Treatment
    a. Hypertension and hyperthermia can be treated with **phentolamine**.
    b. Psychotic symptoms can be treated by **haloperidol,** which antagonizes the dopaminergic properties of stimulants.

D. **Hallucinogens and phencyclidine**

1. Specific substances
    a. Lysergic acid diethylamide (LSD)
    b. Psilocybin
    c. Mescaline
    d. 2,5-Dimethoxy-4-methylamphetamine (STP)
    e. Phencyclidine (PCP)

2. Intoxication depends on the substance.
    a. Most hallucinogen intoxications produce:
        (1) Dilated pupils
        (2) Increased heart rate and blood pressure
        (3) Increased temperature
        (4) Paranoia in a clear sensorium
        (5) Illusions
        (6) Hallucinations
        (7) Depersonalization
        (8) Anxiety
        (9) Distortion of time sense
      (10) Inappropriate affect
    b. PCP intoxication can also cause:
        (1) Violent behavior
        (2) Hyperactivity
        (3) Hyperacusis

        (4) Mutism
        (5) Echolalia
        (6) Analgesia
        (7) Nystagmus
        (8) Ataxia
        (9) Muscular rigidity
      (10) Seizures
      (11) Coma
      (12) Intracranial hemorrhage

  3. Treatment of intoxication and "bad trips" depends on the substance.

    a. The psychological effects of most hallucinogens are usually decreased by reassurance in a quiet setting. Oral administration of diazepam is sometimes a useful adjunct.

    b. Patients intoxicated with PCP may react violently to any environmental stimulation, including attempts at reassurance. They generally should be left alone in a quiet area. If they become violent, they may be sedated with intravenously administered haloperidol or diazepam. Seizures should be treated with intravenous administration of diazepam.

E. **Cannabis.** Specific substances include marijuana, hashish, and Δ-tetrahydrocannabinol (TCH).

  1. Intoxication by marijuana and related substances rarely produces hallucinations. More common effects include:

    a. Euphoria
    b. Anxiety
    c. Increased appetite
    d. Increased suggestibility
    e. Distortion of time and space
    f. Red conjunctivae
    g. No change in pupils
    h. Dry mouth
    i. Tachycardia

  2. Treatment. The psychological effects of the cannabis group of drugs, like those of most hallucinogens, are generally eased by reassurance in a quiet setting. Oral administration of diazepam is sometimes useful.

F. **Opioids.** Many street preparations are adulterated with quinine, procaine, lidocaine, lactose, or mannitol and are contaminated with bacteria, viruses, or fungi.

  1. Specific substances

    a. Morphine
    b. Heroin
    c. Hydromorphone
    d. Oxymorphone
    e. Levorphanol
    f. Codeine
    g. Hydrocodone
    h. Oxycodone
    i. Methadone
    j. Meperidine
    k. Alphaprodine
    l. Propoxyphene
    m. Pentazocine, which has both narcotic antagonist and agonist properties

  2. Mild-to-moderate intoxication may produce:

    a. Analgesia without loss of consciousness
    b. Drowsiness and mental clouding
    c. Nausea and vomiting
    d. Apathy and lethargy
    e. Euphoria

    f. Itching
    g. Constricted pupils
    h. Constipation
    i. Flushed, warm skin due to cutaneous vasodilation
    j. Dysarthria
    k. Impaired attention and memory
    l. Illusions

  3. Severe intoxication is associated with:
    a. Miosis
    b. Respiratory depression, which may recur up to 24 hours after apparent recovery from an overdose with most narcotics and up to 72 hours after apparent recovery from a methadone overdose
    c. Hypotension or shock
    d. Depressed reflexes
    e. Coma
    f. Pulmonary edema
    g. Seizures (with propoxyphene or meperidine)

  4. Treatment
    a. Severe intoxication is primarily treated by **supportive care**.
    b. Naloxone, a narcotic antagonist, can:
      (1) Reverse coma and apnea [The effects of concomitantly self-administered drugs (e.g., barbiturates) are not altered, and detoxification from these drugs should also be undertaken.]
      (2) Precipitate a severe abstinence syndrome in narcotic-dependent patients
      (3) Cause vomiting

G.   **Inhalants.** The act of sniffing ("huffing") inhalants is becoming an increasingly severe problem among children and adolescents. Because brain damage may occur with repeated use, and no antidote or specific treatment of intoxication exists, it is important to identify the problem and institute remedial therapy.

  1. Specific substances
    a. Gasoline
    b. Glue
    c. Paint thinner
    d. Solvents

  2. Intoxication may cause:
    a. Dizziness
    b. Euphoria
    c. Altered states of consciousness
    d. Confusion
    e. Nystagmus
    f. Ataxia
    g. Dysarthria
    h. Lethargy
    i. Depressed reflexes
    j. Psychomotor retardation
    k. Tremor
    l. Muscular weakness
    m. Blurred vision
    n. Delirium

  3. Chronic use may result in dementia.

  4. There is no specific treatment for inhalant dependence and abuse other than to prevent further access to the substance.

H. **Anticholinergic drugs.** A number of psychiatric medications have anticholinergic side effects. Some anticholinergic substances grow wild, and some are included in various herbal medications.

  1. **Specific substances**
     a. Most over-the-counter cold and sleeping preparations
     b. Atropine
     c. Belladonna
     d. Henbane
     e. Scopolamine
     f. Antiparkinsonian drugs (e.g., trihexyphenidyl, benztropine)
     g. Tricyclic and tetracyclic antidepressants and paroxetine
     h. Low-potency neuroleptics (e.g., thioridazine)
     i. Jimson weed
     j. Mandrake
     k. Propantheline

  2. **Intoxication** with anticholinergic substances is coded as "other intoxication" in DSM-IV and may produce:
     a. Confusion
     b. Memory loss
     c. Delirium
     d. Hallucinations
     e. Amnesia
     f. Body image distortions
     g. Drowsiness
     h. Tachycardia
     i. Decreased peristalsis
     j. Fever
     k. Warm, dry skin
     l. Fixed, dilated pupils
     m. Coma

  3. **Treatment** is primarily directed toward protecting the patient and waiting for the drug to be metabolized. Intravenous administration of physostigmine can temporarily reverse coma or severe hyperpyrexia but should be used cautiously. Relief is transient due to the short half-life of the drug, whereas gastrointestinal and cardiac side effects may be significant.

III. **SUBSTANCE WITHDRAWAL** produces substance-specific, physiologically determined syndromes that appear after abrupt withdrawal or decrease in dosage of the drug. Withdrawal from some compounds produces mild syndromes. Withdrawal from others produces phenomena that are uncomfortable but not dangerous. Life-threatening abstinence syndromes result from a few substances. Blood levels are often zero in abstinence syndromes.

A. **Alcohol abstinence syndromes**

  1. **Alcohol withdrawal ("the shakes")** usually appears within a few hours of stopping or decreasing alcohol consumption. Generally, this lasts for 3 to 4 days and occasionally lasts as long as 1 week.
     a. **Signs and symptoms** include:
        (1) Tachycardia
        (2) Tremulousness
        (3) Diaphoresis
        (4) Nausea
        (5) Orthostatic hypotension

(6) Malaise or weakness

(7) Anxiety

(8) Irritability

b. Treatment

  (1) The standard practice has been to administer a benzodiazepine, most frequently chlordiazepoxide or clorazepate, in a tapering dose over 2 to 3 days.

  (2) Recent research demonstrates that administering individual doses of chlordiazepoxide only if autonomic signs are present prevents complications of withdrawal (e.g., seizures and delirium tremens) as effectively as regular dosing.

  (3) Thiamine is usually administered parenterally at 100 mg/day for 3 days.

2. Major motor seizures ("rum fits")

  a. Symptoms. Major motor seizures occur during the first 48 hours of alcohol withdrawal in a small percentage of patients.

  b. Treatment is by means of intravenous administration of diazepam. Phenytoin is not administered unless the patient has epilepsy.

3. Alcohol withdrawal delirium (delirium tremens) begins on the second or third day (rarely later than 1 week) after withdrawal or decrease of alcohol intake. It occurs in fewer than 5% of alcohol-dependent patients, usually after they have been drinking heavily for 5 to 15 years. If seizures also occur, they always precede the development of delirium. With appropriate treatment, mortality is rare.

  a. Symptoms of delirium tremens include:

    (1) Delirium

    (2) Autonomic hyperactivity (e.g., increased pulse rate, blood pressure, and sweating)

    (3) Agitation

    (4) Vivid hallucinations

    (5) Gross tremulousness

  b. Treatment

    (1) Hydration

    (2) Parenteral administration of thiamine for 3 to 4 days

    (3) A benzodiazepine (e.g., chlordiazepoxide) administered in a divided dose (i.e., 200–400 mg/day)

    (4) A neuroleptic, such as haloperidol, in severe cases of agitation or psychosis

    (5) Electroconvulsive therapy, which has been found to lessen the effects of severe withdrawal syndromes from alcohol and other substances

4. Alcohol hallucinosis (alcohol-induced psychotic disorder with hallucinations in DSM-IV) is a rare condition that develops within 48 hours of cessation of drinking or at the end of a long binge with gradual decreases in blood alcohol levels.

  a. The principal symptom is vivid auditory hallucinations without gross confusion. Usually, the patient hears threatening or derogatory voices that discuss the patient in the third person or speak directly to the patient. Command hallucinations are absent. Symptoms usually last a few hours or days but persist for weeks or months in approximately 10% of patients. Occasionally, the syndrome may become chronic, in which case it may be indistinguishable from schizophrenia.

  b. Treatment. Neuroleptics may relieve hallucinations in patients who do not improve spontaneously.

B. **Withdrawal from sedatives, hypnotics, and anxiolytics** produces syndromes that vary in time of onset, duration, and severity. Withdrawal syndromes are likely to occur after chronic use of 400–600 mg/day of pentobarbital, 3200–6400 mg/day of meprobamate, and 40–60 mg/day of diazepam or their equivalents. Milder withdrawal syndromes may develop in individuals taking lower doses for longer periods of time. It is difficult to predict if an individual will develop a withdrawal syndrome and how severe it may be.

1. Symptoms usually begin within 12 to 24 hours, peak at 4 to 7 days, and last about 1 week after withdrawal from short-acting compounds like pentobarbital or alprazolam. Withdrawal from long-acting compounds such as diazepam or phenobarbital begins later (4 to 10 days after drug discontinuation) and reaches its peak more slowly (around the seventh day). Signs and symptoms include:

  a. Anxiety and agitation
  b. Orthostatic hypotension
  c. Weakness and tremulousness
  d. Hyperreflexia and clonic blink reflex
  e. Fever
  f. Diaphoresis
  g. Delirium
  h. Seizures
  i. Cardiovascular collapse

2. **Treatment.** Withdrawal from CNS depressants can be life-threatening, and treatment is mandatory when the syndrome is diagnosed. Whereas some patients with uncomplicated withdrawal may be managed as outpatients, hospitalization is required for the management of more severe and complicated withdrawal to ensure compliance with the treatment protocol and adequate coverage if the condition worsens. Treatment is not as effective if it is initiated after the appearance of delirium.

  a. Because all CNS depressants produce cross-tolerance, a known compound (pentobarbital or phenobarbital) is substituted for the offending substance and is gradually withdrawn to suppress the abstinence syndrome. The amount of phenobarbital or pentobarbital to which the patient is likely to be tolerant, and that therefore will suppress withdrawal, can be calculated by administering 200 mg of pentobarbital or 60 to 100 mg of phenobarbital when the patient no longer appears to be intoxicated (usually within 12 to 16 hours after discontinuation of the offending substance).

    (1) If the patient becomes severely intoxicated or falls asleep with the test dose, he is not tolerant and does not need further treatment.
    (2) If the patient develops moderate symptoms after the test dose (e.g., dysarthria, nystagmus, ataxia without sleepiness), she is moderately tolerant and requires 200 to 300 mg of pentobarbital or 60 to 90 mg of phenobarbital per day.
    (3) Absence of symptoms or nystagmus without other signs of intoxication in response to the test dose indicates significant tolerance. The patient should then be administered a total daily (divided) dose of 600 to 1000 mg of pentobarbital or 180 to 300 mg of phenobarbital every 6 hours to suppress withdrawal.
    (4) Tolerance may also be tested by giving successive 60- to 100-mg doses of phenobarbital every 1 to 4 hours until the patient is intoxicated. The amount necessary to produce definite signs of intoxication, or a maximum of 500 mg/day, is then administered in divided dose every 6 hours to suppress the abstinence syndrome.

  b. Once the patient is stabilized, the dose of pentobarbital is decreased by 10% every 1 to 2 days. Phenobarbital, which is longer acting, may be withdrawn more rapidly. Reappearance of abstinence phenomena indicates that the dose needs to be reduced more gradually. Unexpected intoxication during the phenobarbital protocol indicates accumulation of the barbiturate and a need for faster dosage reduction.

  c. Because cross-tolerance exists between barbiturates and alcohol, phenobarbital or pentobarbital can also be used to suppress alcohol abstinence syndromes, as well as withdrawal from more than one CNS depressant.

C. **Stimulant withdrawal.** There is no observable physiologic disruption; however, psychological and behavioral manifestations may be severe.

1. **Symptoms**
  a. Increased sleep
  b. Nightmares due to rapid eye movement (REM) rebound
  c. Fatigue
  d. Lassitude
  e. Increased appetite
  f. Depression ("cocaine blues")

       g. Suicide attempts
       h. Craving for the drug

    2. Treatment
       a. Antidepressants like bupropion or desipramine are helpful for withdrawal depression.
       b. Hospitalization may be necessary if the patient is suicidal.

D. **Cessation of hallucinogens** does not produce a significant abstinence syndrome.

    1. Symptoms. Flashbacks (brief reexperiences of the hallucinogenic state) may be precipitated by marijuana or antihistamine intake. Serotonin reuptake inhibitors have also been noted to induce flashbacks.

    2. Treatment. Reassurance that symptoms will subside and administration of a benzodiazepine are usually sufficient therapy.

E. **Opioid withdrawal** is not life-threatening; however, it may be extremely uncomfortable.

    1. Symptoms usually appear 8 to 10 hours after cessation of morphine. The onset is slower when long-acting drugs, such as methadone, have been withdrawn. Symptoms peak at 48 to 72 hours and disappear in 7 to 10 days. Disturbances include:
       a. Lacrimation and rhinorrhea
       b. Sweating
       c. Restlessness and sleepiness
       d. Gooseflesh
       e. Dilated pupils
       f. Irritability
       g. Violent yawning
       h. Insomnia
       i. Coryza
       j. Craving for the drug

    2. Treatment
       a. The effects of narcotic withdrawal are lessened by **methadone** substitution. When the patient demonstrates objective signs of withdrawal, a sufficient dose of methadone to suppress abstinence, or a maximum dose of 20–50 mg/day (never more than 100 mg) is administered. The dose of methadone is then decreased by 10%–20% per day.
       b. Clonidine, administered at 0.1–0.3 mg three times per day for 2 weeks may help to suppress withdrawal symptoms, although it can cause hypotension. Clonidine should be tapered rather than abruptly discontinued.
       c. Although any licensed physician may prescribe methadone for pain, the use of methadone to detoxify a narcotics addict (as well as methadone maintenance to prevent relapse of addiction) violates federal law in any setting other than a site approved for the treatment of narcotic addiction.

F. **Anticholinergic drug withdrawal** occasionally produces influenza-like syndromes, depression, mania, or seizures. Discontinuation of clinically significant doses taken for more than 1 month should, therefore, be gradual. Treatment is with **atropine** or reintroduction of the offending agent with more gradual discontinuation.

G. **Nicotine withdrawal** has been found to be a significant impediment to smoking cessation. Symptoms include malaise, irritability, anxiety, and craving for tobacco. Treatment with nicotine patches containing declining doses of nicotine is effective only when it is combined with a behavioral program. Clonidine administered as described in III E 2 b or by means of a patch may be a useful adjunct.

H. **Caffeine withdrawal** produces insomnia, depression, and headaches. Gradual reduction of intake may prevent withdrawal symptoms.

IV. PRINCIPLES OF TREATMENT OF SUBSTANCE-RELATED DISORDERS.
Certain approaches are useful for treatment of abuse and dependence with all substances.

A. **Detoxification.** It is impossible to address the causes of substance abuse and dependence while the patient continues to use the substance. The first goal of treatment, therefore, is to withdraw the substance.

B. **Insistence on abstinence.** There may be a few individuals who can use addicting substances in moderation after successful treatment of dependence or abuse, but it is impossible to identify them. Complete abstinence is safest.

C. **Avoidance of other substances associated with dependence or abuse.** Not infrequently, people who have been dependent on alcohol or another substance ask to be treated with benzodiazepines or related compounds for anxiety or insomnia. Acceding to this request is dangerous for several reasons:

1. It introduces another substance that can be associated with dependence.

2. Taking a pill for rapid relief of dysphoria reinforces the association between drug taking and feeling better, thereby increasing the tendency to go back to the drug of choice for the same result.

3. There is no evidence that tranquilizers decrease the use of alcohol as a self-treatment for anxiety, and some reports suggest that using benzodiazepines increases the risk of relapse of alcoholism.

D. **Involvement of the family.** Family members may encourage use of the substance in the patient, especially if there is family strife that everyone is able to ignore because all attention is focused on the identified patient. For example, a family may ignore or overlook sexual abuse of one child by focusing attention on another child's problem with drugs or alcohol. A spouse may also be drug dependent. The family can be important allies in insisting that the patient deal with the problem.

E. **Toxicology screens.** Despite technical problems that may reduce reliability, periodic urine screens are often essential in identifying relapse and noncompliance.

F. **Self-help groups.** Peer support groups provide credibility and encouragement from individuals who have had similar problems and who are adept at dealing with common resistances to treatment. Twelve-step programs have been developed for most substances.

G. **Sanctioned treatment.** When a patient is forced to remain in therapy by a legal sanction (e.g., loss of driver's license or professional license for relapse), the outcome is better than when the patient is free to withdraw from therapy at any time.

H. **Contingency contracting.** This approach provides a powerful negative contingency for leaving treatment or relapsing and a positive contingency for remaining drug free. In the most widely used form of contingency contracting, the patient agrees in advance that the therapist will notify an employer or licensing body if relapse occurs. The patient may leave a letter with the therapist outlining the problem, which is to be mailed if a urine screen is positive or the patient does not keep an appointment. Some patients deposit a sum of money with the therapist; a certain amount is then paid back to the patient for each week of abstinence. When the contingency for relapse is a report to the appropriate medical licensing authority, the relapse rate of substance-dependent physicians is less than 25%.

V. **ALCOHOLISM** affects approximately 10% of the population. Alcohol abuse or dependence usually develops during the first 5 years of regular use of alcohol.

A. **Three patterns of chronic alcohol abuse** have been described:

1. Regular daily excessive drinking

2. Regular heavy drinking on weekends only

3. Long periods of sobriety interspersed with binges that last days, weeks, or months

B. **Familial influences** seem to play a role in the development of alcoholism. Individuals are at an increased risk of being alcoholic if they have:

1. A family history of alcoholism, especially a son of an alcoholic father

2. A family history of teetotalism (i.e., avoidance of alcohol under any circumstance)

3. An alcoholic spouse

C. **Diagnostic clues** to alcoholism include:

1. Inability to decrease or discontinue drinking

2. Binges lasting at least 2 days

3. Occasional consumption of a fifth of spirits or the equivalent in wine or beer

4. Blackouts (transient amnesia for events that occur while the patient is intoxicated)

5. Continued drinking despite a physical illness that is exacerbated or caused by drinking

6. Drinking nonbeverage alcohol (e.g., shaving lotion)

7. Drinking in the morning

8. Withdrawal syndromes

9. Apparent sobriety in the presence of an elevated alcohol level in the blood, indicating tolerance to the sedative effects of alcohol

D. **Physical, psychiatric, and social complications**

1. **Physical complications,** which may be caused by associated nutritional deficiencies or by a direct toxic effect of alcohol, are not uncommon in patients who drink more than 3 to 6 ounces of whiskey a day or the equivalent. More familiar syndromes include:
   a. Cerebral atrophy
   b. Wernicke encephalopathy
   c. Korsakoff psychosis
   d. Nicotinic acid deficiency encephalopathy
   e. Polyneuropathy
   f. Cardiomyopathy
   g. Hypertension
   h. Skeletal muscle damage of uncertain clinical significance
   i. Gastritis
   j. Peptic ulcer
   k. Constipation
   l. Pancreatitis
   m. Cirrhosis
   n. Impotence
   o. Various anemias
   p. Teratogenicity
      (1) **Fetal alcohol syndrome,** characterized by mental retardation, microcephaly, slowed growth, and facial abnormalities, may be a risk even if moderate amounts of alcohol are consumed during pregnancy.

      (2) Because safe quantities have not been established, complete abstinence from alcohol during pregnancy is recommended. If a patient does drink, she should be advised to do so on a full stomach to minimize rapid rises in blood alcohol levels.

  q. Accidents

      (1) Almost half of all traffic fatalities involve alcohol.

      (2) Drunk drivers who are killed in motor vehicle accidents are 4 to 12 times more likely than drivers who are not killed to have had a previous arrest for driving under the influence, indicating that drinking and driving are recurrent problems.

2. Psychiatric complications. The major psychiatric complication of alcoholism is **suicide.** More than 80% of individuals who kill themselves are depressed, alcoholic, or both.

  a. Seventy-five percent of alcoholics have no other primary psychiatric diagnoses, although depression is a common complication of the direct effects of alcohol on the brain and the consequences of drinking on the patient's life.

  b. Alcoholism may be an attempt at self-treatment of another psychiatric disorder, such as depression, anxiety, mania, psychosis, or posttraumatic stress disorder. This possibility should be considered when psychiatric symptoms clearly preceded heavy drinking. However, the history is often undependable, and only a trial period of abstinence reliably distinguishes between primary alcoholism and alcohol abuse that is secondary to another condition. If psychological distress resolves after a period of abstinence, alcoholism is likely to have been a cause rather than a result of the psychiatric disorder.

  c. Alcoholism is a common comorbid condition with mood disorders, anxiety disorders, and personality disorders. In such situations, both conditions must be treated.

3. Social complications occur with the use of all psychoactive substances. The accident rate on the job is increased 3 to 4 times in workers who use psychoactive substances. Alcohol and other drugs cause sexual, marital, and legal problems.

E. **Specific treatment approaches** result in approximately one third of patients remaining sober, one third enjoying a period of sobriety followed by relapse, and one third continuing to drink. Useful interventions include the following:

1. Confrontation of denial. The major obstacles to therapeutic success are the patient's denial of the severity of the problem and the wish to continue drinking. Repeated statements that the patient is not in control of the drinking and repeated confrontation with the complications of the alcoholism may be necessary before the patient agrees to treatment.

2. Insistence on abstinence. Because it is not possible to identify in advance the very few patients who may be able to succeed with controlled drinking, total abstinence is the only realistic goal.

3. Assessment of motivation. The patient who is willing to consider abstaining completely for 1 month has at least some motivation to give up alcohol completely. If the patient insists on some continued alcohol intake (usually while assuring the doctor that it will be easy to keep from drinking excessively), treatment is less likely to be successful. Further therapeutic efforts may be unsuccessful until the patient is willing to give up alcohol completely for at least a brief period of time.

4. Disulfiram (Antabuse). Many alcoholics' efforts at abstinence are supported by disulfiram, which causes severe nausea and vomiting when it interacts with alcohol. Even if the patient does not need the drug, the patient's willingness to take it is a favorable prognostic sign. The only contraindications to the use of disulfiram are organic brain syndromes or other conditions that might interfere significantly with compliance. The usual dose is 500 mg at bedtime for 5 days followed by 250 mg at bedtime for at least 6 months. Vitamin C and antihistamines may abort the alcohol–disulfiram reaction.

5. Naltrexone has been approved recently to reduce craving for alcohol.

6. **Involvement of family.** The patient's family can be an important source of support, or they may openly or covertly encourage the patient to go on drinking.
   a. A family "intervention," in which all family members confront the patient's drinking, helps the patient to deal with denial.
   b. A spouse's refusal to remain with the patient unless the patient stops drinking may be the only force strong enough to convince the patient to agree to a trial of abstinence. Such threats should be mobilized only when they are a true expression of the spouse's feelings, or they will not be credible.
   c. Contingency contracting that involves remaining in the hospital may be very effective.
   d. Employers and other important individuals in the patient's life should also be involved in treatment whenever possible.

7. **Alcoholics Anonymous.** Alcoholics Anonymous is a highly useful treatment group. Other peer counseling programs also provide peer support and encouragement for the patient to stop drinking.

8. **Behavior therapy.** Punishing drinking (e.g., with disulfiram) and rewarding sobriety, for example by paying the patient for abstinence (i.e., contingency contracting), are useful for patients who consider their drinking a bad habit. Expressive psychotherapy is appropriate for patients who feel that their drinking is motivated by unresolved emotional conflicts.

9. **Ongoing emotional support by the primary physician.** Primary care physicians provide an important source of encouragement for the patient to confront the problem and to maintain sobriety. The physician should accept periodic relapses in a nonjudgmental manner. If the patient refuses specific therapy for alcoholism, the physician should continue to be available to the drinking patient in case a psychosocial crisis precipitates the patient's wishing to become involved in treatment.

VI. **OPIOID DEPENDENCE AND ABUSE** is a major public health problem. The incidence of heroin use increased during the 1960s, and use of this substance is now a problem in smaller communities in the United States, as well as in large cities.

A. **The epidemiology** of narcotic use, particularly heroin, deserves consideration. Two to three percent of adults aged 18 to 25 years have tried heroin at some time in their lives. Abuse of narcotics usually occurs in the context of abuse of other drugs. Using "soft" drugs like marijuana seems to break down a psychological barrier to using "hard" drugs. Approximately 50% of individuals who abuse narcotics become physically dependent. Most addicts tend to become abstinent over time. Often they finally discontinue drug dependence approximately 9 years after its onset.

1. **Patterns of narcotic abuse vary widely.** Some addicts, particularly those who are maintained on methadone, lead productive lives and enjoy good health. For others, the need to obtain illicit drugs and money to buy them leads to prostitution and other crimes. However, the behavior of an opioid abuser is sigificantly determined by his behavior and personality before drug use. Many narcotic abusers lead an antisocial lifestyle that persists until the drug is withdrawn. These individuals differ from those with antisocial personality disorder who are also narcotic abusers in that the antisocial behavior antedated substance abuse. Because of physical complications of abuse and a lifestyle associated with violence, the death rate is 2 to 20 times higher in opioid addicts than it is in the general population (i.e., 10 in 1000 die). Patterns of narcotic use and dependence are as follows.
   a. **Acquired during medical treatment.** A very small percentage of the addicted population becomes dependent in the course of medical treatment. If these individuals continue to receive narcotics from the physician, they are less likely to encounter the problems faced by other dependent individuals, who must obtain the drugs illegally.

    b. Recreational use. More commonly, narcotic abuse develops when an adolescent or young adult who is engaged in experimental or recreational drug use progresses to more intensive use. Since 60% to 90% of adolescents experiment to some extent with drugs (experimentation with drugs has been reported in children as young as 5 years of age), the number who go on to opioid dependence is not great. Later dependence on CNS stimulants and depressants is more common.

    c. Methadone maintenance. A significant number of individuals who have become dependent on opioids receive methadone from organized treatment programs.

    d. Health care personnel. The incidence of narcotic addiction is higher in physicians, nurses, and other health care personnel than in any other group of individuals with comparable education and socioeconomic class. Most physician-addicts initially use a narcotic to relieve depression, fatigue, or a physical ailment rather than for pleasure. The pattern and consequences of the addiction are no different than they are for other addicts, except that health care personnel are more likely to make drugs available to themselves through prescriptions and narcotics ordered for patients in hospitals.

2. Epidemic transmission. Heroin abuse tends to be transmitted in an epidemic fashion among individuals who know each other. These epidemics begin slowly, peak rapidly, and then decline quickly. They tend to abate completely after 5 to 6 years.

    a. Susceptibility to heroin addiction varies in different populations. Young African-American men are at highest risk, and women seem to be at lower risk.

    b. Dependence is initiated in a susceptible individual by someone known to the individual who is already addicted. The risk of such initiators exposing their acquaintances to heroin use continues for about 1 year. Drug "pushers" actually cause few new cases of dependence, although they obviously are a major source of the drug.

    c. Heroin abuse tends to spread until all susceptible individuals within a given group have been exposed. New addicts then tend to expose their friends in other circles, who produce a third generation of abusers.

3. Drug cultures. When cultural norms support heroin use, and relatively pure preparations are available, a large percentage of users become dependent.

    a. More than 40% of the United States Army enlisted men stationed in Vietnam reported trying narcotics at least once, and approximately 50% of these became physically dependent at some time during their stay in Vietnam. However, very few individuals who became dependent on narcotics in Vietnam continued drug use when they returned to the United States. This suggests that removal of peer group support for drug abuse, removal of the easy availability of drugs, and, possibly, removal of major environmental stresses ended the reasons for continued abuse.

    b. Most individuals in the United States who become dependent on narcotics have a psychological predisposition to abuse and tend to remain in peer groups that encourage substance use. Relapse is likely when they return to an environment in which drugs are available and friends and colleagues condone abuse.

4. Psychiatric illness. Approximately 50% to 87% of people with opioid dependence suffer from another psychiatric illness, especially depression, anxiety states, and borderline and antisocial personality disorders. Individuals from disorganized social backgrounds are also more susceptible to narcotic dependence. A combination of a susceptible psychosocial constellation, availability of narcotics, an environment that encourages abuse, and friends or colleagues who already are users may be necessary for the development of addiction.

B. **Medical complications** of narcotic abuse may result from contaminants of illicit preparations and the patient's lifestyle.

1. Venereal disease is common in female drug abusers as a result of engaging in prostitution to obtain the narcotic.

2. Fatal overdose due to fluctuations in the purity of available compounds is not uncommon.

3. **Anaphylactic reactions** may be caused by the intravenous injection of impurities.

4. **Hypersensitivity reactions** to impurities may also cause the formation of granulomata and neurologic, musculoskeletal, and cutaneous lesions.

5. **Infections** commonly caused by contaminated products and shared needles include hepatitis, endocarditis, septicemia, tetanus, and formation of pulmonary, cerebral, and subcutaneous abscesses. Up to two thirds of individuals in narcotic treatment centers test positive for human immunodeficiency virus (HIV).

6. **Suicide and death** at the hands of associates are more common in narcotic abusers than in the general population.

C. **Treatment** of opioid dependence requires a multidisciplinary approach.

1. **Methadone maintenance** for the treatment of addiction can only be carried out by a federally approved program.
   a. If the patient has strong psychosocial supports available and is highly motivated to discontinue drug use, the patient can be withdrawn immediately using methadone (see III E 2).
   b. If supports are weak or motivation to undergo withdrawal is uncertain, a period of methadone maintenance is instituted to strengthen supports, motivation, and the relationship with the treatment team. The usual dose of methadone in this setting is 40–80 mg/day.
      (1) The patient must have clear-cut signs of addiction (e.g., intoxication, needle tracks, and medical or psychosocial consequences of abuse) to qualify for methadone maintenance.
      (2) Periodic unscheduled urine and blood screens are performed to test compliance with the program. Persistent noncompliance (i.e., continued self-administration of narcotics) results in dismissal.
      (3) Very gradual withdrawal from methadone is attempted when the patient seems ready. Most addicts note some abstinence symptoms when the dosage is reduced below 20 mg/day, and reduction in dosage by as little as 1 mg/week below this level may be necessary for the detoxification of long-term methadone users.

2. **L-α-Acetylmethadol (LAAM),** also known as methadyl acetate, a long-acting preparation, suppresses narcotic withdrawal for 72 hours. When it is used instead of methadone for maintenance, less frequent administration of the drug is necessary. However, more patients drop out of LAAM maintenance than methadone maintenance.

3. **Therapeutic communities** play an important role in the treatment of narcotic addiction. Confrontation by fellow addicts of lying and rationalization of drug use has more credibility to an addict than therapies that are administered by professionals.

4. **Residential treatment.** If outpatient therapy is unsuccessful, residential treatment is necessary to remove the patient from easy access to the drug and from associates who encourage continued abuse. Group confrontation and support are used extensively in these settings. Compliance with treatment is higher when it is mandated by the courts than when it is voluntary and the patient is free to withdraw at any time.

5. **Licensure restrictions.** Narcotic-abusing physicians increasingly are being identified by state licensing bodies and medical societies. Treatment programs have been very successful when the problem is identified early and when continued licensure for medical practice is made contingent on documentation of ongoing abstinence (contingency contracting).

6. **Prevention of addiction in a medical setting.** Health care providers should not permit fears of addiction from interfering with the administration of appropriate doses of narcotics to patients in pain. The following guidelines apply to the administration of opioids to patients at risk of dependence.

a. Adequate doses of narcotics should be administered to patients with bona fide acute pain syndromes. Addicts generally require higher doses than other patients.

b. Narcotics should be administered regularly rather than as needed. This approach prevents patients from becoming preoccupied with pain and its relief and provides a constant blood level that results in lower individual doses being necessary.

c. An addict should not be detoxified during an acute physical illness.

d. Prescriptions should not be written for outpatients with suspicious complaints or those with a high abuse potential, as indicated by:

   (1) Losing prescriptions or running out of medication early

   (2) Requests for a specific drug

   (3) History of abuse of alcohol or other drugs

   (4) Physician shopping

   (5) Claims that a physician who originally wrote a prescription is unavailable

   (6) Threats when narcotics are not prescribed

   (7) Dishonesty with the physician

VII. ABUSE OF AND DEPENDENCE ON TRANQUILIZERS AND SLEEPING PILLS
is created or encouraged in everyday medical practice more frequently than opioid dependence and abuse.

A. **Manifestations of dependence and abuse.** Barbiturates and related compounds are particularly prone to pathologic use. Benzodiazepines with short half-lives are more prone to dosage escalation to reduce interdose withdrawal, whereas highly lipid soluble benzodiazepines produce a more rapid effect that may be experienced as a high. Diazepam, which is very lipid soluble, lorazepam, which has a short half-life, and alprazolam, which has both properties, are the most frequently abused benzodiazepines. Dependence may only first be suspected when an abstinence syndrome that responds to phenobarbital or pentobarbital appears in a patient who is admitted to the hospital and is denied access to the abused substance.

1. Because they suppress REM sleep, barbiturates and related sedatives, such as secobarbital, glutethimide, and ethchlorvynol, subject the patient who uses them to a **rebound of REM sleep,** usually in the form of **nightmares,** when the drug is discontinued. Although it seems to the patient that he or she cannot sleep without the drug, continued drug use serves only to prevent withdrawal and suppress REM rebound, and escalating doses often are needed to accomplish this result.

2. When barbiturates and related compounds are used as tranquilizers, drug withdrawal tends to be mistaken for a return of anxiety, which leads to an increase in dosage to suppress the symptoms. Fear of withdrawal symptoms then leads to continued drug use and an inability to function without the drug, as well as other manifestations of dependence.

3. Symptoms of benzodiazepine withdrawal may persist for months after drug discontinuation, leading to prolonged use of the benzodiazepine to suppress withdrawal.

B. **Identification and management of abuse.** Misuse of sedatives and tranquilizers can be minimized if barbiturates are not prescribed for insomnia and anxiety, and benzodiazepines are not prescribed for patients with a history of substance dependence. Identification and management of problems with CNS depressants involve:

1. A **detailed history** of amounts and kinds of all prescription and nonprescription drugs that have ever been taken should be obtained. Often, the patient continues to take drugs that were prescribed by a physician that he or she is no longer seeing.

2. **Prescriptions** for a patient who has terminated treatment should be **discontinued**.

3. **Toxicology screening** in patients who abuse any drug should be performed to identify mixed abuse. Drugs will not be present in the blood of a patient who is experiencing a withdrawal syndrome.

4. **Regular appointments** should be scheduled for the patient who has been taking barbiturates for years and who is reluctant to discontinue them. Assurance of an ongoing relationship with a physician the patient trusts may make the patient more willing to consider tapering drug intake. Insistence on discontinuation of barbiturates and related medications is mandatory for patients who escalate the dose, have withdrawal symptoms, or experience psychomotor impairment.

5. **Hospitalization** should be considered for detoxification of patients with severe or mixed dependence. This permits adequate treatment of what may be life-threatening withdrawal and ensures compliance with the withdrawal protocol.

VIII. COCAINE ABUSE AND DEPENDENCE have become extremely serious public health problems. One fourth of young adults have used cocaine, and adverse consequences are common.

A. **Routes of administration.** There are three routes of self-administration of cocaine.

1. **Nasal** administration is associated with the onset of euphoria over a period of 20 minutes that lasts approximately 1 hour.

2. **Intravenous** administration produces immediate euphoria.

3. Crack, an easily synthesized compound that is not inactivated by high temperature, is **smoked,** producing immediate euphoria.

B. **Addictive potential.** Contrary to the popular wisdom of a few years ago, cocaine is highly addictive. The advent of crack and the flooding of the market with cheap cocaine have made cocaine a drug of abuse at all socioeconomic levels.

1. Animals will choose self-administration of cocaine over food and water until they die.

2. Some patients report feeling addicted from the very first dose of cocaine.

3. Crack is the cheapest and most addictive form of cocaine.

4. Cocaine is frequently used in conjunction with other substances, especially alcohol and tranquilizers.

C. **Psychomotor impairment.** In one recent report, more than 50% of a group of drivers who were stopped by the police for reckless driving and who were not intoxicated with alcohol, were intoxicated with cocaine, marijuana, or both.

D. **Psychiatric disorders.** Cocaine use may be a means of self-treatment for certain psychiatric disorders, especially depression and attention deficit disorder. Some manic individuals abuse cocaine to achieve a sense of control over excitement that occurs spontaneously without the drug. In any of these situations, cocaine is so inherently rewarding that attempts to treat the comorbid condition without treating cocaine abuse are invariably unsuccessful.

E. **Treatment.** The same approaches that have been applied to abuse of opioids and alcohol have been found helpful in the treatment of cocaine abuse and dependence. In addition, three types of medication that enhance dopaminergic transmission in reward centers have been thought to reduce craving for stimulants, which probably act on the same centers through a dopaminergic mechanism.

1. **Imipramine, desipramine,** and **maprotiline** are the antidepressants that have been used to reduce craving. **Bupropion** and possibly **venlafaxine** should be more effective because they are more specifically dopaminergic.

2. **Amantadine** decreases cocaine craving in the first few weeks after withdrawal. It may also be useful in long-term treatment.

3. **Bromocriptine** is a dopamine agonist that has been reported to be useful in a short-term trial.

4. **Cognitive therapy** has been found to have a delayed onset of action in promoting abstinence from cocaine. The benefits of medications tend to dissipate after the medication is discontinued.

DIRECTIONS: Each of the numbered items or incomplete statements in this section is followed by answers or by completions of the statement. Select the ONE lettered answer or completion that is BEST in each case.

1. The feature of addiction that differentiates it from other forms of substance misuse is

(A) overwhelming involvement in seeking and using a drug
(B) physical dependence
(C) use of narcotics
(D) antisocial behavior
(E) tolerance and withdrawal

2. The percentage of United States Army enlisted men who became dependent on narcotics while in Vietnam was roughly

(A) 5%
(B) 20%
(C) 40%
(D) 75%
(E) 90%

3. The most reliably effective treatment of opioid dependence is

(A) administration of narcotic antagonists
(B) use of antidepressants
(C) psychological support
(D) removal from an environment that condones drug use
(E) therapy for comorbid conditions

4. In contrast to the hallucinogens, which one of the following statements best describes phencyclidine (PCP)?

(A) PCP is more likely to produce neurologic signs
(B) PCP causes hallucinations more frequently
(C) PCP intoxication is more likely to respond to reassurance
(D) PCP intoxication is less likely to induce violence
(E) PCP withdrawal is more severe

5. Characteristics of contingency contracting include which one of the following?

(A) Rewards are contingent on avoiding intoxication
(B) Therapy is contingent on paying
(C) Success is contingent on treating comorbid conditions
(D) Negative consequences are contingent on relapse
(E) Participation is contingent on being a professional

6. Which of the following abnormalities is a manifestation of barbiturate intoxication but not of barbiturate withdrawal?

(A) Confusion
(B) Nystagmus
(C) Postural hypotension
(D) Disorientation
(E) Agitation

7. A patient's blood alcohol level is 10 mg/100 ml, but there is no clinical evidence of intoxication. It is a reasonable assumption that the patient

(A) is tolerant to opioids
(B) is dependent on alcohol
(C) has pancreatitis
(D) is impotent
(E) has cerebral atrophy

DIRECTIONS: Each of the numbered items or incomplete statements in this section is negatively phrased, as indicated by a capitalized word such as NOT, LEAST, or EXCEPT. Select the ONE lettered answer or completion that is BEST in each case.

8. Effects of amphetamine intoxication include all of the following EXCEPT

(A) tachycardia
(B) depression
(C) suspiciousness
(D) anorexia
(E) insomnia

9. Opioid overdoses produce all of the following signs EXCEPT

(A) dilated pupils
(B) hypotension
(C) depressed reflexes
(D) coma
(E) decreased respiration

10. The relationship between alcoholism and depression is characterized by all of the following EXCEPT

(A) nonbeverage forms of alcohol cause depression more frequently than other forms
(B) depression can follow sobriety
(C) alcohol and depression frequently are comorbid
(D) the suicide risk is increased in alcoholics
(E) alcoholism runs in the families of depressed people

11. A 40-year-old businessman from another city arrives in the emergency department complaining of severe migraine headaches that are resolved only by meperidine. His primary physician is on vacation. The emergency department physician should ask about all of the following conditions EXCEPT

(A) delusions
(B) legal problems
(C) losing prescriptions
(D) loss of consciousness
(E) use of alcohol

12. Amphetamine psychosis (stimulant-induced psychotic disorder) is characterized by all of the following EXCEPT

(A) depression
(B) loose associations
(C) clear sensorium
(D) tactile hallucinations
(E) paranoia

DIRECTIONS: Each set of matching questions in this section consists of a list of four to twenty-six lettered options followed by several numbered items. For each numbered item, select the ONE lettered option that is most closely associated with it. Each lettered option may be selected once, more than once, or not at all.

Questions 13–17

Match each of the following substances with the symptom it is most likely to cause.

(A) Suggestibility
(B) Insomnia
(C) Miosis
(D) Violence
(E) Postural hypotension

13. Phencyclidine

14. Marijuana

15. Stimulants

16. Barbiturates

17. Opioids

Questions 18–22

Match each of the following substances with the withdrawal syndrome it usually causes.

(A) Anxiety
(B) Hypersomnia
(C) Flashbacks
(D) Piloerection
(E) Influenza-like symptoms

18. Stimulants

19. Anticholinergics

20. Opioids

21. Benzodiazepines

22. Hallucinogens

ANSWERS AND EXPLANATIONS

1. The answer is A *[I C]*. Although the definition of addiction varies, most definitions share the concept of overwhelming involvement in and preoccupation with obtaining and using any type of drug. Addictive behavior may occur with any substance; addiction to placebo has even been reported. Physical dependence is defined as the presence of tolerance and/or withdrawal. Antisocial behavior may play a role in attempts to make enough money to obtain substances, but it is not a defining feature of addiction or any other form of misuse.

2. The answer is B *[VI A 3 a]*. Forty percent of enlisted men tried narcotics while they were in Vietnam, and approximately half of these individuals became dependent. The finding that a small minority of men continued to use narcotics on return to the United States suggests that the easy availability of drugs and the encouragement of a peer group allow opioid abuse to continue.

3. The answer is D *[II F 4; VI C 4]*. Narcotic antagonists precipitate withdrawal in opioid-dependent individuals. Satisfactory long-acting narcotic antagonists analogous to disulfiram in the treatment of alcoholism have not been developed. Although some patients (especially physicians) may use narcotics as self-treatment for depression, and narcotics may cause depression, antidepressants do not stop use of the opioid. Psychologic support is helpful, but it is usually not sufficient to get the patient to abstain from opioids. Removal of the patient from an environment that supports continued drug use is the most reliable way of ensuring abstinence.

4. The answer is A *[II D 1–3]*. Unlike other hallucinogenic substances, phencyclidine (PCP) intoxication can produce neurologic signs that include analgesia, nystagmus, ataxia, seizures, and coma. However, PCP is not more likely to produce hallucinations than any other hallucinogenic substances. Patients who are intoxicated with PCP may become violent, and attempts to reassure them make them more violent. A more effective treatment of intoxication is to leave the patient in a quiet place and use restraint or sedation with a neuroleptic if violence does not abate. No PCP-specific withdrawal syndrome has been identified.

5. The answer is D *[IV H]*. In contingency contracting, the patient agrees in advance that in the event of relapse or noncompliance, the therapist will notify an employer or licensing body or will arrange some other negative consequence. Rewards, such as receiving money back that the patient paid to the therapist in advance, are contingent on abstinence not just avoidance of intoxication. Contingency contracting has been found useful for substance-abusing physicians, but it is useful for any population in which meaningful consequences of relapse can be identified.

6. The answer is B *[II B 1 c, 2 e; III B 1]*. Both intoxication and withdrawal from barbiturates may cause confusion, delirium, anxiety, agitation, and postural hypotension. If caused by withdrawal, these signs improve with administration of a barbiturate. Nystagmus, which is a sign of intoxication but not withdrawal, may appear.

7. The answer is B *[V C 9]*. Absence of intoxication in the presence of a high blood alcohol level indicates that the patient is tolerant to the central nervous system depressant effects of alcohol, which is a major criterion for alcohol dependence. Pancreatitis, impotence, and cerebral atrophy are complications of alcoholism that should be investigated but these are not diagnosed by a blood alcohol level. Since opioids and alcohol are not cross-tolerant, tolerance to alcohol does not provide any information about tolerance to opioids.

8. The answer is B *[II C 2, 3]*. Amphetamine intoxication produces tachycardia, hypertension, paranoia, anorexia, and insomnia. Depression is a more predictable feature of amphetamine withdrawal.

9. The answer is A *[II F 2 g]*. Like alcohol, barbiturates, and benzodiazepines, narcotics can produce depression of consciousness, reflexes, blood pressure, and respiration. Narcotics cause constricted rather than dilated pupils. Opioid intoxication can be diagnosed with intravenous naloxone.

10. The answer is A *[V D 2]*. Any form of alcohol can induce depression as a direct effect of the substance. Alcoholics may drink in an attempt to treat an underlying depression; when they achieve sobriety, the depression becomes more noticeable, or they appreciate their problems more clearly. Alcoholism and depression co-occur in individuals and families. Alcoholics are at increased risk of suicide, and drinking may decrease impulse control sufficiently for a suicidal patient to act on the impulse.

11. The answer is A *[VI C 6 d]*. Suspicion of narcotic abuse is increased by demands for a specific opioid; losing prescriptions; requests for prescription refills, when the physician who allegedly wrote the prescription is unavailable; legal, occupational, or psychosocial consequences of abuse; and threatening behavior when a requested prescription is not written. A history of loss of consciousness might indicate central nervous system (CNS) disease, intoxication with any substance, or abstinence from CNS depressants. Abuse of multiple drugs is common in narcotic abusers. Psychosis is not a common cause or result of opioid use.

12. The answer is A *[II C 3]*. Stimulant psychosis often is associated with paranoia and loose associations in a clear sensorium, which may make it indistinguishable from schizo-

phrenia. Tactile hallucinations and delusions of infestation with parasites also may occur. Depression is usually associated with stimulant withdrawal, not stimulant intoxication.

13–17. The answers are: 13-D, 14-A, 15-B, 16-E, 17-C *[II B 2 g, C 2 g, D 2 b (1), E 1 a, F 3 a]*. Phencyclidine intoxication causes violent behavior more frequently than do other hallucinogens. Marijuana is associated with suggestibility but not hallucinations. Stimulants disrupt sleep. Postural hypotension is commonly caused by barbiturates, whereas opioid intoxication produces miosis.

18–22. The answers are: 18-B, 19-E, 20-D, 21-A, 22-C *[III B 1 a, C 1 f, D 1, E 1 d, F]*. Withdrawal of stimulants causes depression. Abrupt withdrawal of anticholinergic substances leads to cholinergic rebound, with influenza-like symptoms and occasionally mania. Opioid withdrawal causes piloerection (gooseflesh). Withdrawal of benzodiazepines frequently causes anxiety, which may be difficult to distinguish from return of the original symptoms. Flashbacks on withdrawal of hallucinogens may be precipitated by marijuana.

Chapter 7

Somatoform and Associated Disorders
Gordon L. Neligh

I. **DEFINITIONS.** The somatoform disorders are a heterogeneous group that have common presenting features suggestive of physical illnesses, symptoms, or preoccupations. As a feature of this group, the physical symptoms are unexplained by a general medical condition or are disproportionate to symptoms that might be expected from a general medical condition. To establish one of these diagnoses, the clinician must rule out occult physical illnesses or conditions, other psychiatric disorders that might better explain the symptoms (e.g., the patient with major depressive illness who has a delusion of having a fatal cancer), and substance abuse. The condition must be of sufficient severity to impair social and occupational or other important areas of functioning. Disorders and conditions with a mixed picture of physical and psychiatric symptoms might be divided into the following groups.

A. **Disorders involving subjective symptoms unexplained by physical findings.** This group of disorders includes symptoms such as conversion symptoms (see II A 2 d) and may involve many body systems, including the joints, reproductive organs, gastrointestinal tract, nervous system, and special senses. This group does not include disorders involving a conscious or intentional misrepresentation of symptoms (see I F).

B. **Disorders involving unusual attention to and preoccupation with symptoms, organs, and body parts.** This group of disorders includes either preoccupation with a body part or parts that the patient considers defective, deformed, weak, or ugly in contrast with external evidence to the contrary (e.g., body dysmorphic disorder) or unusual degrees of attention to physical symptoms (e.g., a mole that the person incorrectly believes to be malignant) or organ systems (e.g., excessive preoccupation with examining feces for blood or deformity believed to be evidence of malignancy).

C. **Disorders in which psychological symptoms may exacerbate a general medical condition.** Conditions in this group include general medical conditions exacerbated by a psychological factor (e.g., stress), including some cardiovascular disorders, irritable bowel syndrome, psoriasis, and many other medical conditions. Included in this category may be disorders exacerbated or caused by immune and neuroendocrine dysfunctions (associated with affective and anxiety disorders) and mitral valve prolapse (common in panic disorder).

D. **Psychiatric disorders that present with primarily physical symptoms or present physical symptoms as an unusual or atypical form of the disorder.** Disorders in this category include unusual presentations of familiar psychiatric disorders (e.g., the patient with depression who presents with headaches or malaise, the panic disorder patient with symptoms of a myocardial infarction).

E. **Disorders in which psychiatric symptoms are caused or exacerbated by a general medical condition.** Medical conditions can cause psychiatric symptoms resembling almost any psychiatric disorder. Common examples are hypothyroidism mimicking depressive disorders, toxic delirium mimicking schizophreniform disorder, and paroxysmal atrial tachycardia resembling panic disorder.

F. **Disorders in which physical symptoms are incorrectly reported or are created by the patient for the purpose of gaining a specific benefit.** Familiar disorders in this group include **factitious disorder** and **malingering**. The hallmark of these conditions is that the patient consciously fabricates symptoms, such as putting blood from a finger stick into his urine sample and complaining of flank pain.

G. **Disorders of a primarily medical nature that the practitioner mistakes for psychiatric conditions.** The *Diagnostic and Statistical Manual of Mental Disorders*, 4th edition (DSM-IV), emphasizes that clinicians frequently dismiss as psychiatric based unusual physical symptoms and physical disorders early in their course. This mistake may lead to unfortunate consequences for the clinician as well as the patient. Therefore, the clinician should note the formal diagnostic criteria for somatoform disorders to avoid this serious and costly mistake.

II. DIAGNOSIS

A. **Somatization disorder**

1. The **patient's history** includes many physical complaints beginning before age 30, occurring over several years, and resulting in treatment for or significant impairment in social, occupational, or other important areas of functioning.

2. Each of the following **criteria** must be met, with individual symptoms occurring at any time during the course of the disturbance.
    a. **Four pain symptoms:** A history of pain related to at least four different sites (e.g., head, abdomen, back, joints, extremities, chest, rectum) or functions (e.g., during menstruation, sexual intercourse, urination)
    b. **Two gastrointestinal symptoms:** A history of at least two gastrointestinal symptoms other than pain (e.g., nausea, bloating, vomiting, diarrhea, intolerance of several different foods)
    c. **One sexual symptom:** A history of at least one sexual or reproductive symptom other than pain (e.g., sexual indifference, erectile or ejaculatory dysfunction, irregular menses, excessive menstrual bleeding, vomiting throughout pregnancy)
    d. **One pseudoneurologic symptom:** A history of at least one symptom or deficit suggesting a neurologic condition not limited to pain, such as conversion symptoms (e.g., impaired coordination or balance, paralysis or localized weakness, difficulty swallowing or lump in throat, aphonia, urinary retention, hallucinations, loss of touch or pain sensation, double vision, blindness, deafness, seizures) or dissociative symptoms (e.g., amnesia or loss of consciousness other than fainting)

3. **Patient has either of the following:**
    a. After appropriate investigation, each of the symptoms in II A 2 cannot be fully explained by a known general medical condition or the direct effects of a substance (e.g., a drug of abuse, a medication).
    b. If a related general medical condition is present, the physical complaints or resulting social or occupational impairment exceed what would be expected from the history, physical examination, or laboratory findings.

4. The symptoms are not intentionally produced or feigned (e.g., as in factitious disorder or malingering).

B. **Undifferentiated somatoform disorder**

1. **The patient has one or more physical complaints** (e.g., fatigue, loss of appetite, gastrointestinal or urinary problems).

2. **The patient has either of the following.**
    a. After appropriate investigation, the **symptoms cannot be fully explained by a known general medical condition or the direct effects of a substance** (e.g., a drug of abuse, a medication).

     b. If a related general medical condition is present, the physical complaints or resulting social or occupational **impairment exceeds what would be expected** from the history, physical examination, or laboratory findings.

3. **The patient's symptoms cause clinically significant distress or impairment** in social, occupational, or other important areas of functioning.

4. **The duration of the disturbance is at least 6 months.**

5. **The disturbance is not better explained by another mental disorder** (e.g., another somatoform disorder, sexual dysfunction, mood disorder, anxiety disorder, sleep disorder, psychotic disorder).

6. **The symptom is not intentionally produced** or feigned (e.g., as in factitious disorder or malingering).

C. **Conversion disorder** (DSM-IV criteria)

1. There is one or more symptoms or deficits affecting voluntary motor or sensory function and suggesting a neurologic or other general medical condition.

2. Psychological factors are judged to be associated with the symptom or deficit because the initiation or exacerbation of the symptom or deficit is preceded by conflicts or other stressors.

3. The symptom or deficit is not intentionally produced or feigned (e.g., factitious disorder and malingering).

4. The symptom or deficit cannot, after appropriate investigation, be fully explained by a general medical condition, or by the direct effects of a substance, or as a culturally sanctioned behavior or experience.

5. The symptom or deficit causes clinically significant distress or impairment in social, occupational, or other important areas of functioning or warrants medical evaluation.

6. The symptom or deficit is not limited to pain or sexual dysfunction, does not occur exclusively during the course of somatization disorder, and is not better accounted for by another mental disorder.

7. The DSM-IV requires specification of the subtype of conversion disorder:
   a. With motor symptoms or deficits (e.g., impaired coordination or balance, paralysis or localized weakness, difficulty swallowing or "lump in throat," aphonia, urinary retention)
   b. With sensory symptoms or deficits (e.g., loss of touch or pain sensation, double vision, blindness, deafness, hallucinations)
   c. With seizures or convulsions (includes seizures or convulsions with voluntary motor or sensory components)
   d. With mixed presentation (if symptoms are evident in more than one category)

D. **Pain disorder**

1. Pain in one or more anatomic site is the predominant focus of the clinical presentation and is of sufficient severity to warrant clinical attention.

2. The pain causes clinically significant distress or impairment in social, occupational, or other important areas of functioning.

3. Psychological factors are judged to have an important role in the onset, severity, exacerbation, or maintenance of the pain.

4. The symptoms or deficit are not intentionally produced or feigned (e.g., as in factitious disorder and malingering).

5. The pain is not better explained by a mood, anxiety, or psychotic disorder and does not meet criteria for dyspareunia.

6. **Subtypes** are defined as follows.

   a. **Pain disorder associated with psychological factors.** Psychological factors are judged to have a major role in the onset, severity, exacerbation, or maintenance of the pain. If a general medical condition is present, it does not have a major role in the onset, severity, exacerbation, or maintenance of the pain. This disorder is not diagnosed if criteria for somatization disorder are met. **Acute** or **chronic** duration should be specified.

   b. **Pain disorder associated with both psychological factors and a general medical condition.** Both psychological factors and a general medical condition are judged to have important roles in the onset, severity, exacerbation, or maintenance of the pain.

   c. **Pain disorder associated with a general medical condition.** A general medical condition has a major role in the onset, severity, exacerbation, or maintenance of the pain. This category is for medical conditions and for those conditions in which the relationship between anatomic and psychological factors is not clearly established (e.g., low back pain).

E. **Hypochondriasis** is a preoccupation with fears of having (or the idea that one has) a serious disease because the person has misinterpreted bodily symptoms.

   1. The preoccupation persists despite appropriate medical evaluation and reassurance.

   2. The belief in the preoccupation is not of delusional intensity (e.g., as in delusional disorder, somatic type) and is not restricted to a circumscribed concern about appearance (e.g., as in body dysmorphic disorder).

   3. The preoccupation causes clinically significant distress or impairment in social, occupational, or other important areas of functioning.

   4. The duration of the disturbance is at least 6 months.

   5. The preoccupation is not better explained by generalized anxiety disorder, obsessive-compulsive disorder, panic disorder, a major depressive episode, separation anxiety, or another somatoform disorder.

F. **Body dysmorphic disorder** is a preoccupation with an imagined defect in appearance. If a slight physical anomaly is present, the person's concern is markedly excessive.

   1. The preoccupation causes clinically significant distress or impairment in social, occupational, or other important areas of functioning.

   2. The preoccupation is not better explained by another mental disorder (e.g., dissatisfaction with body shape and size as in anorexia nervosa).

G. **Somatoform disorder not otherwise specified.** This category includes disorders with somatoform symptoms that do not meet the criteria for any specific somatoform disorder. Examples include:

   1. **Pseudocyesis.** This false belief of being pregnant is associated with objective signs of pregnancy, which may include abdominal enlargement (although the umbilicus does not become everted), reduced menstrual flow, amenorrhea, subjective sensation of fetal movement, nausea, breast engorgement and secretions, and labor pains at the expected date of delivery. This condition cannot be explained by a general medical condition, such as a hormone-secreting tumor.

   2. A disorder involving nonpsychotic hypochondriacal symptoms of less than 6 months' duration

   3. A disorder involving unexplained physical complaints that are of less than 6 months' duration and are not due to another mental disorder

H. **Factitious disorder** is the intentional production or feigning of physical or psychological signs or symptoms. The motivation for the behavior is to assume the sick role. External incentives for the behavior (e.g., profiting economically, avoiding legal responsibility, improving physical well-being, as in malingering) are absent. **Subtypes** are as noted:

1. With predominantly psychological signs and symptoms
2. With predominantly physical signs and symptoms
3. With combined psychological and physical signs and symptoms

I. **Factitious disorder not otherwise specified.** This disorder includes production of intentional symptoms in another, such as a child, for the purpose of having the other person assume a sick role.

J. **Malingering** is the intentional production of false or grossly exaggerated physical or psychological symptoms motivated by external incentives (e.g., avoiding military duty, avoiding work, obtaining financial compensation, evading criminal prosecution, obtaining drugs). Malingering should be strongly suspected if a combination of the following is noted:

1. Medicolegal context of presentation (e.g., the person is referred by an attorney to the clinician for examination)
2. Marked discrepancy between the person's claimed stress or disability and the objective findings
3. Lack of cooperation during the diagnostic evaluation and in complying with the prescribed treatment regimen
4. The presence of antisocial personality disorder

III. ETIOLOGIC THEORIES

A. **Specificity theory.** The theory of emotional specificity (i.e., the physiologic expression of blocked emotions) has led to personality studies of patients with peptic ulcers, coronary artery disease, and cancer. Although these studies have lent some support to the theory, it has, in general, lost favor as a comprehensive explanation.

1. **Freud** and his followers studied somatic involvement in psychological conflict and were particularly interested in **conversion reactions,** in which a psychological problem is symbolically manifested physically, although physiologic tissue damage cannot be demonstrated.
2. **Dunbar** suggested that **specific conscious personality traits** cause specific psychosomatic diseases.
3. **Alexander** theorized that **specific unconscious conflicts** cause specific illnesses in organs innervated by the autonomic nervous system. These illnesses occur because prolonged tension can produce physiologic disorders, leading to eventual pathology. Alexander also believed that constitutional predisposing factors are involved. His theory led to the concept of the **classic psychosomatic diseases,** including:
   a. **Bronchial asthma**
   b. **Rheumatoid arthritis**
   c. **Ulcerative colitis**
   d. **Essential hypertension**
   e. **Neurodermatitis**
   f. **Thyrotoxicosis**
   g. **Duodenal peptic ulcer**

B. **Stress response theories.** Whatever event is perceived by the patient as stressful can produce stress, whether this event is the death of a loved one, divorce, financial loss, or illness. In each culture, different events may carry different "weights" as stressors. Within a culture, however, stressful life events can be assessed quantitatively for their risk of producing psychophysiologic illnesses in a large group of people. Psychological reactions to stress can alter neuroendocrine, immune, cardiovascular, and other physiologic parameters that can lead to a **nonspecific cause of disease**.

1. **Neurophysiologic reactions to stress** activate the pituitary–adrenal axis and are known as the **general adaptation syndrome**. The nonspecific systemic reactions of the body to stress include:
   a. **Alarm reaction** (shock)
   b. **Resistance** (adaptation to stress)
   c. **Exhaustion** (resistance to prolonged stress, which cannot be maintained)

2. **Physiologic reactions to stress** include the following:
   a. **Fight-or-flight response** is arousal of the sympathetic nervous system, resulting in increased production of epinephrine and norepinephrine, with an increase in pulse and muscle tension. When an affected individual can neither fight nor flee, this state of arousal can lead to organic dysfunction.
   b. **Withdrawal and conservation.** Engel and coworkers have shown that when an individual is threatened with loss (real or imagined), the metabolism can slow down. The individual withdraws, and this action conserves energy.
      (1) Pulse and body temperature decrease.
      (2) The individual may become susceptible to illness, particularly infection. Studies on the psychophysiologic effects of bereavement support this hypothesis: Morbidity and mortality rates are higher during the first year after death of a spouse in a bereaved group compared to those rates in an age-controlled, nonbereaved group. Elderly people removed from their homes and placed in nursing homes have an increased risk of death from cardiovascular causes.

C. **The biopsychosocial model** proposed by Engel offers the interaction of biologic, psychological, and social events as the means for understanding the etiology, pathologic process, and treatment for psychiatric disorders as well as psychophysiologic conditions. This model is reciprocal rather than linear. In other words, a biologic event can alter psychological perceptions and cognitive set. These changes, in turn, can alter social behaviors. The social environment responds by treating the individual differently, and the response to that different treatment is an alteration in physiology.

1. **Biologic factors** reflect the physiologic, neurophysiologic, and pathophysiologic functioning of the person.
   a. **Hereditary and congenital factors** include inherited risks for psychiatric disorders (e.g., affective and anxiety disorders), physiologic vulnerabilities (e.g., risks for heart disease or some cancers), and defects (e.g., malformations, biochemical abnormalities, differences in pain threshold).
   b. **Physical disease processes** can affect the functioning of the brain and other physiologic processes.
   c. **Environmental factors** can affect the brain and body physiology (e.g., exposure to toxic substances, medications being prescribed, substances of abuse, amount of daylight, alterations of circadian rhythms related to a job).
   d. **Normal physiologic responses** to environmental events may place the individual at risk for a variety of additional physical and psychological events.
      (1) **Immune system compromise,** which is reflected in the increased risks of death following significant losses from causes such as infectious illnesses and some neoplasms
      (2) **Cardiovascular responses to stress,** which include hypertension and increased heart rate (which may unmask some arrhythmias)
      (3) **Neuroendocrine systems,** which are altered by environmental stressors, major mental illnesses, and many of the medications used to treat mental illnesses. Many of these abnormalities may reflect changes in hypothalamic–pituitary functioning modulated in the brain. Major systems involved include the following.

(a) **Cortisol** is altered in relation to stress, anxiety, and depression.

(b) **Prolactin** is altered in a variety of psychiatric disorders as well as in normal stress responses. Interestingly, prolactin also may modulate T-lymphocyte function.

(c) **Thyroid function** is variably altered in major mental illnesses, particularly depression. Thyrotropin-releasing hormone has been the focus of recent study, as has depression in mildly hypothyroid people.

(d) **Other hormones,** such as growth hormone, have been studied in relation to psychiatric disorders. Their role in stress response is less clear than the role of those factors just listed.

(4) **Neurohumoral factors** are reported to be altered in major mental illness and stress response. β-endorphin and dynorphin abnormalities are associated with anxiety-related disorders. Somatostatin, corticotropin-releasing hormone, and thyrotropin-releasing hormone also appear to be altered with stress, as do dopamine, γ-aminobutyric acid (GABA), norepinephrine, and serotonin. These neurohumoral factors may be an intermediary mechanism by which stressful events are translated into longer term alterations in brain function. However, any primary role for this function remains unclear.

2. **Psychological factors**

a. **Perception of pain or physiologic events** is the conscious registering of the stimulus or event. Perception of physical events has been shown to be altered by a number of factors, such as a state of arousal, individual differences in threshold, mood, other stimuli (e.g., the gate-control theory of pain), and physiologic events.

b. **Attention to the pain or physiologic event** is perhaps the best example of the conscious effect of the physical event on the person. For example, the chronic pain patient notices the pain very frequently, in spite of efforts to ignore it.

c. **Meaning or context of the symptom.** The meaning or context of the symptom determines how much attention it gets. For example, the literature contains many reports of broken legs and war wounds that go unnoticed by the injured person. In contrast, the patient who believes that a change in a physical symptom is the sign of a worsening or fatal illness pays a great deal of attention to the symptom.

d. **Primary gain from a physical symptom** is the abatement of a psychological symptom that results from the attention demanded by the physical symptom. For example, a broken leg takes attention away from worries about a relationship and may even be more "comfortable."

3. **Social factors** help to determine the meaning of the physical symptom or pain, and they may serve to extinguish or perpetuate attention to the symptom. Following are some of the social factors determining how a physical symptom will be perceived.

a. **The sick role** is defined by the culture, the family group, and the beliefs of the individual. The sick role can be understood as the expected behavior of the person as a result of illness. In some cultures, the sick role is very limited; a person, when sick, is allowed only to lie down and stop eating. In other cultures, the sick role may be highly elaborated on the basis of the type of sickness, chronicity, and the supposed role of the individual in bringing on the illness. Some positive and negative aspects of the sick role follow.

(1) **Secondary gain** results from the social benefits of the sick role. The person may be able to avoid work, gain financial rewards, avoid conflict, and gain sympathy.

(2) The sick role of some **"socially stigmatized" illnesses,** such as human immunodeficiency virus (HIV), mental illness, and epilepsy, may preclude the person from working, finding housing, or enjoying social relationships, all of which are independent of concrete evidence contradicting the need for social isolation (e.g., actual contagiousness of HIV, low evidence of dangerousness).

(3) Some sick roles may create disability independent of or disproportionate to the disability associated with the illness. For example, in mental hospitals and tuberculosis sanitariums, **institutionalism** produced adaptation to the hospital culture, which was often more socially disabling than the condition itself.

b. Interpersonal relationships are often altered by illness.

(1) In families, a member of the family (often a child) may be placed in the sick role to help the family avoid other major issues (e.g., substance abuse by a parent).

(2) Acutely, the sick role normally elicits caring responses from others. As the sick role becomes more chronic, it elicits increasing anger and rejection from others (even from unsophisticated physicians and caregivers).

(3) Development of socially stigmatized illnesses may elicit acute rejection from the social network (e.g., HIV, mental illness, cardiac disease in a sedentary smoker).

(4) Illness and the sick role may upset the power dynamics in a relationship. Individuals may seek to reestablish the power dynamics by precipitating another crisis.

(5) Communication between the ill person and others may become increasingly centered on the illness, creating a cycle in which exacerbation of symptoms becomes the mechanism for eliciting a response from others.

(6) Family communication style involving high levels of **expressed emotionality** is associated with many psychophysiologic disorders, as well as major mental illnesses (see Chapter 2).

c. Health-related behaviors

(1) Social, educational, and psychological factors may contribute to the tendency of an individual to avoid or engage in behaviors that increase risk of disease or injury (e.g., unprotected sex and HIV risk, smoking, substance abuse, motorcycle riding).

(2) Little is known about psychiatric comorbidity of many of these high-risk behaviors.

(3) Public health approaches to the reduction of high-risk behaviors have been largely educational and, in many cases, have been less effective than expected.

(4) Relatively little work has been done on altering lifestyle to reduce health risk using means other than education and substance abuse treatment.

IV. COMORBIDITY AND DIFFERENTIAL DIAGNOSIS. Although somatoform disorders are presented as discrete diagnostic entities, in reality the phenomenologic overlap between these disorders and other physical and psychological disorders is great. Furthermore, in contrast to other groups of psychiatric disorders, such as schizophrenia and major affective disorders, relatively little phenomenologic and diagnostic work has been done. However, the costs of these patients to the health care system in excessive disability, needless diagnostic tests, and poorly justified surgery are enormous. Patients in this group usually have mixed, complex diagnostic and treatment pictures. Some of the diagnostic blurring in the DSM-IV is intentional: It helps clinicians avoid dichotomous thinking about patients, such as, "The patient has somatization disorder; now I can make a psychiatric referral and stop looking for physical disease."

A. Major illnesses with psychological factors

1. Gastrointestinal disorders. Emotional states have long been known to cause a reaction in the gastrointestinal tract. Vague complaints of nausea, indigestion, diarrhea, constipation, and abdominal pain are common in association with psychiatric disorders.

a. Peptic ulcers

(1) **Etiology.** Gastric, duodenal, and acute posttraumatic stress ulcers all have different etiologies. The Mirsky study of United States Army recruits showed that several factors are necessary for the development of ulcers, including high stress, high pepsinogen secretion, and psychological conflict (dependency). Although conflicts involving dependency are noticeable in some ulcer patients, not all individuals affected by these conflicts are prone to developing ulcers, nor are all ulcer patients psychologically distressed.

(2) **Treatment.** Patients who comply with good medical management do not usually require psychotherapy. The physician should help the patient identify those areas of life that seem to cause stress. Also, it may be useful to teach the patient the relaxation techniques in which the patient tenses all muscles, relaxes them in

groups (e.g., arms, hands, legs, feet), then notes the resultant feeling. Hypnotic techniques may also offer good relaxation for some patients. Antianxiety agents are occasionally indicated, as are antispasmodics.

b. Ulcerative colitis

    (1) Etiology. A large proportion of familial occurrence of ulcerative colitis would suggest a genetic cause. However, the exact etiology is unknown. It has been demonstrated that exacerbation of ulcerative colitis is associated with psychological stress, and remission is associated with psychological support. Stress, such as unresolved grief on the anniversary of a death, can precipitate episodes of the disorder. Associated psychological features include:

        (a) Immaturity

        (b) Indecisiveness

        (c) Conscientiousness

        (d) Covertly demanding behavior

        (e) Fear of loss of an important individual

    (2) Treatment. Although psychotherapy cannot guarantee that the condition will not recur, it is useful when it focuses on helping patients develop mature ways of expressing needs, as well as helping them deal with unresolved losses.

c. Irritable bowel syndrome (also termed spastic colon and nervous diarrhea) is disordered bowel motility, including both hypermotility and hypomotility.

    (1) Etiology. Although the syndrome is usually associated with environmental stress, patients tend to have other psychological symptoms, such as anxiety and depression.

    (2) Treatment. Brief psychotherapy to help the patient identify environmental stress and effect changes usually aids in decreasing symptoms. Tricyclic antidepressants are also effective in this disorder.

2. Cardiovascular disorders. Much evidence suggests that the cardiovascular system reacts to the emotional state of the patient.

a. Coronary artery disease is the most common cause of death in the United States.

    (1) Etiology. Multiple nonpsychiatric elements are implicated in the development of coronary artery disease, including genetics, diet, smoking, high blood pressure, obesity, and amount of physical activity. A personality type has also been implicated, according to some studies. The **type A behavior pattern** is only one risk factor out of many, and its exact role in the development of coronary artery disease is unclear. However, men who fall into this type of behavior pattern are at twice the risk for coronary artery disease as those who do not. Characteristics of the type A personality include:

        (a) Competitiveness

        (b) Ambition

        (c) Drive for success

        (d) Impatience

        (e) A sense of time urgency

        (f) Abruptness of speech and gesture

        (g) Hostility

    (2) Treatment. Behavioral methods designed to decrease environmental stress and modify lifestyle when mutable are increasingly common.

b. Essential hypertension

    (1) Etiology. The causes of essential hypertension are unknown, but psychological factors were initially thought to involve conflicts between passive–dependent and aggressive tendencies in patients who repressed their hostility. Unfortunately, no reliable evidence is available to support this theory. On the other hand, a common reaction to stress is an elevation of blood pressure. Patients who have a biologic susceptibility to essential hypertension may react to a stressful situation by exacerbating that hypertension rather than, for example, increasing gastrointestinal motility.

    (2) Treatment of hypertension may involve biofeedback, in which the patient is attached to a machine that provides information about ordinarily unnoticed biologic parameters. For example, a tone sounds when the patient's blood pressure rises. The patient then learns to relax to decrease the tone as well as the blood pressure. Biofeedback therapy, however, tends not to be long-lasting and must be repeated to maintain the effect. Many antihypertensive agents have psychiatric effects, particularly that of producing depression. Care should be taken to avoid administering antihypertensive agents that cause depression when treating depressed patients.

c. Arrhythmias
- **(1) Etiology.** Even in the absence of heart disease, psychological factors can influence the normal rhythm of the heart beat. **Stress** may cause arrhythmias by arousing the sympathetic nervous system (as is evident in the fight-or-flight reaction). Sinus tachycardia, a paroxysmal atrial tachycardia, and ventricular ectopic beats are the most common arrhythmias to arise in reaction to stress. These reactions may be more common in patients who are already fearful of heart disease.
- **(2) Treatment** involves questioning the patient about unreasonable fears of heart disease and helping the patient to identify environmental stresses that precipitate the reaction. The condition may be part of either an anxiety disorder or a depression, which should be treated. Benzodiazepines may be useful for a limited time, as may β-blocking agents (e.g., propranolol). Contrary to a common belief among some physicians, effective treatment of depression with careful use of antidepressant medications (some of which have specific antiarrhythmic properties) may be safer than avoiding treatment for the depressed patient with cardiac disease.

3. Respiratory disorders. Changes in respiration in the normal individual may correspond to an emotional state (e.g., the sigh of boredom, the gasp of surprise). The strongest psychological reactions associated with respiratory disease, however, are those that develop secondary to the illness. The panic associated with shortness of breath can be quite disabling.

a. Hyperventilation syndrome
- **(1) Etiology.** This disorder is often associated with **anxiety,** particularly panic disorder (see Chapter 6), which may cause an increased depth or rate of breathing. In turn, this response leads to **respiratory alkalosis** and then to light-headedness, paresthesias, and carpopedal spasms. These symptoms increase the anxiety in the patient, resulting in a vicious circle of increased hyperventilation and respiratory alkalosis. Typical of hyperventilation are symptoms of shortness of breath; numbness of fingers, nose, and lips; and light-headedness.
- **(2) Treatment.** Educating the patient about the syndrome once the acute event is past may be sufficient treatment. However, if underlying anxieties continue to provoke the syndrome, psychotherapy is indicated. If the patient meets the criteria for panic disorder, pharmacotherapy can be considered as well.

b. Bronchial asthma
- **(1) Etiology.** Once thought to be caused by psychological factors, asthma attacks now are believed to be the result of a genetic vulnerability exacerbated by allergies and infections. Nevertheless, stress and an inconsistent relationship between the asthmatic child and an overly protective mother may be factors in the onset of specific episodes of illness. Both overly dependent patients who react to any slight changes of symptoms and overly independent patients who deny symptoms are at greater risk for hospitalization than are psychologically normal patients.
- **(2) Treatment.** Psychotherapy is usually indicated when anxiety, which may precipitate an asthma attack, is not relieved by the supportive care of a physician. Family therapy may be helpful in separation issues, which may also exacerbate asthma symptoms.

4. Migraine headache
- **a. Etiology.** More than 90% of chronic, recurrent headaches are migraine, tension, or mixed migraine–tension. Whereas muscle tension headaches (often with bilateral occipital or bitemporal distribution) represent muscle spasms, migraine headaches are usually unilateral and represent a period of vasoconstriction (aura) followed by

vasodilitation (headache). Although anxiety and stress commonly precipitate all three types of headache, the theory that specific psychological dynamics (e.g., repressed hostility) lead to migraine headaches has not been proved. Many true migraine patients report development of headaches during a period of relaxation after a stressful period (e.g., examinations in college). Depression should be ruled out as a cause but treated if present.

   b. Treatment of migraine headache includes:

      (1) Drug therapy

         (a) Ergotamine

         (b) Propranolol

         (c) Tricyclic antidepressants

         (d) Calcium channel blockers (e.g., verapamil)

      (2) Biofeedback

      (3) Psychotherapy, in patients with chronic stress

      (4) Hypnosis and **imagery** to increase peripheral blood flow (e.g., imagining that hand is in warm water) to abort progression from aura to headache

 5. Immune disorders. Psychological states affect immune response in complex ways that are not yet fully understood. Stress may depress cell-mediated immune response (via T lymphocytes). Disorders of immune response may involve susceptibility to various conditions.

   a. Autoimmune diseases

      (1) Systemic lupus erythematosus (SLE)

      (2) Rheumatoid arthritis

      (3) Pernicious anemia

   b. Allergic disorders

   c. Cancer. Studies show that the patient who reacts to stress with feelings of hopelessness or depression is at higher risk for cancer.

   d. Although a controversial subject, increasing evidence suggests **immune system dysfunction** in disorders such as depression.

      (1) Evidence also suggests abnormal diurnal variation in circulating natural killer cell phenotypes and cytotoxic activity in patients with major depression.

      (2) Interleukin-1β is produced in increased amounts in patients with depression, which in turn may contribute to hypothalamic–pituitary axis dysregulation.

      (3) Mortality studies, such as record linkage studies, report increased mortality from physical illnesses that are at least indirectly associated with lack of full immunologic competence (e.g., deaths from infectious disease, neoplasms associated with major depression).

      (4) Clinicians have long noted that stresses, loss, and mental illness are associated with flare-ups in disorders kept in some control by the immune system (e.g., melanoma, tuberculosis).

B. | **General medical conditions presenting as somatoform disorders.** In all of the somatoform disorders, the patient may have an undiagnosed physical disorder with inconsistent, vague, or confusing symptoms. Several illnesses should be considered.

 1. SLE and several other autoimmune disorders are associated with multiple organ systems and are characterized by exacerbations and remissions. SLE typically begins in late adolescence or the early twenties, and women are nine times more likely to have SLE than men. The onset may be vague, and psychiatric symptoms (e.g., mood disorders, schizophreniform disorder) may be present.

 2. Endocrine disorders

   a. Hyperthyroidism (thyrotoxicosis) may be present, with complaints of fatigue, palpitations, dyspnea, and anxiety.

   b. Hypothyroidism also may present with fatigue and anxiety. Mood disorders, including depression, are possible. Menstrual problems are commonly seen and may be dismissed as a somatization problem.

    c. Hyperparathyroidism can present with severe anxiety, gastrointestinal symptoms, polyuria, and some pain.

  3. Neurologic disorders. Any physical illness that begins early in life and is associated with an insidious or intermittent onset of symptoms should be considered in the differential diagnosis of somatoform disorder.

    a. Multiple sclerosis (MS) may have transient, remitting neurologic symptoms associated with dysphoric mood and anxiety. It often is misdiagnosed as a psychiatric illness early in its course.

    b. Temporal lobe or **complex partial seizures** may cause a distorted body image as well as mood disorders and changes in personality.

    c. Acute intermittent porphyria (AIP) is rare, but it may mimic somatization disorder with its gastrointestinal pain and neurologic complaints.

    d. Other systemic diseases and toxic or metabolic diseases can present with confusing symptom pictures, particularly early in their course, and should not be dismissed as a somatoform disorder, particularly if the symptoms do not fit into the "classic" picture of the somatoform disorders.

  4. Psychiatric disorders

    a. Major depression is perhaps the most common illness presenting with complaints that are comorbid with or mistaken for somatoform disorders.

    b. Acute adjustment reactions can present with multiple somatic symptoms or preoccupation with symptoms.

    c. Schizophrenia occasionally presents with multiple somatic complaints or delusions.

    d. Panic disorders can present with multiple somatic complaints and extreme preoccupation with symptoms.

    e. Personality disorders frequently coexist with somatoform disorder and should be discriminated from the somatoform disorder for both treatment and diagnosis.

C. | **Substance abuse**

  1. Alcoholism remains the major comorbid substance abuse disorder in various psychosomatic and psychophysiologic illnesses.

  2. Although **opiates** are probably underprescribed for acute pain (e.g., following surgery, acute physical trauma), opiates prescribed for chronic pain in patients with somatization disorder, pain disorder, factitious disorder, or conversion disorder represent a threat for addiction to opiates.

  3. Other substances may become abused by the vulnerable patient. Benzodiazepines, barbiturates, psychomotor stimulants, and others may be abused by substance-abusing, somaticizing patients.

  4. Once the patient has become **habituated to a prescription** medication and uses it for relief of psychological as well as physical symptoms, **secondary drug-seeking behaviors may develop** (e.g., using multiple doctors simultaneously, magnifying or creating symptoms, and using other peoples' medications).

D. | **Dissociative disorders** (see Chapter 11)

  1. Significant association is present among somatization disorder, conversion symptoms, and dissociation symptoms.

    a. An association between somatization disorder and dissociative symptoms is so frequent that they were considered to be in the same diagnostic class in previous editions of the DSM (i.e., "psychoneurotic reactions" in DSM-I, "hysterical neurosis" in DSM-II).

    b. Recent work demonstrates a strong association among somatization, dissociation, and a history of sexual abuse.

  2. Clinically, dissociative symptoms are often found in somatization disorder patients. Some odd symptoms in somatization disorder patients (e.g., picking at skin, pulling own hair) may be mechanisms the patient has learned to keep from dissociating.

E. Major depression

1. A strong tendency exists for **major depression** to present with **somatic complaints** in some cultures, with the patient at the same time denying symptoms of depression (e.g., headaches, malaise, abdominal pain in some Asian and American Indian cultures). In most of these cases, the patient responds well to treatment for major depression.

2. **Major unipolar depression** can present atypically with symptoms resembling almost all of the somatoform disorders, particularly if psychotic and melancholic features are present.

3. In the United States, **hypochondriasis** and **body dysmorphic preoccupations** are not uncommon as features of a major depression.

4. For reasons that remain unclear, major depression is commonly missed and incorrectly treated in primary medical care settings. Even though it is easily treated, depression may be missed in the differential diagnosis in medical clinics.

5. **Depression concurrent with chronic pain** is quite common. In some studies, up to 87% of chronic pain patients suffer from major depression.

6. Somaticized presentations seem to be more common in **unipolar depression** than in bipolar depression. Some investigators propose that no somatization disorder is present in the depressed phase of bipolar disorder.

F. Anxiety disorders

1. **Panic disorder** frequently presents acutely with symptoms resembling a myocardial infarction or a pulmonary embolus. Somatic preoccupations with heart disease, seizure disorders, and brain tumors are quite common, chronically, as patients grope for an explanation of their alarming symptoms.
   a. Some studies report that panic disorder patients have between 10% and 20% comorbid rates of mitral valve prolapse on echocardiogram.
   b. Cardiovascular causes of death increase the risk of premature death in patients with panic disorder.

2. Patients with **obsessive-compulsive disorder** frequently have health-related preoccupations and rituals, which may involve contamination fears and excessive hand washing.

3. **Posttraumatic stress disorder (PTSD)** may involve physical health preoccupations, depending on the nature of the psychological trauma.

G. Psychotic disorders

1. Occasionally, patients with **schizophrenia** and **schizophreniform disorder** may have primarily somatic hallucinations and delusions. These hallucinations tend to be bizarre enough to be distinguished easily from symptoms of somatoform disorders (e.g., organs are being squeezed by someone's telepathic powers).

2. **Mood congruent hallucinations** and **delusions** involving the body rotting or having cancer are not uncommon in patients with psychotic depressions.

3. It may be difficult to distinguish folk beliefs from psychotic and somatoform disorders. If other members of the culture or subgroup share the belief system, beliefs should not be called "psychotic."
   a. **Culture-bound somatic syndromes** include **koro,** a syndrome primarily affecting Asian men, in which the patient believes that the penis is shrinking into the body, with death as the expected result; and **dhat** in India, in which loss of semen is connected to beliefs about spiritual health.
   b. In the United States, **health-related subcultures** have beliefs about such health topics as the cause of disease, nutrition, vitamin use, and crystals. On occasion, these

beliefs lead to behaviors that can cause major health problems and even psychotic symptoms (e.g., fat-soluble vitamin overdose or scopolamine poisoning from too much herbal tea).

c. Patients with limited information about health, physiology, and anatomy sometimes present with physical complaints that are grossly incorrect. This aspect should be seen as an educational problem rather than as a psychotic symptom in the absence of other symptoms of psychotic disorders.

4. **Psychotic physical delusions** and **hallucinations** generally respond to the treatment of the specific psychotic disorder producing the symptom.

H. **Other psychiatric disorders**

1. **Personality disorders** may present with a variety of physical preoccupations, concerns, and symptoms of a psychological etiology.
   a. **Patients with antisocial personality disorder** are likely to produce symptoms of malingering when legal cases promise substantial potential reward, when they can escape the legal consequences of their acts, or when they can otherwise experience profits through "secondary gain."
   b. **Borderline patients** may create injuries or harm themselves in ways that may resemble factitious disorder or malingering. With borderline patients, however, the motivation does not appear to be adopting a sick role, but rather relieving psychological distress through the self-mutilating act.
   c. **Histrionic and narcissistic personality–disordered patients** can be expected to magnify symptoms of physical illnesses as a means of making themselves the center of attention and ensuring what they believe to be adequate commitment from the health care provider.

2. **Social phobics and avoidant personality–disordered patients** may avoid health care settings because of fears of having to disrobe and talk to the doctor. They may even postpone treatment of very serious illnesses (e.g., myocardial infarctions, cancer).

V. **SPECIFIC SOMATOFORM AND RELATED DISORDERS**

A. **Somatization disorder**

1. **Epidemiology.** Approximately 1% of women have somatization disorder, and the ratio of women to men is 10:1. It is thought to be less common in individuals with higher education. Prevalence and incidence differ among cultures and ethnic groups.

2. **Etiology**
   a. Recent studies suggest a significant **genetic component** to somatization disorder. It has been linked to a high incidence of:
      (1) Alcoholism in first-degree male relatives
      (2) Antisocial personality disorder in first-degree male relatives
      (3) Somatization disorder in first-degree female relatives
   b. **Adoption studies** of female children of somatizing women showed a markedly increased rate of somatization disorder compared to control groups.
   c. **Environmental influences** are suggested by an increased rate of somatization disorder when the child is raised in chaotic circumstances, involving parental divorce, poverty, and alcoholism.
   d. Evidence of **dysfunction on neuropsychiatric tests** has led some investigators to hypothesize that patients have an impaired ability to screen out somatic sensations.
   e. **Secondary gains** of the sick role may provide a learned component of the disorder.

3. Complications
   a. Excessive medical evaluations due to frequent consultation with multiple physicians
   b. Unnecessary invasive diagnostic procedures and surgery
   c. Anxiety and depressive symptoms, which are common in this population
   d. A wide range of associated interpersonal difficulties, including marital and parenting problems
   e. Substance abuse, including prescribed medications
   f. Suicidal ideation, particularly in patients with substance abuse problems and depression
   g. Sexual function impairment (i.e., a lack of interest in sex, specific sexual dysfunctions)

4. Differential diagnosis of somatization disorder includes major depression, general medical conditions, schizophrenia, panic disorder, and hypochondriasis.

5. Treatment of somatization disorder is often frustrating for the physician. Physicians should expect and accept their own feelings of frustration and anger when managing patients with this condition. This disorder is best conceptualized as a lifelong disorder rather than a curable condition. Symptoms tend to fluctuate with stress in the patient's life. General principles of treatment include:
   a. Regular appointments, so that the patient is assured of an ongoing supportive relationship with the physician. Appointments should focus on life stresses and the patient's functioning rather than on symptoms. Recent studies have shown that supportive treatment reduces use of health services (e.g., emergency room visits), hospital days, and physician charges. Periodic visits should include a limited but reasonable examination of new symptoms.
   b. Consolidation of care with **one physician** to minimize medications, reduce surgery, and limit diagnostic evaluations to a reasonable level
   c. Avoidance of unnecessary surgery. Surgical procedures should be considered only for clear indications. The physician should thoughtfully consider the expected gains as compared to the potential complications. Frequently, the initial surgery is followed by multiple subsequent surgeries for "adhesions."
   d. Avoidance of habit-forming medications and little or no medications for questionable indications
   e. Appropriate evaluation of new symptoms when they do occur. Patients with somatization disorder are still at risk for organic illness
   f. Adequate use of antidepressant medications (i.e., not a gesture of 50 mg of amitriptyline per day). Outcome studies demonstrate a much improved outcome for somatization-disordered patients with depressive symptoms, in contrast to somatization disordered patients without depressive features.
   g. Monoamine oxidase inhibitors (MAOIs) are reported to be very effective in some cases of somatization disorder. The literature support for this finding is sparse in the United States, but is reported in other countries.

B. **Conversion disorder** (non–DSM-IV criteria)

1. Clinical presentation
   a. Associated features. Conversion disorder involves the unconscious "conversion of a psychological conflict" into a loss of physical functioning, which suggests a neurologic disease or other disease. The symptom is temporally related to a psychosocial stressor.
   (1) An **additional psychiatric diagnosis** (e.g., adjustment disorder, schizophrenia, personality disorder) can be made in 30% to 50% of patients.
   (2) Conversion disorders are also seen in patients with real organic physical illness.
   (3) **"La belle indifférence,"** in which the patient exhibits little concern over the symptoms, is sometimes present. However, it is not a reliable sign of conversion alone because a patient with a physical illness may be stoic about his condition.
   (4) **Modeling is common.** Patients may unconsciously imitate the symptoms observed in important individuals in their lives.

b. Symptoms. Although most conversion symptoms are transient, some can have a chronic course and result in a significant disability. Also, symptoms may be inconsistent with known pathophysiology, such as a stocking–glove anesthesia. The patient classically presents with an acute loss of function, which suggests neurologic disease. Symptoms may be bizarre or unusual, including:

(1) Paresthesias and anesthesias
(2) Gait disturbances (e.g., astasia, abasia)
(3) Paralysis
(4) Loss of consciousness and seizures
(5) Aphonia
(6) Vomiting
(7) Fainting
(8) Visual disturbances (e.g., blindness, tunnel vision)

2. Incidence and prevalence are not known with certainty; however, conversion disorder seems to be less common now than in the past, and it may present with less classic symptomatology than was seen previously. Conversion disorder is seen more frequently in low socioeconomic classes, and some cultures have much greater rates of conversion disorder than others. Although the disorder occurs more commonly in women, it is seen in men. Onset usually is in adolescence through the twenties; however, it can occur at any age.

3. Etiology is thought to be psychological.
  a. Two mechanisms have been described that explain the gains experienced by the patient with conversion disorder.
    (1) The primary gain is that the internal conflict is kept from consciousness.
    (2) The secondary gain is reinforcement from the environment, such as the patient avoiding unpleasant duties because of the symptoms. Some secondary gain is seen in almost all illnesses, however.
  b. Other causes that have been postulated include the following:
    (1) The less powerful individual gains control over her environment by the elaboration of symptoms (i.e., the concern and attention of others are focused on the patient).
    (2) The symptoms are learned and are then reinforced by the reactions of those around the patient.
    (3) For some patients, physiologic contributions are suggested by the fact that the symptoms are seen more frequently in patients with brain injuries and other neurologic defects.

4. Differential diagnosis. It is important to note that between 15% and 30% of patients diagnosed as having conversion disorder have an undiagnosed physical illness (e.g., MS, other neurologic conditions).

5. Prognosis. A good prognosis is associated with:
  a. Good premorbid functioning
  b. Acute onset
  c. An obvious stressful precipitant

6. Treatment
  a. Stressful events in the patient's life should be evaluated and appropriate intervention provided, such as psychotherapy or family therapy. Associated psychiatric illness (e.g., depression) should be treated, which may involve pharmacologic approaches.
  b. Confronting the patient with the fact that the symptoms are psychologically based is not helpful. While some patients come to understand the symbolic aspect of the symptom and gain conscious mastery of the conflict, most patients are receptive to the explanation that the disorder is a reaction to stress and to the reassurance that the condition will resolve over time. These interventions may allow the patient to let go of symptoms without losing face.

    c. Suggestion during hypnosis or an amobarbital (Amytal) interview that the symptoms will improve can result in dramatic resolution. Symptom substitution, suggested in the psychodynamic literature, is relatively rare in actual practice.

    d. Attention to the possibility of organic disease is critical. First, organic causes of the symptom must be considered and ruled out. If an organic condition is present, such as intoxication with anticonvulsants, treatment of the organic condition may often lead to the resolution of the conversion symptom.

C. Pain disorder

1. **Clinical presentation.** The patient complains of pain for which there is no demonstrable physical cause or pain that is excessive given the known organic pathology. Generally, this disorder results in significant impairment and inability to function.

    a. Clinical differentiation of pain disorder from chronic pain itself may be difficult. The distinction between pain disorder and chronic pain itself may not be terribly useful in daily practice. For both, accepting the patient's pain is a good starting place for treatment. Individual differences in pain threshold, depressive and anxiety symptoms, and physical pathology that may have been missed dictate caution in making this diagnosis. As pain disorder patients are followed over time, an organic cause of the pain becomes clear in a portion of the group.

    b. In some cases, **psychological factors** appear to play a role in the symptoms, such as:

        (1) Secondary gain due to financial compensation

        (2) Avoidance of objectionable work

        (3) Control of significant others

    c. In other cases, there is little indication of psychological factors.

    d. Most cases of chronic pain involve both physical and psychological contributions, which can lead to:

        (1) Problems with the physician–patient relationship

        (2) Multiple physical examinations

        (3) Unnecessary surgery

        (4) Substance abuse

2. **Incidence and prevalence** are unknown. However, pain disorder is a common condition in a primary care setting. The disorder occurs more frequently in women than in men.

3. **Etiology**

    a. Psychological factors

        (1) Patients may have learned as children to express emotions physically instead of verbally.

        (2) Patients may be unconsciously reinforced by the sick role.

        (3) When compensation for injury is an issue, patients may be consciously or unconsciously reinforced for illness behavior.

        (4) Many patients report histories of deprivation, neglect, or abuse, which may make them more vulnerable as adults.

        (5) Many patients have a history of working at an early age, holding physically demanding jobs, and centering their lives around work.

    b. Physical theories

        (1) Endogenous opiate substances (endorphins) in the brain, which raise the pain threshold, may be altered genetically, developmentally, or secondarily to stress, making these individuals more prone to continued pain.

        (2) Monoamine neurotransmitters (particularly serotonin) appear to be involved in pain inhibitory fibers in the brain stem. This neurotransmitter system may be altered genetically, developmentally, or secondarily to stress, which results in continued pain perception. This hypothesis is supported by the responsiveness of this disorder to tricyclic antidepressants.

        (3) A possible genetic component to this disorder is suggested by the increased incidence of first-degree relatives with:

            (a) Chronic pain

      (b) Depression
      (c) Alcohol dependence
      (d) Substance abuse

4. **Differential diagnosis** is discussed in IV E. This disorder requires a thorough diagnostic work-up to rule out organic pathology. Other disorders to be ruled out include hypochondriasis, somatization, depression with somatic symptoms, and schizophrenia. When secondary gain (e.g., financial compensation) is evident, conscious simulation of the pain symptom (i.e., malingering) must be considered. When the assumption of the role of a patient is repeatedly the goal of the consciously produced symptom, factitious disorder must be considered. Also, personality and cultural attributes must be taken into consideration; for example, a dramatic, histrionic presentation of organic pain should not be confused with somatoform pain disorder.

5. **Prognosis**
   a. **Duration of illness.** The longer the duration, the less likely the chance of functional recovery. Very few patients with chronic pain of greater than 5 years' duration improve.
   b. **Age.** The older the patient, the less likely the chance of recovery.
   c. **Secondary gain.** The more reinforcement—financial, social, or otherwise—for the symptom, the less likely the chance of recovery. Many clinicians who treat chronic pain refuse to treat their patients with pending litigation because of the poor outcome under these circumstances.
   d. **Coexisting personality disorder** is also a negative prognostic factor.
   e. Prominent depressive features are considered a good prognostic feature, if the patient consents to treatment for the depression. (Surprisingly, few patients actually consent.)

6. **Treatment.** This condition is notoriously difficult to treat; and although many patients can make significant improvements in functioning, few are cured.
   a. **Medications**
      (1) **Chronic narcotic use,** paradoxically, is not helpful in chronic pain because the patient becomes habituated to the narcotics, which results in a loss of the analgesic effect and a vulnerability to withdrawal symptoms. Because of the peaks and valleys of short-acting narcotic blood levels, these agents can actually exacerbate chronic pain symptoms. Detoxification can improve pain symptoms. For a minority of chronic pain patients who appear to require chronic narcotic treatment, a long-acting preparation, such as methadone, is preferable.
      (2) **Sedative–hypnotics** depress the nervous system and increase pain perceptions as well as inactivity. Therefore, they should be avoided.
      (3) **Antidepressants.** From 50% to 60% of patients report improvements in sleep, sense of well-being, and pain perception with tricyclic antidepressants (up to 87% in some studies). Some controversy exists in terms of what doses of antidepressants to use. Doses lower than antidepressant doses may be adequate for treatment of chronic pain (e.g., 75–125 mg amitriptyline or equivalent per day) versus an antidepressant dose (150–225 mg per day for adults). Antidepressant doses must be adjusted carefully because of the other medications these patients may be taking.
   b. **Therapy**
      (1) **Psychotherapy.** Supportive approaches are useful in helping the patient deal with life stresses that may exacerbate pain symptoms. Cognitive and interpersonal therapy are indicated if the patient has prominent depressive or anxiety symptoms.
      (2) **Behavioral therapy** focuses on reinforcing wellness instead of sick role behavior. Although this approach may not affect the patient's perception of pain, it is effective in improving the patient's level of functioning. By reducing the

secondary gain from the symptoms, the patient may devote less attention to the pain.

(3) **Family therapy** is a useful adjunctive approach when family dynamics reinforce the patient's sick role and undermine attempts to improve functional capacity.

(4) **Group therapy,** where available, is a useful adjunct in supporting the patient's efforts to improve functional capacity.

c. **Multidisciplinary approaches,** which are usually available in pain clinic settings, allow a comprehensive treatment plan, which some patients may need to maximize their functioning. It may involve the previously mentioned strategies, as well as:

(1) Physical therapy

(2) Occupational therapy

(3) Biofeedback training

(4) Relaxation techniques

(5) Hypnosis

(6) Acupuncture

(7) Neurosurgical ablation of pain tracts

(8) Transcutaneous electrical stimulation

7. Prevention

a. Information about preventing pain disorder is inadequate.

b. Some pain experts suggest that, paradoxically, inadequate treatment of acute pain may lead to the development of chronic pain. These experts suggest adequate prescription of narcotics following surgery or physical trauma, but they avoid chronic narcotic prescriptions.

c. Adequate screening and treatment of major depression and other psychiatric disorders are helpful in people whose pain complaints extend beyond the expected time or severity following surgery or trauma.

D. | **Hypochondriasis**

1. Clinical presentation. Patients are chronically preoccupied with fears that they have an illness despite thorough evaluation and reassurance from the physician that no organic problems can be found. Some experts on this disorder divide the cases into **primary hypochondriasis,** which exists secondary to only a stressor, and **secondary hypochondriasis,** which occurs in the course of another psychiatric illness. Primary hypochondriasis is relatively rare.

a. **Normal physical sensations,** such as sweating and bowel movements, **are misinterpreted. Minor ailments,** such as cough or backache, **are exaggerated.** Minor physical symptoms are interpreted as being of sinister health significance, and vigilance may become a form of autosuggestion. In primary hypochondriasis, the fear and misperception become a cyclic, self-reinforcing pattern. For example, a cough or a mole may be feared to be cancerous, and close observation of the cough or mole convinces the patient that the fear is realistic.

b. **"Physician shopping"** is common and is a frustration for both the patient and physician. Simple reassurance that the feared symptom is not serious is interpreted by the patient as evidence that the physician is not taking the situation seriously. The patient then seeks another doctor.

c. **Anxious and depressed mood** as well as obsessive-compulsive features are commonly observed, and suggest a good prognosis with treatment of the primary condition.

d. **Impairment** can be mild or so severe as to result in invalidism.

e. In general, these patients do not accept the idea that they have a psychiatric disorder.

2. Incidence and prevalence

a. As many as 1% of the population may be hypochondriacal, and it is commonly seen in medical practice. Equal numbers of men and women are affected.

b. Usual age of onset is 20 to 30, but patients most commonly present to the physician in their forties and fifties.

3. **Etiology.** Secondary hypochondriasis is thought to be a part of the familiar symptoms that develop in the primary illness, such as the foreboding of anxiety, the hopelessness of depression, or the delusional beliefs of schizophrenia. **Cognitive and behavioral theories** suggest the cyclic pattern of fear, vigilance, and distorted reasoning, which are also common to the development of phobias. **Psychodynamic theories** focus on possible developmental contributions. Patients with the primary disorder may have been raised in homes where excessive concern about illness or little parental warmth was shown except when the child was ill.

4. **Differential diagnosis.** Other conditions that must be ruled out are:
   a. Depression
   b. Panic attacks
   c. Obsessive-compulsive disorder
   d. Schizophrenia
   e. Somatization disorder
   f. Actual physical pathology
   g. Personality disorders (if comorbid condition, a poor prognostic feature)

5. **Treatment**
   a. Physician reaction to hypochondriacal patients is often negative. The physician who is unaware of such feelings may act on them in an antitherapeutic way, such as over-prescribing medication or performing unnecessary diagnostic procedures.
   b. The fact that the patient is concerned and wants assistance should be acknowledged early in treatment. A sympathetic, educational approach to the patient is ideal. Once rapport is established, screening for other conditions, particularly depression, anxiety, and obsessive-compulsive disorder, should be undertaken. Regular follow-up appointments to evaluate new symptoms are often helpful and reassuring.
   c. It may be necessary to prescribe medication; however, the patient should be told that it will help but not "cure" the ailment. Narcotics and other habit-forming drugs should not be prescribed in the absence of physical pathology (although hypochondriacal patients can also get broken legs, for example, which should be treated normally).
   d. Pimozide is reported to be dramatically effective in some patients with hypochondriasis of a delusional intensity, but is not approved for this use in the United States. It is approved in the United States only for the treatment of Tourette disorder.

E. Body dysmorphic disorder

1. **Clinical presentation.** The hallmark of this disorder is preoccupation with some imagined defect in the body, usually of the face. Usually a history shows frequent visits to doctors, especially dermatologists or plastic surgeons. Depressive mood and obsessive-compulsive traits are common.

2. **Incidence and etiology** are unknown. Even epidemiologic studies admit probable underestimation of the prevalence of the disorder, because most of these patients have shame about reporting their symptoms.

3. **Differential diagnosis**
   a. If the symptom is of delusional intensity, it should be classified as a **delusional disorder, somatic subtype,** which may be responsive to antipsychotic medication.
   b. Major depression and schizophrenia should be ruled out. This process may be difficult if distorted ideas about the body reach delusional proportions. Many patients with body dysmorphic disorder have symptoms such as ideas of reference related to their symptoms.
   c. Recent evidence suggests strong links between obsessive-compulsive disorder and body dysmorphic disorder, and also that they sometimes co-occur.

    d. Anorexia nervosa and body dysmorphic disorder should be differentiated.

    e. Personality disorders in the context of this disorder represent a poor prognostic feature.

4. Treatment

    a. Invasive diagnostic procedures or unnecessary surgery should be avoided. When reconstructive surgery is undertaken, the patient is unlikely to be satisfied with the results.

    b. Recent literature reports good response from **fluoxetine** and **clomipramine** for many with this disorder.

    c. Canadian and European literature suggest that **pimozide** may be effective in treating this disorder.

    d. Insight-oriented psychotherapy has been ineffective; an educational–supportive approach has been reported to have some success.

F. **Environmental illness.** A relatively new phenomenon, environmental illness is a poly-symptomatic disorder that some think is associated with immune system dysfunction and allergy-like sensitivity to many compounds in food and air. Early studies suggest an association with increased somatic, mood, and anxiety symptoms suggestive of personality disorders. Clinicians working with this population report very high levels of depression and anxiety in this population. This phenomenon may represent the emergence of a new culture-bound disorder in the United States and Europe, as was found with people who compulsively exercise to the point of physical damage.

VI. FACTITIOUS DISORDER

A. **Clinical presentation.** Patients are in voluntary control of their symptoms of physical illness in that, although their behavior is deliberate, what precipitates this behavior is not.

    1. Symptoms may range from complaints of pain when patients feel no pain to self-inflicted infection, such as that arising from self-injection with feces or saliva, which can develop into life-threatening illness. The medical knowledge of patients is often highly sophisticated. By complaining of bizarre or unusual symptoms, these patients may encourage invasive diagnostic procedures, such as laparotomy or angiography. Patients may lie about any aspect of their history with a dramatic flair (**pseudologia fantastica**). Narcotic abuse and addiction are associated findings in about one-half of these patients.

    2. History. At hospital admission, patient behavior is disruptive and demanding. Symptoms change as work-ups prove negative. Eventually, patients are confronted with evidence of faking, and they usually react angrily and leave against medical advice. This pattern of behavior can become chronic and involve multiple admissions to different hospitals. It is then called **Munchausen syndrome**.

B. **Incidence and prevalence.** The disorder may seem to be more common than it actually is because a single patient may interact with many physicians in different hospitals. It usually begins in adulthood and is a lifelong condition.

C. **Etiology.** Although an illness or operation in early childhood may be a contributing factor, the disorder is considered to be entirely psychological. There may have been an experience with a physician in early life either through a family relationship or through illness. A significant portion of these patients are employed in the health care field as paraprofessionals. Masochism has been considered an important feature in a patient who seeks unnecessary surgery. The illness has also been conceptualized as a variant of the borderline syndrome in that the physician becomes the perpetual object of transference; patients continually reenact with the physician the disordered relationship with their parents. Studies suggest relatively frequent electroencephalogram (EEG) abnormalities in this group, suggesting some central nervous system (CNS) dysfunction.

D. Differential diagnosis

1. **Physical illness.** A patient with a true physical disorder may present the symptoms with an unusual or dramatic flair, which makes the physician suspicious of faking and which is more likely to occur if the patient also has a personality disorder, including one of the following types:
   a. Histrionic
   b. Borderline
   c. Schizotypal

2. **Somatization disorder.** The symptoms are not under the patient's voluntary control, and the patient does not usually insist on hospitalization. Conversion disorder also may be present.

3. **Hypochondriasis.** The essential feature of this disorder is the patient's preoccupation with the illness in general rather than with symptoms. The symptoms are not under the voluntary control of the patient. Hypochondriasis starts later in life than factitious disorder, and the patient is less likely to insist on hospital admission or submit to dangerous diagnostic procedures.

4. **Malingering.** Although it is difficult to differentiate malingering from factitious disorder, the goals in malingering are clear to both patient and physician, and the symptoms can be stopped when they no longer serve an end. In patients with factitious disorder, the goal of the behavior seems to be the patient role itself, in contrast to other secondary gain features of malingering.

E. Treatment. A patient with factitious disorder with physical symptoms rarely receives psychiatric treatment. The physician's reactions are usually strongly negative, which also prevents psychiatric evaluation. Until the patient is willing to face the reality of a psychiatric illness and agrees to psychiatric hospitalization or treatment, the prognosis is likely to be poor. The approach to the patient is one of management rather than cure, and unnecessary diagnostic procedures should be avoided. The patient should be confronted in a calm, noncondemning manner, and the cost of the illness emotionally as well as financially should be discussed.

VII. MALINGERING

A. Clinical presentation. Malingering is **not considered a mental disorder or an illness**. Malingering individuals will fully and deliberately fake or exaggerate illness with the conscious intent to deceive others. Their reasons for faking illness (e.g., monetary and legal concerns) can be understood by examining the circumstances affecting these individuals rather than their psychological constitution. Individuals are often evasive and uncooperative upon examination, and a marked discrepancy appears between their claimed disability and the physical findings. Individuals who malinger may have an antisocial personality disorder (see Chapter 11).

B. Incidence and prevalence. True malingering is rarely seen. A physician is more likely to misdiagnose this condition in a patient with one of the somatoform disorders because the physician has a negative reaction to the patient and is unable to see that another disorder, such as hypochondriasis, is not consciously faked by the patient.

C. **Differential diagnosis.** In **factitious disorder** with physical symptoms, the goals of the patient cannot be clearly understood, as they can in the case of malingering, even though the patient is voluntarily causing the symptoms of illness.

D. **Treatment.** Because malingering is not an illness, it has **no medical or psychiatric treatment**.

VIII. **PLACEBO RESPONSE** has been defined as any effect attributable to a medication, procedure, or other form of therapy but not to the specific pharmacologic property of that therapy. For instance, 30% to 40% of patients in pain respond as well to placebos as they do to morphine. No particular personality type responds to a placebo (e.g., a histrionic patient is no more likely to have a placebo response than is any other patient). Physicians use the placebo response (mistakenly) to help differentiate "real" from "psychological" symptoms in their patients. The placebo response is a powerful aspect of most medical care. It operates commonly, even when the physician is unaware of it. However, **it does not differentiate physical from psychological symptoms**. Recent findings suggest that the placebo response to pain is a **physiologic phenomenon**. Placebo response can be blocked by a narcotic antagonist, naloxone, which suggests that the analgesic effect of a placebo may be based on the action of endorphins, the naturally occurring opioid substances in the brain, which raise the pain threshold. Training in hypnosis can help the physician take maximum advantage of placebo effect in the treatment of patients.

DIRECTIONS: Each of the numbered items or incomplete statements in this section is followed by answers or by completions of the statement. Select the ONE lettered answer or completion that is BEST in each case.

1. A 63-year-old man presents to his internist with a preoccupation with his bowel movements. He is convinced that his irregularity represents an occult cancer. Repeated examinations and a lower gastrointestinal series reveal no abnormalities. No occult blood is present in the stool. He has not had this symptom until the past year. What is the most likely diagnosis?

(A) Hypochondriasis
(B) Somatization disorder
(C) Conversion disorder
(D) Major depression
(E) Panic disorder

2. A 54-year-old pipe fitter has been unable to work for 2 years because of chronic back pain caused by lifting a heavy toolbox. Repeated neurologic and neuroradiologic examinations reveal muscle spasm and pain in the L4–L5 area, which occasionally is referred in the expected distribution. No herniations, tears, or fractures have been found. Which one of the following would be a single best intervention for this patient?

(A) Narcotic analgesics
(B) Benzodiazepines
(C) Family therapy
(D) Antidepressants
(E) Antiinflammatory agents

3. A 53-year-old Navajo man is brought to the clinic with the belief that he is ill because a witch sprinkled "corpse powder" on the door to his home, and he was contaminated by it. He now has headaches, abdominal pain, and no energy. He believes that he may eventually die from this problem. The patient believes that he saw the witch in the form of a dog or coyote at sunset one night. Which one of the following diagnoses is most appropriate for this patient?

(A) Somatization disorder
(B) Psychotic disorder not otherwise specified
(C) Conversion disorder
(D) Major depression
(E) Diagnosis deferred on Axis I

4. Which one of the following is unlikely to be found in relatives of patients with somatization disorder?

(A) Antisocial personality disorder
(B) Schizophrenia
(C) Alcoholism
(D) Somatization disorder
(E) Conversion disorder

DIRECTIONS: Each of the numbered items or incomplete statements in this section is negatively phrased, as indicated by a capitalized word such as NOT, LEAST, or EXCEPT. Select the ONE lettered answer or completion that is BEST in each case.

5. A developmentally disabled patient is being treated for grand mal seizures. A new anticonvulsant is being tried for better control of these seizures. While in the clinic, the patient falls forward out of a wheelchair onto the floor and has what appears to be a false or sham seizure. When the residential facility staff is contacted, they say that this new type of "seizure" is quite recent, corresponding roughly with the new anticonvulsant. A reasonable approach to managing the patient includes all of the following EXCEPT

(A) a tight behavioral program to negatively reinforce the sham seizures
(B) a review of the choice of anticonvulsants and their levels
(C) a review of the recent changes in the patient's living situation
(D) a psychiatric examination
(E) a case manager for the patient

6. Which one of the following is NOT typical of type A behavior?

(A) A pervasive sense of time urgency
(B) Competitiveness
(C) Ambition
(D) Halting, guarded speech
(E) Hostility

DIRECTIONS: Each set of matching questions in this section consists of a list of four to twenty-six lettered options (some of which may be in figures) followed by several items. For each numbered item, select the ONE lettered option that is most closely associated with it. To avoid spending too much time on matching sets with large numbers of options, it is generally advisable to begin each set by reading the list of options. Then, for each item in the set, try to generate the correct answer and locate it in the option list, rather than evaluating each option individually. Each lettered option may be selected once, more than once, or not at all.

Questions 7–11

Match the following symptoms to the disorder most likely to be associated with it.

(A) Somatization disorder
(B) Conversion disorder
(C) Major depression
(D) Panic disorder
(E) General medical condition

7. Unilateral temporal headache, parietal headache, or both

8. Sudden loss of sensation and flaccid paralysis of the entire left arm in a 20-year-old woman

9. Multiple chronic joint pains in a 35-year-old man with a negative work-up

10. General malaise in a 50-year-old man with a negative work-up

11. Complaints of episodic chest tightness and breathing difficulty in a 28-year-old woman with a negative work-up

ANSWERS AND EXPLANATIONS

1. The answer is D *[IV B 4; V A, B, D]*. Major depression is likely to be the diagnosis on the basis of prevalence in the population, age of the patient, and symptoms. The most significant issue is the age of onset. For all of these disorders except major depression, an onset beyond age 35 is very unusual. At the specific age of the patient, it is likely that he is facing retirement, which might be a major stressor and a threat to his identity. Given the mono-symptomatic nature of his presentation, somatization disorder is not possible. Conversion symptoms are usually neurologic in focus and usually represent a sensory or motor loss. Conversion disorder is highly unlikely. No evidence of a panic disorder is present, and the age of onset is wrong. Hypochondriasis is possible; but if it is present, it is unlikely to be primary hypochondriasis because of the onset. If it is hypochondriasis, it is likely to be secondary to major depression, which receives diagnostic priority.

2. The answer is D *[V C 6]*. One would never treat a patient on the basis of such limited information or limit treatment to a single intervention. However, given the chronicity of the pain, the disproportionate level of disability, and the stability of the condition, antidepressants would probably be the best choice. The only bad choice of the group would be a narcotic analgesic. Although effective in the treatment of acute pain, the role of narcotics in chronic pain is quite limited. The chances are that this patient would become habituated without long-term benefit from narcotics. The doses of antidepressant are controversial; some clinicians believe that a non-antidepressant dose is adequate, whereas other clinicians advocate an antidepressant dose.

3. The answer is E *[IV G 3]*. Without culture-specific information, the clinician has no idea whether this man's beliefs are associated with the beliefs of his cultural group. In this case they are. A common error is to assume that the man's seeing the dog or coyote is a psychotic symptom and to treat him with a neuroleptic. Not only would this not help him, it exposes him to unnecessary additional risk. The patient may have a major depression on the basis of his symptoms, but his depression may have been triggered by his belief that he has been the victim of a witch. The symptoms do not follow the pattern of a conversion or somatiza-

tion disorder. In this case, the clinician's best choice is to defer the diagnosis and to seek consultation from another member of the culture, ideally a health care provider or traditional healer.

4. The answer is B *[II A 4; IV B 4 c, C; V A]*. Somatization disorder, conversion disorder, alcoholism, and antisocial personality disorder are found in the families of patients with somatization disorder. Schizophrenia is not reported to have a familial link to somatization disorder.

5. The answer is A *[III C 1 c; IV B 3; V B 6 d]*. This new symptom may be caused by a number of etiologies. Particularly in the developmentally disabled, an anticonvulsant that significantly impairs thinking or level of consciousness may cause the sham seizures to appear, either at therapeutic or toxic levels. This anticonvulsant is the most likely cause given this patient's history. However, negative events in the patient's living situation may cause the appearance of conversion symptoms, particularly in patients with limited verbal abilities. The patient may have been sexually abused in the residential setting, for example. In addition, other psychiatric disorders (e.g., major depression) could readily cause the symptoms. A case manager might be helpful both for determining what changes in the patient's life may explain the symptoms and for changing the patient's care plan if necessary.

6. The answer is D *[IV A 2 a]*. A pervasive sense of time urgency, competitiveness, ambition, and hostility are typical of the type A behavior pattern of increased risk for myocardial infarction; guarded, halting speech is not. In fact, the person with type A behavior has pressured, rapid speech and tends to interrupt before the other person has finished a sentence. Although this profile indicates a greater risk for myocardial infarction, recovery from a myocardial infarction is generally better for a type A person than for a person with type B behavior.

7–11. The answers are: 7-E *[I E; III C 3 a; IV A, B]*, **8-B** *[II A 4; IV D; V B]*, **9-A** *[II A; IV D; V A]*, **10-C** *[IV E]*, **11-D** *[IV F 1]*. Unilateral presentations of headache usually represent organic pathology, specifically migraine headaches. It is also possible that on the basis of the limited data, several other forms of organic illness might be the cause. It is unlikely to be a conversion symptom or a symptom of somatization disorder because of the unilateral presentation, and it is not likely to be the headache associated with depression, which is commonly bifrontal, nor the occipital headache of muscular headache associated with anxiety.

The sudden onset of a sensory and motor loss in the left arm could be caused by a neurologic illness (e.g., multiple sclerosis, stroke, cervical injury) but would be unlikely given the overlapping distribution of the sensory and motor losses, which do not follow more specific nerve distributions. If it is a conversion symptom, it could also be associated with somatization disorder. However, the unexplained joint problems are much more characteristic of somatization disorder, leaving conversion disorder as the best diagnosis in this case.

Although the sudden loss of neurologic function in the left arm could certainly occur in a patient with conversion disorder, a better match is the joint pains, which are more unique to somatization disorder, in the absence of physical and laboratory findings.

Once again, the process of elimination helps to make this match. A unilateral headache is unusual in a patient with either depression or the somatoform disorders. General malaise could easily be caused by any number of medical illnesses, ranging from hypothyroidism to hypokalemia. However, general malaise is also a common complaint in patients with major depression, making this the best answer.

Complaints of difficulty breathing and tightness in the chest can certainly be caused by general medical conditions, such as a myocardial infarction. The episodic nature of the complaint makes an arrhythmia possible, as well as several more exotic conditions. However, the age of the patient and the type of presentation make this case relatively typical of early panic disorder.

Chapter 8

Sexual and Gender Issues
Gordon L. Neligh

I. **NORMAL SEXUAL RESPONSE**

A. **General issues**

1. **Sexuality is a part of the human condition** and involves all aspects of the biologic, psychological, and social framework. It concerns not only the mental and physical aspects of an individual's life but the cultural, social, and religious aspects as well. In the past decade, much has been learned about the complexity of human sexuality, making many of the assertions of 10 years ago much less certain.

2. **Assessment of sexual functioning by the physician** should be routine in the complete medical evaluation, but often is not because of the physician's attitude and anxiety. Psychiatrists also may be less eager than in the past to inquire about sexual functioning. Media attention to sexual abuse by trusted caregivers may cause some physicians to fear that questions about sex will be misperceived by the patient. However, to understand sexual disorders, the physician must be comfortable with sexual issues and must understand normal sexual function, including the stages of sexual response.

B. **Stages of sexual response.** Physiologic studies have greatly increased the understanding of both healthy and impaired sexual functioning.

1. **Arousal**
   a. **Physical stimulation** of the genitals, bowel, or bladder may produce an involuntary sexual response via spinal reflex through sacral parasympathetics.
   b. **Psychic stimulation** is mediated through a complex neural pathway involving at least the limbic system, the hypothalamus, and the lateral spinal cord.
   c. **Physiologic response**
      (1) **Erection and lubrication** are influenced by several **neurotransmitter systems**.
         (a) **Cholinergic nerves** were believed to be responsible for erection in the male and pelvic vasocongestion in the female. The failure of atropine (an anticholinergic) to block these responses suggests that cholinergic nerves are only a part of this response.
         (b) The ability of β_2-adrenergic stimulants and α-adrenergic blocking agents to enhance erection suggests that **adrenergic neurons** are involved in sexual arousal and focus attention on vascular mechanisms of arousal in both sexes.
         (c) **Vasoactive intestinal polypeptide (VIP)** is found in high concentrations in male and female erectile tissues and may enhance cholinergic neurotransmission, accounting for the inability of atropine to block vasocongestion and erection.
      (2) **Vascular mechanisms** for vasocongestion and erection have been the focus of recent attention.
         (a) **Classic studies** suggest that polsters, which are pads located between erectile bodies and arterioles, may permit increased blood flow into erectile tissues.
         (b) **Recent studies** focus on the role of pelvic musculature in controlling both arterial inflow and venous outflow as primary mechanisms for erectile tissue function.

2. Excitement
  a. Men. Approximately 20 to 30 seconds after stimulation, erection of the penis begins as blood flow into the erectile tissue increases.
    (1) Physiologic changes. The urethral meatus dilates, the testes elevate slightly, skin temperature increases, the heart rate increases to 100 to 180 beats per minute, and diastolic pressure increases by 20 to 40 mm Hg.
    (2) Measurement of arousal. Penile tumescence (as measured by plethysmometry) is considered the most reliable measure of arousal state.
  b. Women
    (1) Physiologic changes. The breasts increase in size, and the nipples become erect. The labia majora and minora engorge with blood and spread. The clitoris lengthens. The skin flushes, and skin temperature increases. Heart rate and blood pressure increase.
    (2) Measurement of arousal. Physiologic changes may not correlate with a subjective sense of arousal. Arousal in women may be most reliably measured by vaginal blood photometric devices.

3. Plateau
  a. Men. The testicles elevate and become engorged with blood. Secretions from Cowper gland appear on the glans of the penis. The scrotum thickens and looses all the skin folds. There is general muscle tension and hyperventilation.
  b. Women. The clitoris becomes very sensitive and retracts. The labia deepen in color. The orgasmic platform develops, in which the outer one-third of the vagina narrows due to swelling and muscle tension, and the inner two-thirds lengthen and widen. The vagina becomes lubricated, general muscle tension increases, and there is hyperventilation.

4. Orgasm
  a. Men. The sensation of ejaculating inevitably occurs before orgasm. The muscles of the perineum contract rhythmically, and the prostate gland, seminal vesicles, and urethra also contract, causing the emission of semen.
  b. Women. There may be a variety of experiences in women. The orgasmic platform contracts rhythmically, and the rectal and urethral sphincters close. The controversy of whether there are one or two types of female orgasms (i.e., clitoral and vaginal) remains unresolved.

5. Resolution
  a. Men. Detumescence of the penis occurs. There is general muscle relaxation. The testes become uncongested and descend. There is a refractory period during which the male cannot have an erection. The length of the refractory period increases from approximately 1 or 2 minutes in adolescents to several hours in older men.
  b. Women. There is a general relaxation. Vasocongestion is lost, and the labia return to their original size, shape, and color. The inner vagina remains distended for several minutes. Women do not have a refractory period and are able to achieve another orgasm immediately.

II. NORMAL SEXUAL FUNCTION AND GENDER IDENTITY DEVELOPMENT

A. Definitions

  1. Gender identity is the psychological sense of being masculine or feminine rather than the biologic state of being masculine or feminine.

  2. Gender role is the social behavior that allows others to categorize the person as male or female.

  3. Sexual orientation is the erotic attraction felt toward persons or objects of a particular type.

4. **Sexual identity** refers to biologic sexual characteristics, such as genitalia, hormonal composition, and secondary sexual characteristics.

B. **Sexual development**

1. **Sexual differentiation.** The early embryo is undifferentiated sexually. The Y chromosome is necessary for the development of complete male genitalia, although male-appearing genitalia may be formed in the presence of high levels of androgens in XX fetuses. If the fetus is XX and is not exposed to excessive androgens, female external genitalia will develop. Genetic problems and changes in hormones during embryonic development may lead to intersex conditions, hermaphroditism, pseudohermaphroditism, and other conditions that are beyond the scope of this chapter.
   a. **Androgens** are produced by the fetal testicles and by the adrenal glands. The androgens influence the organization of the developing brain, which later influences "male" behavior.
   b. Among other effects, **testosterone** may be associated with changes in brain structure, including the relative size increase of the nondominant hemisphere and of the interstitial nuclei of the anterior hypothalamus, and in reduction in intrahemispheric connections.
   c. **Estrogen.** It was previously believed that only androgens were important in sexual differentiation of the brain (i.e., a developing brain without androgen exposure would develop into a "female" brain). It is now known that estrogen also has a masculinizing effect upon the brain and appears to be necessary for the normal development of both male and female brains.

2. **Gender designation.** An infant is assigned a gender on the basis of genitalia and is reared with all of the parents' and society's attitudes regarding that gender. Gender identity appears to be set by 3 years of age.

C. **Sexual development and gender identity theories.** In humans, behavior that is masculine or feminine appears to be determined more by learning and culture than by biology. Theories about the development of sex roles have undergone major revisions in recent years.

1. **Sexual development theories**
   a. **Prenatal factors.** In addition to chromosomal makeup, the amount of androgen present or absent in the fetus determines whether male or female genitalia will develop. Testes begin to develop at the fetal age of 6 weeks if fetal testicular androgens are present. External genitalia are morphologically complete by 14 weeks of fetal life.
   b. **Infancy (0 to 18 months).** Masturbation is common and normal between the ages of 15 to 19 months. Parental attitudes about the infant's sex influence the parents' interaction with the infant. For example, encouragement of aggressive behavior, rough play, and role-related social play may all be affected by attitudes regarding sexual roles.
   c. **Toddler (18 months to 3 years).** According to some theories, core gender identity is set by the end of the toddler years. Major developmental tasks of this phase include emergence of control over bodily functions. Children become aware of the anatomic differences between the sexes.
   d. **Preschool (3 to 6 years).** Masturbation appears to be recognized as pleasurable by the child. The child appears to be aware of anatomic differences as they relate to gender roles. Some theorists believe that gender role is largely determined during this period.
   e. **School age (6 years to adolescence).** Little is known about sexuality during this period. It was called "latency" age because of what appears to be a lack of sexual development and new sexual behavior in the age group. However, identity issues related to gender, peer group, and self-esteem are clearly issues in this age group.
   f. **Adolescence.** A great deal of sexual behavior occurs during adolescence, including experimentation with heterosexual, homosexual, and masturbatory experiences. Peer group identity, which is of major importance in adolescents, may contribute to the

types of sexual experiences to which the adolescent is exposed. On average, boys report having had their first sexual experience at 16 to 17 years of age, whereas girls reportedly have their first sexual experience at 18 years of age.

g. Adulthood. Changes in gender role, relationships, and expressed sexual orientation may occur throughout much of the life cycle. For example, a middle-aged man or woman may "come out" as gay in relation to a mid-life existential crisis, or a previously isolated person may find a relationship that kindles or rekindles sexual behavior.

h. Late adulthood. Sexual behavior continues throughout the lifecycle. Although the deleterious effects of medical illnesses on sexual function may increase with age, it is not normal for sexual functioning to stop in the elderly.

2. Psychodynamic theories follow the thinking of Sigmund Freud and subsequent psychoanalysts.

a. Much has been written about how disturbances of certain phases of development affect the formation of sexual identity and paraphilias. There is a lack of prospective research supporting many of these ideas, and they have largely been abandoned by psychoanalysts.

b. Newer schools of thought also explain both normal and pathologic sexuality as effects of developmental problems, but they emphasize different psychodynamic models (e.g., separation–individuation, formation of a stable self). For example, a patient suffering from borderline personality disorder may be expected to demonstrate "polymorphous perversity" in having indiscriminate sex of many types because of an unstable self, seeking intense relationships at any cost.

3. Learning theory models are less associated with the developmental phase than with patterns of imitation, fantasy, and reinforcement. For example, according to these models, when a child is able, he may **imitate the gender role behavior** of individuals of the same sex or opposite sex encountered in his environment.

a. Patterns of positive, negative, or absent **reinforcement of these behaviors** may lead to gender role-specific patterns of behavior.

b. Likewise, in adolescence or later, a person may be exposed to a sexual stimulus (either internally or externally generated) and may masturbate using the fantasy as a stimulus for arousal. If the pattern is not interrupted, a cycle of self-reinforcing, erotic orientation can be created.

c. For example, the adolescent who has an experience experimenting with sex with younger children may masturbate to this fantasy and, over time, consolidate a pedophilic sexual orientation. This model has been particularly useful in understanding the more unusual paraphilias as well as socially sanctioned, "normal" sexual orientation.

4. Biologic theories. Much of the research over the past decade has focused on the biology of sexuality and sexual behavior. Current controversies focus on whether neuroanatomic and endocrinologic differences exist between homosexuals and heterosexuals. The extent to which endocrine and neuroanatomic differences between men and women contribute to a wide range of social and sexual behaviors has also been controversial.

a. Attempts to show biologic differences between heterosexuals and homosexuals have been inconclusive.

(1) Family pedigree and twin studies suggest that male homosexuality may have some genetic component, although data in this area is not extensive.

(2) Le Vay's finding of smaller anterior hypothalamic nuclei in homosexual men and women than in heterosexual men is subject to methodologic concerns raised by Le Vay himself.

(3) Early reports of higher testosterone in heterosexual than in homosexual men have not been proved. The finding may have resulted from higher marijuana use by the homosexual men in the sample.

(4) Early reports of higher luteinizing hormone (LH) response to estrogen administration in homosexual men than in heterosexual men (similar to the LH response in women) failed to replicate in later studies.

(5) Theories that homosexuals are more associated with **maternal stress** (and possibly maternal high levels of stress hormones) have not survived well-designed studies of recent years.

(6) **Animal models** of homosexuality, particularly the rat, have been disreputed for a number of methodologic reasons.

b. A variety of hormones regulate the aspects of sexuality in both men and women.

(1) **Men.** In a number of experiments in males, the administration and withdrawal of testosterone are clearly associated with frequency of sexual thoughts and desires but not with erectile function. In aging males, the levels of testosterone and human chorionic gonadotropin (hCG) decrease, and the levels of estrogen, LH, and follicle-stimulating hormone (FSH) increase. Reportedly, prolactin decreases and luteinizing hormone–releasing hormone (LHRH) increases sexual desire and functioning.

(2) **Women.** Androgens are associated with increased coital frequency, higher sexual gratification ratings, and more intense and prolonged responses to erotic stimuli. However, androgens are also associated with fewer sexual partners, lower partner-related activity, and higher masturbation frequency.

(a) There is some evidence that **progesterone** decreases and estrogen increases sexual interest. Progesterone also appears to have behavioral effects; low levels of this hormone are associated with postpartum sadness and "blues" in some women.

(b) **Estrogen** is responsible for "masculinizing" sexual behavior in animal models. In humans, estrogen stimulus produces an LH response in women but not in men. Estrogen may be responsible for a number of human behaviors, including reports of exogenous estrogen precipitating panic attacks in some women and creating a sense of well being in others.

(c) **Prolactin** levels are at least indirectly associated with reduced interest in sex.

5. **Social factors.** People may form social groups based on their sexual orientation, such as homosexuals or sadomasochists. There is remarkably little psychiatric literature about these groups and their role in the lives of those individuals. This may be a result of the persecution by religious or political groups of people with certain sexual orientations.

III. **SEXUAL AND GENDER IDENTITY DISORDERS** as defined in the *Diagnostic and Statistical Manual of Mental Disorders,* 4th edition (DSM-IV) are a larger group than described under earlier diagnostic systems. Nevertheless, the DSM-IV does not describe all the sexual disorders and gender identity disorders encountered in clinical practice. The DSM-IV has a more descriptive approach, and it contains less of presumed etiology than in earlier diagnostic approaches.

A. **Descriptions.** The DSM-IV diagnostic groups include the following disorders.

1. **Hypoactive sexual desire disorder** is described as an absence or deficiency of sexual fantasies and a lack of desire for sexual activity that is persistent or recurrent. The judgment of deficiency or absence is made by the clinician, who accounts for factors that affect sexual function, including the age and the context of the person's life (i.e., issues of interpersonal conflict, grief, isolation).

   a. The disturbance causes marked distress or interpersonal difficulty.

   b. The sexual dysfunction is not better acounted for by another Axis I disorder (e.g., major depressive episode, panic disorder, somatization disorder) and is not due exclusively to direct physiologic effects of a substance of abuse, a medication, or a general medical condition.

2. **Sexual aversion disorder** is described as a persistent or recurrent extreme aversion to, and avoidance of, all (or almost all) genital sexual contact with a partner.

   a. The disturbance causes marked distress or interpersonal difficulty.

   b. The sexual dysfunction is not better accounted for by another Axis I disorder.

3. **Female sexual arousal disorder** is described as a persistent or recurrent inability to attain or to maintain an adequate lubrication–swelling response until completion of the sexual activity.
   a. The disturbance causes marked distress or interpersonal difficulty.
   b. The sexual dysfunction is not better accounted for by another Axis I disorder, a substance, or a general medical condition.

4. **Male erectile disorder** is described as a persistent or recurrent inability to attain or to maintain an adequate erection until completion of the sexual activity.
   a. The disturbance causes marked distress or interpersonal difficulty.
   b. The erectile dysfunction is not better accounted for by another Axis I disorder, a substance, or a general medical condition.

5. **Female orgasmic disorder** is described as a persistent or recurrent delay in, or an absence of, orgasm following a normal sexual excitement phase. Women exhibit wide variability in the type or intensity of stimulation that triggers orgasm. The diagnosis of female orgasmic disorder should be based on the clinician's judgment that the woman's orgasmic capacity is less than would be reasonable for her age, sexual experience, and the adequacy of sexual stimulation she receives.
   a. The disturbance causes marked distress or interpersonal difficulty.
   b. The sexual dysfunction is not better accounted for by another Axis I disorder, substance abuse disorder, or general medical condition.

6. **Male orgasmic disorder** is described as a persistent or recurrent delay in, or absence of, orgasm following a normal sexual excitement phase. The clinician accounts for the person's age when judging that the sexual activity is adequate in focus, intensity, and duration.
   a. The disturbance causes marked distress or interpersonal difficulty.
   b. The sexual dysfunction is not better accounted for by another Axis I disorder, substance abuse disorder, or a general medical condition.

7. **Premature ejaculation** is described as an ejaculation that occurs with minimal sexual stimulation before, on, or shortly after penetration and before the person wishes it. This disturbance persists or recurs. The clinician must account for factors that affect the duration of the excitement phase, including age, novelty of the sexual partner or situation, and recent frequency of sexual activity.
   a. The disturbance causes marked distress or interpersonal difficulty.
   b. The sexual dysfunction is not better accounted for by the direct effects of a substance.

8. **Dyspareunia (not due to a general medical condition)** is described as recurrent or persistent genital pain associated with sexual intercourse. This condition can occur in both males and females.
   a. The disturbance causes marked distress or interpersonal difficulty.
   b. The disturbance is not caused exclusively by vaginismus or lack of lubrication and is not better accounted for by another Axis I disorder (except another sexual dysfunction). It also is not due exclusively to the direct physiologic effects of a substance. Medications associated with dyspareunia include amoxapine and thioridazine.

9. **Vaginismus (not due to a general medical condition)** is described as recurrent or persistent involuntary spasm of the musculature of the outer third of the vagina that interferes with sexual intercourse.
   a. The disturbance causes marked distress or interpersonal difficulty and is not better accounted for by another Axis I disorder, substance abuse disorder, or general medical condition.
   b. The following **subtypes** include:
      (1) **Lifelong** type, which has been present since the onset of sexual functioning
      (2) **Acquired** type, which has an onset after a period of normal functioning
      (3) **Generalized** type, which is not limited to certain types of stimulation, situations, or partners

(4) **Situational** type, which is limited to certain types of stimulation, situations, or partners

(5) **Vaginismus due to psychological factors,** which is the subtype diagnosed when psychological factors are judged to have the major role in the onset, severity, exacerbation, or maintenance; this subtype can also be used when the sexual dysfunction, a general medical condition, or substance abuse are not the cause.

(6) **Vaginismus due to combined factors,** which is the subtype diagnosed when psychological factors as well as a general medical condition or substance contribute to the sexual dysfunction but are not separately sufficient to account for it

10. **Sexual dysfunction due to a general medical condition.** This category represents clinically significant sexual dysfunction that results in marked distress or interpersonal difficulty and predominates in the clinical picture. There is evidence from the history, physical examination, or laboratory findings that the sexual dysfunction is fully explained by the direct physiologic effects of a general medical condition. The disturbance is not better accounted for by another mental disorder (e.g., major depressive disorder). In addition to specifying the particular medical condition responsible for the dysfunction, the type of dysfunction should be specified.

11. **Substance-induced sexual dysfunction** describes clinically significant sexual dysfunction, with marked distress or interpersonal difficulty predominating in the clinical picture. The disturbance is not better accounted for by a sexual dysfunction that is not substance-induced.
    a. There is evidence from the history, physical examination, or laboratory findings that the sexual dysfunction is fully explained by substance use by either of the following:
       (1) The symptoms of Criterion A, which develop during or within a month of substance intoxication
       (2) Medication use, which is etiologically related to the disturbance
    b. The type of dysfunction should be specified (e.g., substance-induced sexual dysfunction with impaired desire).

12. **Sexual dysfunction not otherwise specified** includes sexual dysfunctions that do not meet the criteria for any specific sexual dysfunction (e.g., absence of subjective erotic feelings despite physiologically normal arousal and orgasm).

13. **Exhibitionism.** Over a period of at least 6 months, recurrent, intense, sexually arousing fantasies, sexual urges, or behaviors involving the exposure of one's genitals to an unsuspecting stranger occur. The fantasies, sexual urges, or behaviors cause clinically significant distress or impairment in social, occupational, or other important areas of functioning.

14. **Fetishism.** Over a period of at least 6 months, recurrent, intense, sexually arousing fantasies, sexual urges, or behaviors involving the use of nonliving objects (e.g., female undergarments) occur.
    a. The fantasies, sexual urges, or behaviors cause clinically significant distress or impairment in social, occupational, or other important areas of functioning.
    b. The fetish objects are not limited to articles of female clothing or to devices designed for the purpose of tactile genital stimulation.

15. **Frotteurism.** Over a period of at least 6 months, recurrent, intense, sexually arousing fantasies, sexual urges, or behaviors involving touching and rubbing against a nonconsenting person occur. The fantasies, sexual urges, or behaviors cause clinically significant distress or impairment in social, occupational, or other important areas of functioning.

16. **Pedophilia.** Over a period of at least 6 months, recurrent, intense, sexually arousing fantasies, sexual urges, or behaviors involving sexual activity with a prepubescent child or children (generally 13 years of age or younger) occur. The fantasies, sexual urges, or behaviors cause clinically significant distress or impairment in social, occupational, or other important areas of functioning.

   a. The pedophile is at least 16 years of age and at least 5 years older than the child or children in Criterion 1.
   b. Subtypes include:
      (1) Sexually attracted to males
      (2) Sexually attracted to females
      (3) Sexually attracted to both sexes
      (4) Limited to incest
      (5) Exclusive type
      (6) Nonexclusive type

17. **Sexual masochism.** Over a period of at least 6 months, recurrent, intense, sexually arousing fantasies, sexual urges, or behaviors occur that involve the act (real, not simulated) of being humiliated, beaten, bound, or otherwise made to suffer. The fantasies, sexual urges, or behaviors cause clinically significant distress or impairment in social, occupational, or other important areas of functioning.

18. **Sexual sadism.** Over a period of at least 6 months, recurrent, intense, sexually arousing fantasies, sexual urges, or behaviors occur that involve acts (real, not simulated) in which the psychological or physical suffering (including humiliation) of the victim is sexually exciting to the person with this disorder. The fantasies, sexual urges, or behaviors cause clinically significant distress or impairment in social, occupational, or other important areas of functioning.

19. **Transvestic fetishism.** Over a period of at least 6 months, a heterosexual male has recurrent, intense, sexually arousing fantasies, sexual urges, or behaviors involving cross-dressing, which cause clinically significant distress or impairment in social, occupational, or other important areas of functioning. This disorder is coded as **transvestic fetishism with gender dysphoria** if the man has persistent discomfort with gender role or identity.

20. **Voyeurism** occurs over a period of at least 6 months and is described as recurrent, intense, sexually arousing fantasies, sexual urges, or behaviors involving the act of observing an unsuspecting person who is naked, in the process of disrobing, or engaging in sexual activity. The fantasies, sexual urges, or behaviors cause clinically significant distress or impairment in social, occupational, or other important areas of functioning.

21. **Paraphilia not otherwise specified** is reserved for paraphilias that do not meet the criteria for any of the specific categories (e.g., telephone scatologia, necrophilia, partialism, zoophilia).

22. **Gender identity disorder** is described as a strong and persistent cross-gender identification, not merely a desire for any perceived cultural advantages of being the other sex.
   a. Symptoms manifest as:
      (1) Insisting that he or she is of the other sex
      (2) Cross-dressing
      (3) Preferring other-sex roles in play
      (4) Having an intense desire to play stereotypical games of the other sex
      (5) During childhood, strongly preferring playmates of the other sex
      (6) During adolescence and adulthood, having a conviction that he or she has feelings typical of the other sex
      (7) Stating a desire to be the other sex
      (8) Frequently passing for the other sex
   b. The patient has a persistent discomfort with his or her sex or sense of inappropriateness in the gender role of that sex. During childhood, boys may assert that the testicles or penis will disappear or that he would be better without them; a girl may reject urinating in the sitting position. During adolescence and adulthood, the disturbance is manifested by symptoms such as a preoccupation with getting rid of primary and secondary sex characteristics or believing that he or she was born the wrong sex.
   c. The disturbance is not concurrent with a physical intersex condition (i.e., an inconsistency between genitalia and chromosomal makeup, or external genitalia is inconsistent with internal structures).

d. The disturbance causes clinically significant distress or impairment in social, occupational, or other important areas of functioning.

e. Subtypes are classified according to whether the disorder occurs in children, adolescents, or adults, and whether the person is sexually attracted to males, females, both sexes, or neither sex.

23. Gender identity disorder not otherwise specified includes conditions of gender identity disorder that are not classifiable as a specific gender identity disorder (e.g., intersex conditions; transient, stress-related cross-dressing behavior; persistent preoccupation with castration or penectomy, without a desire to aquire the sex characteristics of the other sex).

24. Sexual disorder not otherwise specified is a diagnosis of exclusion made when a sexual disturbance does not meet any criteria for a specific sexual disorder and is neither a sexual dysfunction nor a paraphilia. This diagnosis may apply to feelings of inadequacy concerning sexual performance or other traits related to gender role, or to persistent and marked distress about sexual orientation.

B. **Diagnosis of sexual and gender identity disorders**

1. Eliciting the sexual complaint may occur in response to asking the patient about his chief complaint, or by asking sexual history screening questions. If the patient has a complaint, it is necessary to **obtain baseline information,** including:
   a. Subjective distress
   b. Frequency of occurrence
   c. Effect of the condition on other areas of the patient's functioning

2. Sexual history. A thorough discussion of sexual functioning is particularly necessary for patients whose medical problems (e.g., diabetes, heart disease) predispose them to sexual problems. A sexual history should be taken at the time of the complete patient history and physical examination or the initial psychiatric interview.
   a. If sexuality is related to the presenting illness, the physician should ask, "How has your sexual functioning been affected by the illness?" or "Many patients experience changes in sexual functioning as a result of this problem. How has it affected you?" The physician should convey openness and a willingness to discuss the subject of sex.
   b. If sexuality is not addressed during the history of the presenting illness, it can be reviewed during the **review of systems**.
   (1) Pathology involving the genital organs, including venereal disease, pain, and discharge should be evaluated as well as the interest in and capacity for sexual functioning.
   (2) If a sexual dysfunction is present, a detailed sexual history is needed for further evaluation, addressing the following points:
   (a) First childhood awareness of sexuality, including attitudes and punishment
   (b) Problems with gender identity
   (c) First sexual experience, including masturbation
   (d) Age of and reaction to puberty, including menarche in women
   (e) History of sexual abuse
   (f) Patient knowledge about sex and how knowledge was acquired
   (g) First experience with a sexual partner, including intercourse
   (h) Homosexual, sadomasochistic, and other experiences and interests
   (i) Current sexual functioning, including frequency and satisfaction
   (j) Questions about extramarital partners if the patient is married
   c. Problems that may be uncovered in the sexual history include:
   (1) Concern about normal sexuality or sexual development secondary to the patient's lack of knowledge or misinformation
   (2) Sexual aspects of a pervasive problem in the relationship with the sexual partner
   (3) Sexual problems that result from the presenting medical or surgical problem
   (4) Primary sexual dysfunction that needs further evaluation and treatment

C. Etiology and differential diagnosis

1. **Medications** prescribed for medical and psychiatric conditions may have obvious or subtle effects on sexual functioning.

2. **Substances of abuse** are common causes of sexual dysfunction.
   a. **Alcohol.** Acutely, alcohol may have a culture-related, disinhibiting effect on sexual behavior. However, alcohol frequently causes acute sexual dysfunctions in both males and females and can have negative long-term effects (e.g., testicular atrophy).
   b. **Cocaine** may increase sexual behavior and interests acutely because of dopaminergic effects. With long-term use, cocaine decreases interest and performance because of depletion of central nervous system (CNS) dopamine stores.
   c. **Amphetamines** have an effect similar to that of cocaine.
   d. **Sedative hypnotics** produce a range of sexual dysfunctions during states of intoxication and withdrawal. Despite the propensity to inhibit sexual response, benzodiazepines are frequently prescribed for anxiety related to sexual performance.
   e. **Narcotics** produce sexual dysfunction with long-term use, possibly as a result of dopamine depletion.

3. **General medical conditions** may account for more than 50% of patients suffering from certain sexual dysfunctions, such as male impotence.

4. **Psychiatric disorders** that may cause sexual dysfunction or performance problems include the following:
   a. **Major depression**
   b. **Panic disorder with agoraphobia**
   c. **Somatization disorder**
   d. **Bipolar affective disorder**
   e. **Personality disorders**

D. Treatment

1. **Sexual dysfunctions**
   a. **Evaluation** is the first, most critical step in devising a treatment plan. A **medical examination,** and, if appropriate, **urologic or gynecologic examination** are indicated. **Substance abuse and psychiatric screening examinations** are the next steps in the evaluation.
   b. **Education** may be among the most effective available treatments for general sexual dysfunctions. The clinician should gently assess the patient's knowledge of sexual function and his beliefs about sex. Interventions should be tailored to the information deficits identified.
      (1) Patients may need to learn the stages of sexual arousal to solve misinterpretation problems.
      (2) A couple may need to be taught details of sexual activity to improve sexual "dysfunction."
      (3) Teaching each partner about the sexual responses of both sexes is often a major step in helping couples deal with sexual dysfunction.
      (4) Desensitizing the discussion of sexual issues for individuals and couples by teaching a language to discuss sex, provides a useful communication tool for sexual partners, or for the therapist and patient.
      (5) **Specific physiologic and anatomic education** may be helpful for some patients. For example, some patients may not know that most women cannot have an orgasm without some clitoral stimulation. These patients can be taught that in some women, sexual positions that pull down on the labia minora can provide strong, indirect stimulation of the clitoris. Often, this type of simple suggestion solves much of a patient's or couple's sexual dysfunction.
   c. **Communication training** of the couple to talk about sex and about their own wishes and needs can lead to greater intimacy. Getting both partners to agree to tell the

other partner what they enjoy and what is unpleasant is a critical step in working with the couple (if they can agree to express needs and wishes in a nonthreatening manner and learn to accept feedback nondefensively). Steps to better communication include the following:

(1) **Exploration of cultural and religious beliefs**

(2) **Examination of the "goals" of sex,** which can lead to a productive renegotiation of these goals

(3) **Teaching the couple to talk during sex,** which is often a major step in resolving minor difficulties

d. **Behavioral therapy** is also an effective group of techniques for "simple" sexual dysfunctions. Behavioral interventions usually involve education and a behavioral technique designed to address a specific problem.

(1) **Relaxation training** may be helpful for both men and women whose dysfunction is related to anxiety.

(2) **Sensate focus (male).** Couples are instructed to explore noncoital caressing, focusing on the discovery and enjoyment of sensual feelings. These exercises should have a pleasuring quality rather than a demanding quality. This allows rediscovery of sensual feelings, which may have been suppressed by the sexual problem.

(a) **Managing anxiety.** Fear of failure and pressure to perform are common in men with erectile dysfunction. Prohibition of intercourse during sensate focus sessions removes this anxiety and allows the patient a feeling of success in enjoying arousal.

(b) **Regaining confidence.** As sensate focus exercises continue, the stop–start technique may be used. After the erection has occurred, the couple ceases the sexual stimulation and allows the erection to subside. They then continue the pleasurable activity, which allows recurrence of the erection. With this technique, the man gains a sense of control of his own arousal level.

(c) **Gradual resumption of coitus.** As the couple feels more confident, gradual approximation of coitus can occur. The man first achieves vaginal containment of the penis but then withdraws so that anxiety is managed and the sense of success can continue. As the couple feels confident, active thrusting can be added with stopping and starting as needed to control anxiety.

(3) **Sensate focus (female).** Exercises are initially used for the woman to explore her own sensuality. The activities are designed to progress at the patient's own rate and to be nondemanding.

(a) The woman starts by touching her skin, breasts, and genitals and noticing the pleasurable sensations. She then progresses to caressing the genitals while noting pleasurable sensations. She is then encouraged to explore clitoral and vaginal sensations and masturbation. A vibrator may be used to provide a high level of stimulation and assist in the experience of orgasm.

(b) **Anxiety management.** Prohibiting orgasm during sensate focus exercises reduces performance anxiety. Relaxation techniques, hypnosis, and, occasionally, antianxiety agents may be used.

(c) **Strengthening pubococcygeal muscles** is associated with a high rate of orgasmic competence. This is accomplished by having the woman consciously tighten the pelvic floor muscles several times a day.

(d) **Experiencing orgasm with a partner.** After the woman has gained confidence in her ability to experience orgasm by herself, she then learns to experience it with a partner. The woman is encouraged to educate her partner about activities that she finds stimulating. She is, thus, given permission to obtain pleasure for herself in the relationship.

e. **Combined educational and behavioral techniques.** Most physicians use the **P-LI-SS-IT model** developed by Annon for the treatment of sexual dysfunction. For several sexual dysfunctions, these techniques may be effective in approximately 90% of cases.

(1) **Permission (P).** The physician's relaxed manner and interest facilitates the discussion of sexual concerns. Approval for enjoying sexual activity should be conveyed. The authority of the physician's role contributes to the effectiveness of this approach.

(2) **Limited information (LI).** In the many cases of sexual dysfunction resulting from lack of information or misinformation about sex, the physician can reassure as well as educate the patient about "normality."

(3) **Specific suggestion (SS).** This type of intervention requires physician skill, and the level of intervention depends on the complexity of the problem. Masters and Johnson, among others, have developed therapy programs for couples that employ short-term behavior approaches. After an extensive history is taken and physical and laboratory examinations are conducted, the couple is taught sensate focusing.

(4) **Intensive therapy (IT).** Patients who do not respond to the basic therapy described in permission, limited information, and suggestion may require psychotherapy and should be referred accordingly. In these cases, there are usually more complex problems in the relationship, or there is associated psychopathology.

(a) **Relationship problems** may be addressed for the individual patient through **interpersonal therapy** or **psychodynamic therapy**. Trouble with sexual relationships usually extends to other nonsexual relationships in the patient's life (e.g., a fear of abandonment may infiltrate relationships with coworkers, friends, and extended family).

(i) The therapist may focus on overcoming the fear of abandonment by exploring past relationships, by exploring feelings about current relationships, and by testing the reality of assumptions about these relationships.

(ii) Psychodynamic approaches may focus on the patient's fears and feelings about the therapist to illustrate the patient's relationship problems with people in general.

(b) **Cognitive therapy** may be particularly useful for anxious and depressed patients, whose routine styles of thinking create a pattern of incorrect interpretations of events and expectations (see Chapter 3).

f. **Couples therapy (conjoint therapy).** As with individual psychotherapy, couples therapy has a long history of use in the treatment of sexual dysfunctions, starting with Masters and Johnson. Some of the issues dealt with in couples therapy include the following:

(1) **Communication problems**

(2) **Conflict management,** in which rules for productive arguing are set

(3) **Power and control issues,** which are solved by power-sharing arrangements or, if needed, individual psychotherapy

g. **Group therapy** is reported to be effective for people with sexual dysfunctions. People with similar problems gain a great deal from sharing with each other.

h. **Medications.** In some cases of sexual dysfunction, the clinician may take advantage of a secondary effect of a medication, whereas in other cases the medication may be prescribed for its direct effects on sexual performance.

(1) **Estrogen replacement** is indicated for inadequate lubrication, atrophy of the vaginal epithelium and related pain on intercourse, and other symptoms associated with menopause. Oral and topical estrogens are effective and are commonly prescribed for these conditions.

(2) **Testosterone** is widely prescribed in the United States. This anabolic steroid increases sexual interest and functioning in testosterone-deficient males and in females.

(a) **Men.** Testosterone has no beneficial effects in males with normal testosterone levels; in fact, it may reduce secretion of endogenous testosterone. Its use may stimulate existing testicular and prostatic cancers in males.

(b) Women. For some women, testosterone may have virilizing effects, which may preclude its use.

(c) Although there is a clear use for testosterone in clinical practice, it should be used with more care than is often currently practiced.

(3) Yohimbine is a central α_2-antagonist that stimulates postsynaptic norepinephrine effects. It has been shown to be effective in the treatment of some cases of male impotence; however, it can cause cardiac problems and anxiety.

(4) LHRH, which is also known as **gonadotropin-releasing hormone (GnRH),** is a hypothalamic hormone with controversial uses. Its effects are very complex, including improving sexual characteristics in hormonally deficient men and inhibiting its own effects if used chronically in high doses. When used in pulsatile doses, it stimulates ovulation in women and testosterone production in men.

(5) Dopaminergic medications have a variety of effects on sexual performance. In some cases, L-dopa is reported to enhance sexual performance in older men, as is **bromocriptine**. The dopaminergic antidepressant **bupropion** has been shown to improve both sexual drive and performance in men and women, but increases the speed of ejaculation in men. Dopamine-blocking medications (e.g., neuroleptic medications) increase ejaculatory time and may interfere with sexual interest. Dopamine inhibits prolactin secretion and may cause amenorrhea in women.

(6) Serotonergic medications may increase prolactin secretion, decrease sexual interest, and increase time to ejaculation. Whereas patients taking serotonergic medications often find these effects disturbing, patients with premature ejaculation and depression may consider these to be beneficial effects.

(7) Phenylethylamine, a substance found in chocolate, has sexually stimulating effects in the rat. Its precise effects in humans are unknown.

2. Gender identity disorders

a. Psychotherapy. Sometimes pervasive identity problems can cause confusion and doubt about sexual and gender roles.

(1) For example, patients with **borderline personality disorder** may have histories of a variety of paraphilias and sexual dysfunctions.

(2) In other cases, the patient may experience specific **conflicts about sexuality** (e.g., patients whose parents had rigid morals and condemned sex, patients with homosexual wishes who try to perform heterosexually).

(3) In patients with **secondary gender identity disorder,** the fluctuations in the patient's dissatisfaction with his or her assigned sex allows the clinician to get a sense of the permanent versus temporary issues of the patient's gender identity.

(a) For example, the patient may be most rejecting of his or her gender in relation to conflicts with a significant person, or as a result of a depressive illness.

(b) In these cases, helping the patient to cope better with relationships or treating the depression may give the psychiatrist a better sense of the stable versus unstable parts of the patient's gender identity issues.

b. Behavioral therapies for children with primary gender identity disorder involve a number of methods of reinforcing desired gender-specific behaviors without reinforcing nondesired behaviors.

(1) Techniques range from therapeutic communities to specific rewards for desired behaviors.

(2) Many of these techniques are highly effective for modifying patterns of gender-specific play and behavior. Critics argue that they may not alter "core identity" as a person of the other sex. There is little evidence that psychotherapy, pharmacotherapy, or other psychiatric interventions can reverse established patterns of gender dysphoria in people with primary gender-identity disorder.

(3) Long-term outcome data for these approaches are sparse.

    c. Psychodynamic and psychoanalytic approaches for children with gender identity disorder focus on establishing appropriate parenting roles for parents whose relationships with each other and with the child are disordered.

        (1) For example, the therapist may help strengthen the role of the father (who is reportedly usually the weak parent) in relation to the mother.

        (2) Another therapeutic task may be to help the child form a sense of self that is separate from the mother, father, and others in the environment.

    d. Gender reassignment surgery may be indicated for patients with a stable, long-term dissatisfaction with their assigned gender.

        (1) Male-to-female reconstruction surgery is performed approximately four times more than female-to-male reconstruction.

        (2) As expected, many patients with primary gender identity disorder adapt well after surgery. Perhaps unexpectedly, a number of those with secondary gender identity disorders also do well after surgery. In general, patients who are well adapted prior to surgery tend to be well adapted after surgery.

        (3) Patients with gender identity disorder and other concurrent psychiatric disorders (e.g., borderline personality disorder) may have an increased risk of suicide after surgery (when the surgery does not solve all of the patient's problems).

            (a) Ethical problem. The psychiatrist can encourage the patient to prepare for surgery if he suspects that the patient is at risk for suicide. Or, the psychiatrist can encourage the patient to postpone surgery until the patient has reduced comorbid factors, so that the risk of suicide will be decreased after surgery. The latter option is often viewed by the patient as paternalism.

            (b) The psychiatrist may be confronted with the problem of having to continue estrogen therapy for a patient who has no intention or means of having gender reassignment surgery. In some cases, the patient prefers the half-way changes of estrogen therapy to either a purely male or female state.

                (i) Some clinicians feel that supporting this person in a half-way state is humane and appropriate.

                (ii) Other clinicians are concerned about the medical risks of this practice and may believe that this half-way state is not adaptive.

3. Paraphilias. Generally, treatment outcomes for patients with paraphilias are not impressive; mainly because this patient population often does not want treatment.

    a. Psychodynamic and psychoanalytic approaches do not seem to provide significant results in patients with paraphilias.

    b. Behavioral therapies, consisting of aversive conditioning, conditioning to heterosexual stimuli, penile plethysmometry to measure arousal, and other techniques, have been the mainstay of treatment for convicted sexual offenders for over a decade. Unfortunately, the positive results first reported from these techniques tend to be only temporary.

    c. Pharmacologic treatments have included female sex hormones, antiandrogens, and, more recently, serotonin-reuptake inhibitors. However, these treatments appear to reduce sexual drive rather than alter the patient's focus of sexual interest. As a result, these treatments may be most effective in hypersexual patients.

    d. Multimodal treatment currently appears to be the treatment of choice for patients with paraphilias.

        (1) There appears to be an almost pervasive lack of appropriate social skills among many patients with paraphilias. Group therapy is often included in the therapeutic program to teach social skills and empathy for other people. Patients in these programs may also be given medications, and they may be involved in individual therapy, behavorial therapy, or other structured programs. Coexisting psychiatric diagnoses are also treated.

        (2) Treatment outcomes are not impressive, particularly when public systems are overwhelmed by the number of patients, limited funds, and high polictical expectations for postitive outcomes in patients who do not want treatment.

IV. PREMENSTRUAL DYSPHORIC DISORDER (DSM-IV), PREMENSTRUAL SYNDROME (PMS), OR LATE LUTEAL PHASE DYSPHORIC DISORDER (DSM-III-R)

A. **Definition.** This disorder has been relegated to criteria sets and axes provided for further study in the DSM-IV, implying that it is no longer an official diagnosis. Researchers question whether it is a distinct entity, a cultural belief pattern, or an artifact of other disorders, particularly affective disorders. PMS is defined as **physical or psychological symptoms that begin the week prior to menstruation and resolve shortly after the onset of the menstrual flow.** The symptoms must be of such severity as to impair functioning.

B. **Diagnosis.** To make this diagnosis, symptoms must be charted prospectively because retrospective reports have been shown to be invalid. Up to 80% of women who complain of PMS do not meet the criteria when prospective charting is used.

1. Most women who complain of PMS without meeting the charting criteria exhibit an affective disorder, anxiety disorder, or substance abuse disorder. Of the women whose cyclical symptoms are verified by prospective charting, a subgroup meets the criteria for other DSM-IV diagnoses and should receive treatment for those disorders.

2. The diagnosis of PMS should be reserved for women with cyclic symptoms who do not meet other psychiatric diagnostic criteria.

C. **Symptoms.** Women who expect to have PMS symptoms are more likely to report symptoms, whether or not the symptoms are actually premenstrual. Although a multitude of symptoms have been described for PMS, typical complaints include:

1. **Psychological complaints**
   a. Tension
   b. Irritability
   c. Depression
   d. Anxiety
   e. Lability
   f. Food cravings
   g. Concentration difficulty
   h. Lethargy

2. **Physical complaints**
   a. Breast tenderness
   b. Weight gain
   c. Bloating
   d. Fatigue

D. **Etiology.** The cause of PMS is not well established.

1. Theories about an imbalance of estrogen and progesterone levels have not been validated.

2. There is an increasing interest in the effect of **female gonadal hormones** on CNS monoamine activity, particularly serotonin.

3. **Thyroid abnormalities** have been noted in some groups that meet the rigorous definition of PMS.

4. **Endorphin activity** may be altered by the menstrual cycle.

5. **Aldosterone** levels may be elevated, leading to water retention.

6. **Prostaglandin** levels may be elevated, leading to water retention, pain symptoms, and dysphoria.

E. **Treatment.** Since the etiology of PMS is unclear, various empirical approaches are used.

1. **Education.** The patient can be taught to recognize her cyclic fluctuations and anticipate problems. The process of charting the symptoms is helpful in promoting self-awareness.

2. **Nonspecific approaches**
   a. **Diet** should consist of regular, small meals low in sodium, sugar, and caffeine.
   b. **Substance use,** especially alcohol, should be avoided.
   c. **Regular physical exercise** reduces tension and stress.

3. **Medications** have been shown to be helpful for some patients.
   a. **Bromocriptine** is useful in alleviating breast tenderness.
   b. **Diuretics** are useful for weight gain and edema.
   c. **Prostaglandin inhibitors** are useful for dysmenorrhea pain. Some patients report that prostaglandin inhibitors help with mood, although this has not been tested.
   d. **Ovulation suppressants** (e.g., oral contraceptives) are useful for some patients.
   e. **Antianxiety medication** is useful for alleviating symptoms of tension and irritability.
   f. **Progesterone suppositories** were a popular treatment for PMS, but numerous well-designed studies have proved them to be no more effective than placebo.
   g. **Pyridoxine (vitamin B$_6$)** and **magnesium supplementation** were popular, but their efficacy is unclear.
   h. **Selective serotonin reuptake inhibitors** may have specifically beneficial effects on PMS.

DIRECTIONS: Each of the numbered items or incomplete statements in this section is followed by answers or by completions of the statement. Select the ONE lettered answer or completion that is BEST in each case.

1. A 38-year-old man presents to his family physician complaining that he has had no interest in sex for the last 4 months. There have been no significant changes in his life circumstances in the last year (e.g., divorce, death in the family, loss of job). With no additional information, the most likely cause of this patient's loss of interest in sex is

(A) personality disorder
(B) generalized anxiety disorder
(C) paranoid schizophrenia
(D) sexual aversion disorder
(E) major depressive episode

2. A 47-year-old woman presents to her primary care physician complaining of pain during intercourse. The pain has become increasingly problematic over the last 6 months. The first item in the differential diagnosis should be

(A) vaginismus
(B) atrophic vaginitis
(C) dyspareunia
(D) major depression

3. A 25-year-old man is brought to the emergency room by police. He has been rubbing his penis against unsuspecting young women in the subway. He was apprehended by police and became suicidal, saying that his arrest would ruin his job and the relationship with his family. The most likely diagnosis is

(A) major depression
(B) pedophilia
(C) frotteurism
(D) paraphilia not otherwise specified
(E) none of the above

DIRECTIONS: Each of the numbered items or incomplete statements in this section is negatively phrased, as indicated by a capitalized word such as NOT, LEAST, or EXCEPT. Select the ONE lettered answer or completion that is BEST in each case.

4. A 32-year-old woman presents with a history of difficulty reaching orgasm with her male partner, despite her initial feelings of arousal. She says that her partner attempts to keep stimulating her after his orgasm, but that when she senses his frustration, she loses her arousal. All of the following are reasonable components of treatment EXCEPT

(A) providing information for the patient
(B) sensate focus exercises
(C) assessment of medical causes
(D) couples therapy
(E) telling the patient that the problem will resolve with time

5. All of the following physiologic changes are associated with the excitement phase of sexual response in women EXCEPT

(A) erection of the nipples
(B) increase in sensitivity and withdrawal of the clitoris
(C) increase in size of the breasts
(D) engorgement and spreading of labia minora and majora
(E) increase in skin temperature

DIRECTIONS: The set of matching questions in this section consists of a list of four to twenty-six lettered options (some of which may be in figures) followed by several numbered items. For each numbered item, select the ONE lettered option that is most closely associated with it. To avoid spending too much time on matching sets with large numbers of options, it is generally advisable to begin each set by reading the list of options. Then, for each item in the set, try to generate the correct answer and locate it in the option list, rather than evaluating each option individually. Each lettered option may be selected once, more than once, or not at all.

Questions 6–9

Match each of the behavioral effects with the corresponding substance.

(A) Dopamine
(B) Prolactin
(C) Testosterone
(D) Progesterone
(E) Estrogen

6. Inhibits prolactin secretion

7. In high levels, inhibits sexual interest and performance

8. Responsible for inducing asymmetric fetal brain development

9. Administration produces a surge of luteinizing hormone (LH) in women but not in men

ANSWERS AND EXPLANATIONS

1. The answer is E *[III A 1–2]*. A major depressive episode is the most likely cause of the patient's loss of interest in sex. On a statistical basis, with a recent onset of the problem and no major life events, depression is the most likely cause of this symptom. The diagnosis of sexual aversion disorder requires ruling out Axis I disorders; therefore, sexual aversion disorder is a less appropriate choice for the starting point in the differential diagnosis.

2. The answer is B *[III A 8–9]*. On a statistical basis and on the basis of the patient's age, the physician may suspect that menopause may have decreased this woman's circulating estrogen levels, resulting in atrophic vaginitis. However, the physician must perform a pelvic examination before making a diagnosis because of the possibility that a neoplasm or other disease may be causing the pain. Diagnoses such as dyspareunia and vaginismus require that general medical conditions be excluded before making these diagnoses. Although dyspareunia is a symptom of somatization disorder, a late onset of the symptom is unusual in a patient suffering from somatization disorder.

3. The answer is C *[III A 15]*. This case is a typical example of frotteurism, although the patient is at the upper limit of the usual age range. Major depression is unlikely because there is no evidence that the patient was depressed before the police arrested him. His suicidal impulses are likely in response to his stiuation, although they must be taken very seriously.

4. The answer is E *[III A 5, D 1 b–d]*. Telling the patient that the problem will resolve spontaneously is unacceptable. The problem is just as likely to get worse with time and may endanger the couple's relationship. Although medical conditions affect a woman's ability to experience arousal more often than the ability to experience orgasm, spinal cord problems and other medical conditions may contribute to the inability to achieve orgasm. Information is often very effective in helping a woman learn to interpret physical sensations more accurately. Sensate focus exercises are both primarily helpful in getting the couple to coordinate their arousal levels and foreplay and in helping to reduce performance anxiety. Couples therapy may help the couple develop reasonable expectations of sex and decrease disappointment and performance anxiety.

5. The answer is B *[I B 3 b]*. The clitoris withdraws during the plateau phase of sexual response. Erection of the nipples, increases in breast size and skin temperature, and engorgement and spreading of the labia majora and minora are associated with the excitement phase.

6–9. The answers are: 6-A, 7-B, 8-C, 9-E *[III D 1 h]*. Dopamine inhibits prolactin secretion.

Hyperprolactinemia is characterized by a markedly diminished interest in sex and a reduction in sexual performance in both men and women. Hyperprolactinemia can be the result of medications, neoplasms, and other conditions.

Testosterone is believed to be the agent responsible during and after fetal development for the increase in the size of the nondominant hemisphere and for the reductions in interhemispheric connections commonly found in male brains.

The luteinizing hormone (LH) response to estrogen has been believed by some to be a marker of "feminized" brains. It is not present in homosexual men, despite early assertions to the contrary.

Chapter 9

Impulse Disorders

Donald W. Bechtold

I. **ANOREXIA NERVOSA** is an eating disorder characterized by obsessional weight loss without an identifiable organic cause.

A. **Diagnostic criteria** (Table 9-1)

B. **Clinical features and associated findings**

1. **Onset.** The average age of onset of the illness is 13 to 14 years; the onset often is preceded by a period of mild obesity or mild dieting. It is interesting to note that a relatively high percentage of anorectics lose a parent within the year preceding the onset of the illness.

2. **Behavioral features** are varied, but commonly include:
   a. Overactivity
   b. Obsessions and rituals with food and food preparation
   c. Purging (self-induced vomiting, diuretic abuse, laxative abuse)
   d. Secretiveness
   e. Extreme behavioral rigidity and inflexibility
   f. Cognitive preoccupations and distortions regarding body image and weight.

3. **Associated findings** that accompany the onset of illness are listed in Table 9-2. In general, these findings reflect metabolic slowing, fluid and electrolyte disturbances, alterations in multiple endocrinologic axes, and organic brain symptoms. In addition, three **personality styles** are classically cited as preceding the onset of anorexia nervosa.
   a. **Obsessive-compulsive (perfectionistic).** An individual who is perfectionistic about other areas of life may focus this compulsivity on eating.
   b. **Histrionic** individuals overly sexualize relationships because of conflicts about sexuality. Such conflicts may also play a role in the etiology of anorexia nervosa (see I D 2 a).
   c. **Schizoid or schizotypal** individuals are prone to odd behavior and are therefore more likely to have unusual eating behavior.

TABLE 9-1. *DSM-IV* Diagnostic Criteria for Anorexia Nervosa

Refusal to maintain weight at or above minimal weight for age and height (85% of ideal body weight or developmentally expected body weight)

Fear of gaining weight or becoming obese, even when significantly underweight

Disturbed body image, such that appropriate body weight is perceived as excessive or low body weight is perceived as appropriate

Amenorrhea (the absence of at least three consecutive menstrual cycles)

Two distinct types:
  Restricting—weight maintained largely by caloric restriction
  Bingeing/purging—both binge eating and purging (vomiting, laxatives, diuretics, enemas)

TABLE 9-2. Associated Findings in Anorexia Nervosa

Peripheral edema
Lanugo hair development
Heightened activity level
Skin changes (dryness, scaling, yellow tinge due to carotinemia)
Lowered metabolic rate (bradycardia, hypotension, hypothermia)
Normal TSH levels; possible low T3 levels
Normal or overstimulated adrenal axis; possible loss of normal diurnal variation in cortisol secretion
Normal serum protein and albumin concentrations
Increased serum carotene (rare in other causes of weight loss)
Possible increase in growth hormone levels
Abdominal pain
Organic brain symptoms (e.g., cognitive slowing, apathy, dysphoria)

4. **Clinical subgroups.** Recent research suggests that anorexia nervosa is a syndrome that can be subclassified. Subclassification is useful prognostically and, possibly, in treatment.

   a. The **anorexia nervosa** subgroup is characterized by strict self-starvation.

   b. Patients with **anorexia accompanied by bulimia** may form a distinct subgroup. As such, these patients seem to be more extroverted, present with the disorder later in life, and have a worse prognosis than patients who indulge only in persistent self-starvation.

   c. **Vomiters** may form another subgroup; they tend to herald a more chronic course with a poorer prognosis.

   d. **Male anorectics** may form yet another distinct subgroup.

5. **Medical complications** (Table 9-3)

C. **Epidemiology.** Anorexia nervosa is 10 to 20 times more common in girls than in boys; within the United States and Western Europe, approximately 1 in 200 adolescent girls are affected. The disorder is more common in Western cultures. Caucasians have the highest rate of anorexia nervosa, particularly girls of Jewish and Italian families. Middle- and upper-class families are at the greatest risk. The disorder is increasing, probably as a result of the high value placed on thinness in Western societies.

D. **Etiology and pathogenesis.** Although no single cause is known, various biologic and psychological factors are implicated in the etiology of anorexia nervosa.

1. **Biologic factors.** Certain mental disorders, endocrine abnormalities, and genetic problems occur with increased frequency in anorectic patients.

TABLE 9-3. Medical Complications of Anorexia Nervosa

Metabolic abnormalities (e.g., hypokalemia, hypochloremic alkalosis)	Gastric dilatation and rupture
	Chronic sore throats and esophagitis
	Anemia
Parotid gland swelling	Leukopenia
Dental erosion and caries	Endocrinologic changes
Menstrual irregularities	Electrocardiogram changes

a. **Temperament.** Many anorectics are high achievers with above average intelligence. Many also tend toward rigid self-control and affective constriction. Interpersonal conflict is more likely to be expressed through passive-aggressive modalities than through direct confrontation.

b. **Mental disorders.** Unipolar and bipolar mood disorders occur at a greater rate in anorectics than in the general population. These disturbances tend to occur later in life and probably are not the underlying cause of anorexia nervosa. The risk for **suicide** is increased in anorectic patients.

c. **Endocrine disorders**

   (1) **Alterations in catecholamine activity** at various central nervous system (CNS) sites could account for some of the clinical features of the illness. Because much of this activity normalizes after weight gain, causality is difficult to determine.

   (2) **An alteration in normal hypothalamic–pituitary function** may account for some of the endocrine abnormalities that occur in anorexia.

d. **Genetic disorders.** Some research (e.g., twin studies) suggests a possible genetic role in the transmission of anorexia nervosa.

2. **Psychological factors.** Three theories have been proposed in the etiology of anorexia nervosa.

   a. **Fear of sexuality.** A classic theory holds that anorectics have a fear of impregnation and an accompanying fantasy that impregnation occurs orally. They defend themselves against pregnancy by not eating. A corollary to this theory is that affected adolescents fear sexuality, menarche, and pregnancy, and starve themselves to remain prepubertal.

   b. **Parent–child conflict.** The **transactional theory** purports that a series of parent–child interactions may cause slight changes in the family system, which, in turn, may lead to a new and more deviated set of interactions. The child's request not to eat or refusal to eat is overridden by the parent's need to feed the child. Eventually, the child cannot regulate her own eating and becomes dependent on her environment for cues concerning this and other areas of self-regulation.

   c. **Dysfunctional family.** The **family system model** also considers parent–child interactions and asserts that family systems seek to maintain a dynamic equilibrium. Changes in any part of the system cause disequilibrium and require compensatory changes elsewhere in the system. An adolescent's attempt to begin the process of separation and emancipation in an overinvolved family, or to exert developmentally appropriate autonomy and self-control in a rigid, autocratic family is seen as disrupting the family system. Therefore, the regression of the child from normal adolescent strivings to a preadolescent developmental posture (through the symptoms of anorexia nervosa) represents an accommodation within the family system, resulting in a more tenable, albeit pathologic, equilibrium.

   (1) **The mother–daughter relationship** could play a role in the etiology. Mothers of anorectic girls are often controlling, allowing their daughters little autonomy. Mothers of anorectic girls may also be fragile in terms of feminine identity and self-esteem, perceiving their pubescent daughters as competitive and threatening. Regression of the child to a prepubertal body morphology may serve to relieve this disequilibrating force in the family system.

   (2) **Fathers** of anorectics are often obsessive-compulsive. They may participate in quasi–weight-control activities, such as distance running, and may transmit their attitudes about weight to their daughters. ("Obligate running" among males has been considered by some to be a male equivalent to anorexia nervosa.) Fathers of anorectic girls may also be fearful of their own sexual impulses toward their daughters, which are heightened by their pubertal development.

E. Differential diagnosis

1. **Medical conditions.** Essentially, the differential diagnosis for unexplained weight loss in adolescence is included. An adequate medical assessment must include consideration of each of the following:

   a. **Addison's disease** may present as weight loss, anorexia (loss of appetite), vomiting, and electrolyte and endocrine abnormalities (low sodium concentration, high potassium concentration, and suppressed serum cortisol levels). Listlessness and depression are frequent findings, in contrast to the hyperactivity of anorexia nervosa.

   b. **Hypothyroidism** may present as intolerance to cold, constipation, bradycardia, low blood pressure, and skin changes similar to those seen in anorexia nervosa (i.e., dry, scaling skin). Obsessional food handling, weight loss (and accompanying fear of weight gain), and hyperactivity are not usual, however.

   c. **Hyperthyroidism** presents as elevated vital signs, hyperactivity, and, sometimes, weight loss. However, patients with hyperthyroidism usually are not obsessive about food.

   d. **Any chronic illness** (e.g., Crohn's disease, ulcerative colitis, rheumatoid arthritis, tuberculosis) can cause progressive weight loss but should be readily identifiable as a physical disorder.

   e. **Neoplasms, especially CNS tumors,** can cause endocrine malfunction (e.g., tumors of the hypothalamus or third ventricle) with accompanying weight loss of either a primary or secondary nature. Other symptoms of the tumor, such as visual disturbances or panhypopituitarism, should be evident.

   f. **Superior mesenteric artery syndrome** can cause vomiting and anorexia. The mechanism apparently involves compression of the duodenum by the superior mesenteric artery, particularly when the patient is supine and especially in individuals who are thin. When found concomitantly with anorexia nervosa, it is often difficult to ascertain whether superior mesenteric artery syndrome is primary (causative) or secondary to the weight loss of anorexia nervosa.

2. **Psychiatric conditions**

   a. **Schizophrenia.** Although schizophrenics may be delusional about food, the delusions are more bizarre than those seen in anorectics (e.g., "there's poison in this" versus "this will make me fat"). Other features of schizophrenia should be present.

   b. **Bulimia nervosa** involves binge eating usually followed by some form of purging in a patient who otherwise maintains her weight.

   c. **Depression** is often accompanied by anorexia. In this case, the anorexia is a so-called vegetative sign of depression, and a depressed mood is usually pronounced.

   d. **Hysterical noneating** is distinguishable by the absence of a morbid concern with weight and calories.

F. Treatment

1. **Medical assessment.** The anorectic patient must be protected from the potentially lethal complications of starvation (i.e., metabolic disturbances, fluid and electrolyte disturbances, and cardiac dysrhythmias). Medical management always begins with assessment for and treatment of potentially life-threatening medical complications of the disorder. Intervention for a medical emergency is sometimes necessary; therefore, immediate assessment requires a determination of how much weight has been lost and over what period of time, as well as an assessment of cardiac, metabolic, and hydration status. Only when medical stability has been attained does treatment for the underlying disorder begin.

2. **Psychotherapeutic modalities**

   a. **Individual therapy. Psychotherapy** usually is a useful adjunct to other treatment modalities but is rarely effective alone. **Psychoanalysis** can be particularly ineffective in anorexia nervosa if it is the only treatment intervention. Both therapies can foster a regression in patients, which, in treatment, is useful only when the patient has the ability and strength to pull out of the regression at the end of the session. Neither treatment provides enough structure for the patient (e.g., anorectics may need to be watched and instructed most of the day).

(1) Initially, the therapeutic work should be aimed at forming an alliance with the patient to work on particular problems. The foci need not include weight or eating habits so long as physiologic stability is maintained.

(2) Gaps in the patient's ego should be clarified (e.g., when the patient is obviously angry about something but is unaware of this, her affect can be pointed out to her).

(3) Transference reactions should be interpreted if and when they interfere with the patient's ability to work on and talk about her problems.

(4) An empathic stance should be maintained with the patient at the same time that issues of physiologic stability and compliance with medical treatment are treated as nonnegotiable. A close partnership must be maintained between the child, the psychiatrist, and the pediatrician in the collaborative management of these patients.

b. Hospitalization. In some cases, the child cannot be effectively treated within the dysfunctional home environment and adequate, less restrictive alternatives are not available. **Out-of-home placement** is indicated if the patient loses weight despite outpatient intervention, if the patient is suicidal, or if vomiting and purging are causing acid–base, electrolyte, or cardiac complications.

(1) Therapeutic approach reflects the understanding that anorectics have a propensity to deny and conceal the severity of their condition.

(a) Careful attention must be paid to the **accuracy of weight measurements**. Serial weights should be obtained at the same time of day, on the same scale, in the same garb (preferably a hospital gown only), and after voiding. Attempts to artificially pad weight by drinking large quantities of water or concealing objects on the body are typical of anorectics.

(b) Splitting (pitting one staff member against another) and manipulations concerning eating are also common and should be discussed at staff meetings and with the patient. Flexibility is important. These patients can be extraordinarily manipulative.

(2) Behavioral techniques may be necessary with refractory adolescents.

(a) The patient should be **weighed every other day**. Urine should be **monitored regularly for ketones,** sometimes as often as daily before each meal.

(b) Alimentation should be provided by a nasogastric tube if the patient steadfastly refuses to eat, and should be readministered if the food is vomited. Alternatively, **hyperalimentation** may be provided through a central intravenous line if all of the above measures fail.

(c) The patient's privileges (e.g., freedom to leave the ward versus confinement in a locked unit) should be tied to the behavioral approach and commensurate with the patient's ability to regulate her own activity and eating. Such a program may take the following form.

(i) The patient's weight should be the target symptom, not the eating behavior, amount of exercise, or vomiting. Reinforcers should be tied to weight fluctuation.

(ii) Once the patient is stable medically and has some weight reserve, urine can be monitored for ketones before each meal as part of a behavioral treatment approach. Monitoring ketones provides information about starvation state, provides the patient with immediate feedback, and offers her the opportunity to alter her starvation state immediately. If the patient's urine contains ketones, her activities and privileges should be completely restricted until her urine reverts to normal.

c. Group therapy. Peer interaction and feedback should be sought and emphasized, since adolescents often pay more attention to their peers than to adults. Adolescents respond to peers with more trust and less suspicion, such that the perception of empathy is enhanced. In addition, the realization that others share the same symptoms helps adolescents feel less isolated. Although many types of groups have been used, self-help groups have been increasing in number and prominence.

   d. Family therapy. Some form of **family intervention is nearly always indicated,** especially for adolescents. Styles of family interaction should be clarified, and projections and vicarious pleasures that family members derive from the patient's symptoms should be interpreted and restructured. Individual therapy for either or both of the parents may be indicated; when marital issues contribute to the symptomatology of the child, marital therapy for the parents may also be indicated. Parent education concerning the normal developmental tasks and transitions of adolescence may be necessary. In general, the family should be allied with the staff, working toward the patient's improvement, and not with the patient to her detriment.

   e. Medications. There is no pharmacologic treatment for anorexia nervosa. Medications may be useful therapeutic adjuncts, but only when targeted at specific, underlying symptoms.

   (1) Cyproheptadine may be of some value because it has appetite-stimulating properties.

   (2) Antidepressants may benefit when depressive symptoms are prominent.

   (3) Likewise, prominent anxiety symptoms may respond to **anxiolytics**.

   (4) When eating and food preparation are excessively ritualized, or other symptoms of obsessive-compulsive disorder (OCD) are present, **anti-OCD agents** may prove beneficial.

   (5) Because of potentially severe side effects, **antipsychotic medication** should be used only when the patient suffers from a psychotic illness.

G. **Prognosis.** On average, 30%–40% of patients have a relatively complete recovery; 30% or more demonstrate partial improvement (some may undergo a period of obesity); and up to 30%–40% continue to demonstrate bizarre eating habits, weight loss, and a severe disease course.

1. **Positive prognostic indicators** include early onset of disease, decreased denial of a problem, gainful employment, and admitting to feeling hungry.

2. **Negative prognostic indicators** include a long disease course, a schizoid personality, and recurrent bulimia, vomiting, and laxative abuse.

3. **Mortality rates** are reported to be 5%–15%. Death, when it occurs, is due to electrolyte abnormalities, suicide, cardiac dysrhythmias, or possibly sudden rehydration and weight gain.

II. **BULIMIA NERVOSA** is a disorder characterized by ravenous overeating followed by guilt, depression, and anger at oneself for doing so. During the episode, a sense of lack of control over eating exists, despite which there is no significant loss of weight below the normal for age and size.

A. **Diagnostic criteria** are listed in Table 9-4. Bulimia nervosa patients fall into two distinct categories.

1. Patients with the **purging type** engage in regular vomiting and use of diuretics or cathartics.

2. Patients with the **nonpurging type** compensate for high-calorie binges with subsequent caloric restriction or exercise; they do not regularly purge.

B. **Clinical features and associated findings**

1. **Onset.** This is most commonly a disorder of adolescent and young adult females.

TABLE 9-4. *DSM-IV* Criteria for Bulimia Nervosa

Two distinct types ("purging" and "nonpurging")

Recurrent episodes of bingeing, characterized by:
— Consumption of a quantity of food that exceeds what a normal person would eat during a given time period, under similar circumstances, and
— A feeling of not having control over eating during the episode

Recurrent inappropriate weight-controlling behavior (e.g., self-induced vomiting, use of cathartics, excessive exercise)

Bingeing and inappropriate weight-controlling behavior both occur at least twice weekly for 3 months

Self-evaluation unduly influenced by body shape and weight

Disturbance does not occur exclusively during episodes of anorexia nervosa

2. **Behavioral features.** Individuals with this disorder have an increased frequency of mood and anxiety symptoms and of substance abuse and personality disorders. Other symptoms of impulsivity, such as stealing, are common. Stealing may be necessary to support an expensive eating habit.

3. **Associated findings** are listed in Table 9-5.

4. **Medical complications** are listed in Table 9-6.

C. **Epidemiology.** Primarily a disorder of adolescent girls, the disorder is probably very common, existing in gradations from mild (perhaps a variant of normal) to severe. Prevalence may be as high as 5%–10% of college-age females. It is many times more common in females than in males.

D. **Etiology.** Very little is known about the cause of the disorder, although theories have been proposed.

1. **Psychological theories**
   a. Bulimia could be caused by a need to take in something orally—perhaps as a substitution for some degree of maternal deprivation.
   b. Some children of short stature fantasize that eating ravenously can help them grow.
   c. Bulimia has been described in children with psychogenic dwarfism (retarded growth due to emotional neglect).
   d. Bulimia could be a disorder of self-regulation. There are high rates of coexistent substance abuse and stealing.

2. **Biologic theories.** A lesion of the satiety center in the hypothalamus could contribute to bulimia, but such a lesion has not been defined or discovered.

TABLE 9-5. Associated Findings in Bulimia Nervosa

Ingestion of high-calorie food

Bingeing episodes occur in secret

Wide fluctuations in weight

Persistent overconcern with weight and body shape

Attempts to lose weight (through dieting, exercise, or use of cathartics, diuretics, enemas)

Bingeing episodes terminated by sleep, abdominal pain, social interruption, or self-induced vomiting

Lengthy phases of normal eating

TABLE 9-6. Medical Complications of Bulimia Nervosa

Metabolic abnormalities (e.g., hypokalemia, hypochloremic alkalosis)
Parotid gland swelling
Dental erosion and caries
Menstrual irregularities
Gastric dilatation and rupture
Chronic sore throats and esophagitis
Anemia

E. **Differential diagnosis**

1. **Prader-Willi syndrome** is characterized by continuous overeating, obesity, mental retardation, hypogonadism, hypotonia, and diabetes mellitus. It is apparently a genetic syndrome, but the mode of transmission is unknown. It is thought to be due to a hypothalamic lesion.

2. **Klüver-Bucy syndrome.** Objects are examined by mouth, and hypersexuality and hyperphagia are characteristic. Visual agnosia, compulsive licking and biting, and hypersensitivity to stimuli are common as well. The condition may result from temporal lobe dysfunction.

3. **Kleine-Levin syndrome** manifests as hyperphagia and hypersomnia, both of which occur in spurts of 2 to 3 weeks at a frequency of 2 or 3 cycles per year. Loss of sexual inhibitions may occur as part of the syndrome. This disorder is more common in boys and appears to represent a limbic or hypothalamic dysfunction.

4. **Hypothalamic lesions** should be considered.

5. **Anorexia nervosa.** A component of anorexia nervosa may be binge eating, but simple bulimia nervosa does not include significant weight loss.

6. **Binge eating in obesity.** In obesity, binging represents a pattern of overeating, is not terminated by purging, and is not accompanied by a preoccupation with body shape.

7. **Epileptic seizures**

8. **CNS tumors**

F. **Treatment.** Long-term efficacy of any one treatment modality has not been established. Bulimia traditionally has been viewed largely as a treatment-resistant condition. However, mixed modality treatment appears to offer promising results.

1. **Individual psychotherapies** of psychodynamic, behavioral, and cognitive orientations have been variably helpful. Individual therapy that combines elements of the various therapeutic orientations in conjunction with supportive group psychotherapy offers promising results.

2. **Medications** are not universally indicated. However, drugs that have been reported to be useful include tricyclic antidepressants, monoamine oxidase inhibitors, lithium, carbamazepine, and phenytoin.

3. **Hospitalization** is indicated for the management of serious medical complications, relentless binging and purging (several times daily), and for the severely depressed or suicidal bulimic patient.

III. **OTHER IMPULSE CONTROL DISORDERS.** Eating disorders may be recognized as falling within a broader spectrum of disorders of self-regulation or impulse control, which also includes substance-related disorders and paraphilias. The following disorders also fall within this spectrum and are clustered within the *Diagnostic and Statistical Manual of Mental Disorders,* 4th edition (DSM-IV) as **impulse control disorders not elsewhere classified**.

A. Intermittent explosive disorder

1. **Diagnostic criteria**
   a. **Repeated, discrete episodes of loss of behavioral control characterized by aggression toward persons or property** are the hallmark of this disorder. Most commonly, the aggression toward persons assumes the form of a physical assault, whereas the aggression toward property manifests as destruction of property.
   b. **Precipitating events** may be variably present or absent but, when present, **are disproportionately insignificant** when compared with the extent of the aggressive behavioral outburst.
   c. Whether the disorder exists independent from the conditions that must be ruled out in a differential diagnosis is controversial. Consequently, the condition may best be considered a **characteristic symptom constellation deriving from multiple etiologies,** rather than as a distinct and discrete disorder.

2. **Epidemiology.** Intermittent explosive disorders apparently are more common in men than in women. Men with these disorders reportedly are more likely to be seen in correctional facilities, whereas women are more likely to be seen in mental health facilities.

3. **Differential diagnosis** includes a variety of psychological and organic etiologies. Regardless of the etiology involved, victimization by or exposure to violence and aggressive behavior likely contributes to the expression of this symptom constellation.
   a. **Psychological etiologies** may include personality disorders (especially antisocial and borderline), psychotic disorders (schizophrenia), mood disorders (manic episodes), and disruptive behavior disorders (especially conduct and attention deficit hyperactivity).
   b. **Organic etiologies** may include seizures (especially with temporal lobe foci), psychoactive substance intoxication, structural lesions (trauma, infarct, tumor, hemorrhage, abscess), normal pressure hydrocephalus, CNS infection, metabolic disorders (hypoglycemia), and hormone disturbances (elevated androgen levels).

4. **Treatment** is best aimed at the underlying condition(s).
   a. **Incarceration, institutionalization, seclusion, and restraint** have all been employed, although these measures likely control rather than alter aggressive behaviors.
   b. **Behavior modification** techniques have met with only modest success, as have conventional psychotherapies.
   c. Various **psychosurgical procedures** have been applied, although currently these are used rarely and reserved for the most dangerous and refractory cases.
   d. A variety of **medications** have also been used with some symptomatic benefit. Mood stabilizers (lithium), anticonvulsants (phenytoin, carbamazepine, valproic acid), β-blockers (propranolol), minor and major tranquilizers (benzodiazepines and neuroleptics), and more recently the selective serotonin reuptake inhibitors (SSRIs) have been used with favorable responses in appropriately selected cases.

B. Kleptomania

1. **Diagnostic criteria**
   a. **Multiple episodes of impulsive stealing in the presence of pertinent negatives** are the hallmark of this disorder. Specifically, the stealing is *not*:
      (1) For monetary value or to satisfy a personal need
      (2) An expression of anger, retribution, or retaliation
      (3) Symptomatic of an underlying psychotic disorder (in response to a hallucination or delusion)
   b. Individuals experience a **mounting sense of tension or anxiety before the stealing episode**. Pleasure, then, is derived from easing this internal tension and anxiety after

gratifying the impulse to steal, not from the object(s) stolen. This contrasts sharply with shoplifting, robbery, burglary, and other stealing behaviors where the secondary gain derives from the object(s) stolen rather than from the impulse gratification itself. In fact, it is common for the objects stolen in kleptomania to be hidden, stored, discarded, returned, or given away.

2. **Epidemiology and etiology.** Kleptomania is believed to be extremely rare. Many reported "cases" must be carefully evaluated in light of the secondary gain afforded by conscious attempts to avoid criminal prosecution (malingering). Because the disorder is rare, little is known of its epidemiology or its etiology.
   a. **Organic etiologies** related to behavioral disinhibition have been suggested but remain poorly defined.
   b. **Psychological etiologies** have been suggested, largely by psychoanalytic theorists who tend to view the behavior as an attempt to restore wishes, drives, and pleasures that were lost, or at least frustrated, during infancy and childhood. These theories also remain poorly defined.

3. **Treatment.** The literature is largely devoid of systematically controlled treatment studies and, instead, includes mostly single-case, anecdotal reports of either psychoanalytic or behavioral therapeutic modalities. There is no clearly defined role for pharmacotherapy in this disorder, unless an underlying organic state has been identified.

C. Pyromania

1. **Diagnostic criteria**
   a. **Multiple episodes of willful and intentional fire setting in the presence of pertinent negatives** are the hallmark of this disorder. Specifically, the fire setting is *not*:
      (1) For financial gain (e.g., insurance reimbursement)
      (2) An act of sociopolitical insurrection
      (3) One of a series of related criminal activities
      (4) An act of vandalism or an expression of retaliation or revenge
      (5) A symptom of an underlying psychotic disorder
   b. Individuals experience a **mounting sense of tension or anxiety before the fire-setting episode,** which sometimes may be in the form of a building sexual tension and excitement (**pyrolagnia**). Relief of tension and anxiety, or sexual pleasure, is derived when the fire-setting impulse is gratified as well as during the aftermath of the fire setting.
   c. Afflicted individuals maintain an **obsessional preoccupation with fire,** in much the same way individuals with eating disorders maintain obsessional preoccupations with food.

2. **Epidemiology.** Pyromania is a rare disorder accounting for only a fraction of all cases of fire setting. The disorder appears to be more common in males than in females, and a childhood onset is common. Individuals with pyromania appear to lack empathic recognition of the physical destructiveness of their actions and the consequences of their actions to its victims.

3. **Etiology.** Specific etiology tends to be obscured by the infrequent nature of the disorder.
   a. An underlying **organic factor** is suggested by long-standing observations of high rates of fire setting in organically impaired populations. This correlation has not been specifically evaluated within the pyromania subset of the fire-setting population, however.
   b. **Psychological theorists** have focused on the intrapsychic representation and meaning of fire. Such theories have emphasized issues related to sexuality, power, rage, and aggression as psychodynamic determinants, which may underlie this disorder.

4. **Treatment.** The nature of the disorder is such that "treatment" most often occurs in penal institutions. No systematically controlled studies have been done to describe the differential efficacies of various treatments that have been applied in this population. There is no clearly defined role for pharmacotherapy in this disorder unless an underlying organic state has been identified.

D. **Pathological gambling**

1. **Diagnostic criteria.** As with alcohol consumption, some degree of gambling is viewed as falling within a wide spectrum of normality.
   a. The **chronic, progressive, and maladaptive nature of the gambling behavior** is the hallmark of this disorder as evidenced by:
      (1) An obsessional, cognitive preoccupation with gambling
      (2) Impaired personal, social, educational, and occupational functioning as a consequence of the gambling
      (3) An overly determined, out-of-control quality that drives, perpetuates, and escalates the gambling despite the derivative functional impairment and adverse consequences
   b. In this context, pathological gambling may be viewed as a variant of an **addictive** disorder. Whether the disorder represents an inability to inhibit the gambling impulse or a volitional failure to do so remains controversial.

2. **Epidemiology.** This is a relatively common disorder. Prevalence studies estimate rates as high as 3% of the American adult population. The disorder is considerably more common in men than in women.
   a. **Predisposing factors** may include extremes in parental discipline styles (either overly indulgent or overly rigid), childhood exposure to parental gambling, parental substance abuse, or parental sociopathy.
   b. **Associated conditions.** Associations between pathological gambling and mood disorders, anxiety disorders, psychoactive substance use disorders, and personality disorders have been described.

3. **Etiology.** Only theories exist.
   a. **Psychoanalytic theories** attempt to connect the behavior with various disturbances in psychosexual development (from the oral stage through latency) as well as with aggressive and libidinal drives. There is no consensus among psychoanalytic theorists.
   b. **Behavioral theories** attempt to explain the behavior largely according to learning theory (i.e., that most pathological gamblers are exposed to the behavior through others and ultimately "learn" it through powerful patterns of reinforcement).
   c. **Other.** It has also been suggested that the behavior may be propagated through the activation of endogenous opioid systems.

4. **Treatment approaches** derive from the theoretic framework applied to explain etiology. Both individual and group modalities have been applied.
   a. The earliest **individual modalities** tended to be conventional, psychodynamic approaches. **Behavioral techniques** have assumed more prominence recently, including both aversive and desensitizing models.
   b. **Group modalities** have also played a more prominent role, particularly self-help groups such as Gamblers Anonymous, which have been structured consistent with a 12-step addictions model.
   c. **Pharmacotherapy** does not play a significant role, unless an underlying organic state has been identified.

E. **Trichotillomania**

1. **Diagnostic criteria**
   a. **Recurrent episodes of pulling out one's own hair in quantities sufficient to result in identifiable hair loss** are the hallmark of this disorder.
      (1) This must be distinguished from stroking, twirling, and fidgeting with hair, all of which fall within a spectrum of normal behavior for many individuals.
      (2) Scalp hair most commonly is involved; facial hair, eyebrows, eyelashes, truncal hair, limb hair, axillary hair, and pubic hair may also be involved.
   b. **Hair-pulling episodes are preceded by a sense of increasing internal tension and anxiety.** When the impulse to pull has been gratified, the individual experiences a

pleasurable sensation, or at least relief from the internal perception of tension and anxiety. Of note is that hair pulling in this context does not typically induce pain.

    c. Obsessional thoughts and other compulsive behaviors may be described. In particular, specific rituals related to the disposition of the hair, including ingestion (**trichophagy**), may exist. Other forms of self-injurious behaviors may be associated as well.

2. Epidemiology. The prevalence of the condition is unknown. The disorder usually begins in childhood and is believed to affect females more frequently than males.

3. Etiology. All etiologic theories are considered tentative and speculative at present.

    a. One view holds that the behavior represents a form of **self-stimulation** in response to emotional deprivation. Significant disturbances in parent–child interactions are commonly described.

    b. Other theorists emphasize the dimension of **self-mutilation** as a form of self-punishment in response to rejection, trauma, and loss.

    c. Some features of the disorder are consistent with a learned behavior, similar to the **habit disorders of childhood**. An association with OCD has been suggested.

    d. Finally, it is possible that an underlying **organic substrate(s)** might exist.

4. Treatment

    a. Psychodynamic and behavioral individual approaches have been described. Psychodynamic approaches were more common historically, but behavioral interventions have been more frequently discussed in recent times. Desensitization, aversion, and habit reversal have all been described. Therapeutic efficacy of all individual modalities has been limited in breadth and scope, however.

    b. A variety of psychopharmacologic agents have been used. Neuroleptics, anxiolytics, mood stabilizers, and recently antiobsessional medications (clomipramine, fluoxetine) have met with only limited success as well.

BIBLIOGRAPHY

American Psychiatric Association: *Diagnostic and Statistical Manual of Mental Disorders,* 4th ed. Washington, DC, American Psychiatric Association, 1994.

Halmi KA, Falk JR: Anorexia nervosa: A study of outcome discriminators in exclusive dieters and bulimics. *J Am Acad Child Psychiatry* 21:369, 1982.

Kaplan HI, Sadock BJ (eds): *Comprehensive Textbook of Psychiatry/V.* Baltimore, Williams & Wilkins, 1989.

Lesser LI, Ashenden BJ, Debuskey M, et al: Anorexia nervosa in children. *Am J Orthopsychiatry* 30:572, 1960.

Sameroff AJ, Chandler M: Reproductive risk and the continuum of caretaking causality. In *Review of Child Development Research,* vol 4. Edited by Horowitz F. Chicago, University of Chicago Press, 1975, pp 187–244.

DIRECTIONS: Each of the numbered items or incomplete statements in this section is followed by answers or by completions of the statement. Select the ONE lettered answer or completion that is BEST in each case.

1. The Prader-Willi syndrome is characterized by which constellation of symptoms?

(A) Overeating, mental retardation, and stealing food
(B) Hypersexuality, overeating, and mouthing objects
(C) Wide fluctuations of weight with lengthy phases of normal eating
(D) Overeating and hypersomnia
(E) None of the above

2. Which of the following statements regarding pyromania is true?

(A) It is a common disorder involved in most cases of arson
(B) Afflicted individuals typically regret, but cannot control, the fire-setting impulse
(C) It is mainly an adult disorder seen only rarely in childhood
(D) Fire-setting behaviors are over-represented among organically impaired populations

3. A 15-year-old girl presents to the emergency room with severe weight loss. On physical examination, she is cachectic with a weight of 68 lb; her heart rate is 36, and her blood pressure is 72/50. The first intervention should be to

(A) evaluate the family to determine the family dynamics
(B) immediately administer a high-protein and carbohydrate diet via a nasogastric tube
(C) draw blood for a serum electrolyte determination and then start intravenous feeding
(D) arrange to have the patient admitted to the psychiatric service
(E) arrange for electroconvulsive therapy

DIRECTIONS: Each of the numbered items or incomplete statements in this section is negatively phrased, as indicated by a capitalized word such as NOT, LEAST, or EXCEPT. Select the ONE lettered answer or completion that is BEST in each case.

4. Which of the following is NOT conceptualized as an impulse control disorder?

(A) Alcohol abuse
(B) Sexual masochism
(C) Mania
(D) Pyromania
(E) Kleptomania

5. Medical complications of bulimia nervosa include all of the following EXCEPT

(A) dental disease
(B) metabolic acidosis
(C) menstrual abnormalities
(D) parotitis
(E) esophagitis

6. All of the following statements concerning intermittent explosive disorder are correct EXCEPT

(A) the etiology is most likely multifactorial
(B) precipitating events are invariably present
(C) precipitating events are disproportionately related to the extent of the behavior
(D) the disorder may derive from hormonal abnormalities
(E) exposure to aggression and violence contributes to this disorder

7. All of the following are true statements regarding kleptomania EXCEPT

(A) it is a relatively common disorder more often seen in men than in women
(B) malingering is prominent within the differential diagnosis
(C) little pleasure is derived from the stolen object
(D) the stolen object is frequently returned to its owner
(E) there is no well-defined treatment for the disorder

8. Which of the following statements regarding bulimia nervosa is FALSE?

(A) There is a prominent focus on body image
(B) Wide fluctuations in weight are common
(C) "Binges" may be separated by prolonged periods of normal eating
(D) Ten percent of college-age women may be affected
(E) Documentation of some form of purging behavior is necessary to establish diagnosis

9. Parental disorders that may contribute to the development of pathological gambling include all of the following EXCEPT

(A) exhibitionism
(B) gambling
(C) drug abuse
(D) sociopathy

DIRECTIONS: Each set of matching questions in this section consists of a list of four to twenty-six lettered options (some of which may be in figures) followed by several numbered items. For each numbered item, select the ONE lettered option that is most closely associated with it. To avoid spending too much time on matching sets with large numbers of options, it is generally advisable to begin each set by reading the list of options. Then, for each item in the set, try to generate the correct answer and locate it in the option list, rather than evaluating each option individually. Each lettered option may be selected once, more than once, or not at all.

Questions 10–13

For each disorder listed below, select the association most consistent with it.

(A) Sexual excitation
(B) Psychosis
(C) Malingering
(D) Obsessive-compulsive disorder
(E) Addiction

10. Trichotillomania

11. Pathological gambling

12. Pyromania

13. Kleptomania

1. The answer is A *[II E 1–3]*. The Prader-Willi syndrome is characterized by ravenous overeating and is accompanied by obesity, mental retardation, and hypotonia. It is probably due to a hypothalamic lesion. Examining objects by mouth, hypersexuality, and hyperphagia are attributed to the Klüver-Bucy syndrome, and overeating and hypersomnia are associated with the Kleine-Levin syndrome. Wide fluctuations in weight with lengthy phases of normal eating may be seen in bulimia nervosa.

2. The answer is D *[III C 2, 3 a]*. High rates of fire-setting have repeatedly been documented among organically impaired populations. This suggests a possible underlying organic contribution to the disorder. Nonetheless, it is a rare disorder that accounts for only a small fraction of all cases of fire-setting. Although it is true that individuals with the disorder struggle to control the impulse to set fires, they tend neither to regret the destruction they have caused, nor to experience empathy on behalf of their victims. Although the disorder may be seen in adulthood, its onset is typically in childhood.

3. The answer is C *[I F 1, G 3]*. Anorexia nervosa may be a life-threatening illness. There is a significant mortality that accompanies this condition, most commonly due to the metabolic or cardiac complications secondary to starvation. The first intervention with anorectic patients is always an assessment of the medical state by drawing blood for serum electrolyte determination, followed by supportive or emergency medical intervention, such as starting intravenous feeding. A too rapid hydration or weight gain should be avoided as it may lead to further complications and even death. A high-protein and carbohydrate diet by nasogastric tube would not correct fluid and electrolyte problems quickly. Evaluation and treatment of the individual and family dynamics are always secondary to the emergency medical management.

4. The answer is C *[III B 1 b]*. The hallmarks of impulse control disorders are the failure to resist impulses that are harmful to self or others; mounting tension before discharging the impulse; and relief or pleasure following gratification of the impulse. In alcohol abuse, the impulse is to drink alcohol; in sexual masochism, it is to suffer physically or emo-

tionally during sexual activity; in pyromania, it is to set fires; and in kleptomania, it is to steal. Mania, by contrast, refers to the predominantly elevated or irritable phase of bipolar mood disorder.

5. The answer is B *[Table 9-6]*. Frequent exposure of the teeth, parotid salivary gland, and esophagus to gastric acid (as occurs in the purging type of bulimia nervosa) can result in irritation, inflammation, and damage to each of these tissues. Menstrual irregularities may relate to disturbances in the hypothalamic-pituitary-ovarian axis. Loss of gastric acid in the purging type of bulimia nervosa results in metabolic alkalosis rather than metabolic acidosis.

6. The answer is B *[III A 1 b, 2]*. Multiple etiologies likely underpin this disorder including psychologic and organic states. When present, precipitating events are disproportionately minor when compared with the extent of the aggressive behavioral outburst. Nonetheless, precipitants may not be identifiable with each explosive outburst. Regardless of the underlying etiology, exposure to violence and aggression likely contributes to the behavior. Elevated androgen levels have been implicated in some cases.

7. The answer is A *[III B 1 b, 2]*. Kleptomania is believed to be an extremely rare disorder. It is qualitatively different from most forms of stealing in that secondary gain is not derived from the object stolen, but rather from gratifying the impulse to steal. Consequently, the objects stolen are frequently returned to their owner. Many "cases" may be false positives secondary to malingering in an attempt to avoid criminal prosecution. All treatments are relatively speculative at this point. There is no clearly defined treatment for the disorder.

8. The answer is E *[II A 2, C]*. An almost obsessional focus on weight and body image is present. There may be large fluctuations in weight, although weight loss substantially below normal does not occur as it does in anorexia nervosa. Binges may occur regularly, or only sporadically, with lengthy intervals of normal eating habits. Prevalence studies indicate that as many as 10% of college-age females may have the disorder. Purging, however, reflects only one of the two subtypes of the disorder. In the nonpurging subtype, weight is controlled through fasting or excessive exercise, and not through purging activities.

9. The answer is A *[III D 2 a]*. Childhood exposure to parental gambling, substance abuse, and sociopathic or antisocial behavior have all been suggested as predisposing factors. Although exhibitionism also represents an impulse control disorder, it has not been linked with the development of pathological gambling.

10–13. The answers are: 10-D *[III E 1 c, 3 c]*, **11-E** *[III D 1 b]*, **12-A** *[III C 1 b]*, **13-C** *[III B 2]*. In addition to compulsive hair pulling, other obsessions or compulsions may be noted in trichotillomania. In addition, trichotillomania may be a symptom of an obsessive-compulsive disorder.

Pathological gambling bears much in common with the addictive disorders. Both involve continuing the maladaptive behavior in spite of chronic, progressive, adverse consequences. Likewise, peer support groups utilizing a 12-step approach have been of benefit in both disorders.

Pyromania is frequently precipitated by sexual tension that builds prior to setting a fire, which is gratified sexually both by setting the fire and during the ongoing aftermath of the fire.

Kleptomania must be distinguished from other forms of stealing by the distinction that the stolen object does not bring secondary gain or gratification as it does in other forms of stealing. When stealing brings secondary gain by way of the value of the object stolen, the attempt to invoke "irresistible urge" as in true kleptomania more likely represents malingering as a means of avoiding criminal prosecution.

Chapter 10

Child Psychiatry

Donald W. Bechtold

I. **INTRODUCTION.** Child and adolescent psychiatry is the study and treatment of the mental, developmental, and behavioral problems of childhood. As such, it overlaps with a variety of pediatric subspecialties. An understanding of standard childhood development is essential to the understanding of childhood psychopathology, since seemingly major difficulties may be normal at certain ages (e.g., negativism is usual at 2 years of age and again at adolescence, but it is problematic during the latency period and in adulthood).

A. **Overview of childhood psychopathology**

1. **Most disorders are more common in boys** than in girls. This may reflect an inherent increased vulnerability of the male to stress and trauma.

2. **Psychopathology is usually the result of chronic, maladaptive interactions** between the child and the environment, often combined with some genetic, physiologic, or temperamental propensity toward developing a mental illness. Isolated traumatic events (e.g., a single episode of brief, sexual fondling by a nonfamily member) can cause transient anxiety, anger, and depression; however, they generally do not cause psychopathology unless they generate long-lasting changes in the child's interactions with his or her environment.

3. **Misbehavior may be the result of the parents' conscious or unconscious prompting.** Children usually behave in a way that is consistent with the parents' desires.

B. **Developmental concepts**

1. **Epigenesis.** There is a natural and unalterable sequence in which development must occur (e.g., in Freudian psychology, the anal period must follow the oral stage and cannot be reversed; in Eriksonian psychology, the autonomy stage must follow the stage of basic trust). Later stages are necessarily viewed as "advances" from earlier stages. In all individuals there is a natural impetus toward development that progresses normally unless adversely influenced by extraneous variables. These variables may include in utero or perinatal insults, physiologic or genetic vulnerabilities, as well as a host of environmental stressors.

2. **Developmental continuities.** Some childhood personality traits and experiences may be "continuous" with and have ramifications for adulthood; others do not.
   a. For example, children who are abandoned at 3 years of age by their parents may feel depressed every time someone leaves them later in life. Children who experience persistent deprivation and neglect throughout childhood may manifest excessive dependency and neediness in their adult relationships. Thus, some childhood experiences may be "continuous" with adult behaviors or personality traits.
   b. Other characteristics, such as cognition and intellect, would be grossly oversimplified if they were thought of as continuous variables derived completely from experiences in early infancy because obvious genetic, physiologic, and individual differences (temperament) would be overlooked.
   c. In general, development is best viewed from a **multifactorial model** in which genetically determined capacities, individual temperamental differences, physiologic variables, and environmental interactions all contribute. The relative weight of

contribution from each of the variables differs for various personality traits and lines of development.

3. **Critical phases.** Particular phases of development must occur at certain ages.
   a. For example, a 4-year-old child who suffered a severe psychological trauma that arrested his development might not experience a normal oedipal period (although the trauma is overcome, and his development recommences at 7 years of age). This distorted oedipal phase might result in irrational fears of physical or psychological harm in competitive situations—a fear that could persist into adulthood. This example is hypothetical; very little evidence for its inevitability is available.
   b. The concept of critical phases has been largely supplanted by that of **"sensitive" phases,** in which development is most efficient but not limited to that phase of development.

4. **Temperament.** Certain children are able to negotiate seemingly overwhelming psychological trauma with minimal overt effect on their subsequent personality development. Others, however, manifest marked symptomatology in the face of considerably less trauma and stress. This dimension of relative vulnerability/invulnerability is referred to as temperament, although it is poorly understood at the present time. What is known to be important is the match or fit between a child's needs and the ability of his environment and caregivers to meet those needs.
   a. For example, temperamentally difficult children may do well developmentally if they have highly competent parents, whereas they do poorly if they have limited or marginal parents.
   b. By contrast, children whose temperaments are characterized by flexibility and adaptability may demonstrate marked resiliency even in the face of recurrent and catastrophic life events.

C. **Approach to the child and adolescent patient**

1. **The physician must be an advocate for the child,** rather than for the parents. To do otherwise is to subject the child to the parents' wishes, even when they are unrealistic, inappropriate, or to the detriment of the child. Nevertheless, the child psychiatrist must deal respectfully and attempt to develop a working relationship with the parents. Often, the effectiveness of work with the child is measured by the effectiveness of the work with the parents. Ineffective work with the parents may substantially limit the therapeutic progress of the child.
   a. In general, parents should be seen frequently, especially at the beginning of treatment.
   b. Preadolescents should usually be seen alone, but, in most cases, after the parents have been seen.
   c. An attempt to communicate with the child patient by talking should be made. If this is difficult, a small assortment of toys, including a dollhouse, paper and crayons, games, puppets, modeling clay, and building materials, can help a child communicate through play.
   d. Adolescents should usually be seen alone. Often, their emerging and developmentally appropriate autonomy should be supported by seeing them before the parents are seen. Use of unnatural slang to bridge the "generation gap" should be avoided. An attitude of sincerity and concern for the adolescent usually establishes rapport with the patient.

2. **The following should be observed during the patient interview:**
   a. The child's reaction to separation from the parents
   b. The child's behavior toward the interviewer (e.g., anxious, very open, shy)
   c. The child's perception of people in general (e.g., trustworthy or dangerous, reliable or neglectful, kind or hostile)
   d. The choice of verbal versus play communication
   e. The clarity of the child's thought processes
   f. The level of development (i.e., social, language, motor, psychosexual, cognitive, moral) of the child and its appropriateness to the child's age

g. The ability of the child to identify different affective states and to discharge these states in an age-appropriate manner

h. The ability of the child to tolerate frustration and to control his impulses (In most cases, this may be observed through naturalistic circumstances such as setting a limit on an inappropriate behavior, declining an inappropriate request, announcing the end of a session, or requiring the child's assistance in cleaning up toys.)

i. The child's perception of himself (e.g., competent or ineffectual, master or victim) and the relative strength of his self-esteem

j. The child's reaction to rejoining the parents after the interview

3. **Gathering information from the child** can be facilitated by requesting that the child:
   a. Make three wishes and elaborate on each wish
   b. Make drawings and elaborate on each drawing (Drawings of people and families are especially helpful.)
   c. Describe the family
   d. Describe important nonfamily members
   e. Describe favorite television shows, movies, and musicians, noting with whom the child identifies
   f. Describe the problem that initiated therapy and how the family told her of the appointment
   g. Describe hopes and wishes for the future

II. BONDING AND ATTACHMENT

A. Definitions

1. **Bonding** describes the **parent's affective relationship with the child**. Bonding develops over time. There appears to be no critical phase of bonding in humans as has been described in animal studies. Bonding likely commences long before the birth of the child and is apparent in the parents' attitudes, fantasies, and wishes for the child.

2. **Attachment** describes the **child's affective relationship with the parents**. Attachment, like bonding, develops over time. There is no critical phase for the development of attachment relationships, which may be formed at any time throughout the life cycle.

B. Assessment of bonding

1. Ask the parents **when and how a name was chosen** for the child. This may suggest when they began planning for the new arrival. The name may also have special meaning. It may indicate how the family perceives the child or suggest attributions made to the child. For example, a son named after his father may be dealt with harshly by his mother when an acrimonious relationship exists between the parents.

2. Determine what sort of **dreams and fantasies the parents had** about the child **during pregnancy**. Frequent, realistic, and hopeful reflection about the baby enhances the outcome related to bonding and attachment.

3. Determine **how the parents' relationship toward each other changed during the pregnancy**. The husband often assumes a maternal role toward his wife when she is pregnant. If, however, he begins abusing her, has affairs, or grows distant or uninvolved, a more difficult relationship between the parents and the new baby is likely. In addition, this is a time in which the parents' own unmet or inadequately met dependency needs and needs for nurture from childhood may complicate their relationships both with each other and with their new child.

4. Determine the **early reactions of the parents to the child in the delivery room and in the nursery**. Ambivalence of the parents concerning their child may be communicated behaviorally. It is important, however, to distinguish ambivalence from uncertainty,

anxiety, and lack of confidence, all of which are normal reactions to childbirth and are particularly common to first-time parents.

5. **Determine of whom the child reminds the parents.** This question assesses for transferences and preconceived attitudes about the infant. Inappropriate attributions to the child must be identified, clarified, disconnected from the child, and reconnected with the original object of attribution.

6. **Determine the mental health of the parents.** Depression, psychosis, personality disorders, and drug abuse are examples of problems that can distort the way the parent perceives, responds to, and interacts with the child.

7. **Special problems** are posed if the newborn spends extra time in the nursery due to illness (e.g., a child born 3 months premature who spends his first 2 months of life in a neonatal intensive care unit). A family with a child in the critical care nursery should be evaluated before discharge to ensure adequate care for the child.

C. **Disorders of bonding and attachment**

1. **Hospitalism** is an extreme example of failure of any affective relationship to develop.
   a. **Symptoms.** Affected infants suffer from:
      (1) Susceptibility to infection
      (2) Apathy
      (3) Retarded development
      (4) Failure to thrive
   b. **Treatment. Parents should be counseled to spend time with the newborn.** In situations in which the parents have not visited a sick infant or have been reluctant to see a newborn, a structured plan to facilitate parent–child interactions should be implemented.
      (1) There should be a **mandatory visitation of at least 12 consecutive hours**.
      (2) **Nursing support** should be available when the parents have questions.
      (3) **Psychiatric intervention** may be required when the grief over a child's prematurity or illness is thought to contribute to the lack of parental involvement.
      (4) **Follow-up** in a special clinic for premature infants is indicated.
      (5) **Referral to a child protective agency** is necessary if the parents cannot demonstrate a bond to their child or when they do not understand their child's needs.
      (6) **Foster home placement** may be necessary to protect the child while attempts are made to correct parental deficits.

2. **Anaclitic depression** results when an attachment relationship is disrupted during a sensitive phase of development (e.g., 18 to 36 months; see V A 1).

3. **Child abuse** may occur if parents have not adequately bonded with the child. This may reflect a deficiency in the development of parental empathy. Not surprisingly, **premature infants** are at increased risk both for complications of bonding and attachment and, concomitantly, for child abuse and neglect [see II C 1 b (5)–(6)]. Psychopathology in either parent should be evaluated and treated.

4. **Vulnerable child syndrome** was originally described by Green and Solnit. These children, who have been ill and have recovered, have parents who may continue to treat them as though they are still vulnerable.
   a. **Symptoms** in this disorder derive from stifling and oppressive affective relationships of the parents with the child. Such children may later show a variety of psychological traits resulting from parental overprotectiveness, including:
      (1) Hypochondriasis
      (2) Hyperactivity
      (3) Separation anxiety
      (4) Learning difficulties
   b. **Management** of vulnerable child syndrome involves informing the parents that the child has recovered and is doing well. Surprisingly, parents may not realize this, and their attitude toward the child may change with this reassurance.

(1) **If reassuring the parents fails,** psychotherapy for the parents is indicated.
(2) **If the child has internalized this sense of fragility and vulnerability,** and it has become part of his identity, psychotherapy for the child is indicated. Affective distance between the parents and the child must be increased, and the age-appropriate autonomy of the child must be reinforced.

5. **Separation anxiety** in toddlerhood and childhood may derive from ambivalent or insecure attachments formed during infancy.

III. FEEDING AND EATING DISORDERS OF INFANCY AND EARLY CHILDHOOD

A. **Pica** is a disorder involving the persistent (for a period of at least 1 month) eating of non-food products (e.g., dirt, clay, paper, plaster). This behavior is developmentally inappropriate and must be differentiated from the practice of mouthing inanimate objects, which is normal between 6 and 12 months of age.

1. **Epidemiology.** Pica may be more common in lower socioeconomic groups.

2. **Etiology**
   a. Children with **mental retardation** mouth objects more than normal children.
   b. **Nutritional deficiencies** may play a role in some cases. Both vitamins and minerals have been suggested. In particular, iron deficiency can cause a craving for ice and nonfood items.
   c. **Parent–child problems** (especially where repeated, traumatic separations are involved) are etiologic in some cases. In these cases, the ingestion most likely represents a response to deprivation and unfulfilled oral needs.
   d. A variety of **rare, neurologic conditions** can cause children to mouth nonfood items (e.g., Klüver-Bucy syndrome).
   e. **Cultural factors** may play a role in some cases, where the ingested substance is believed to have magical or medicinal properties.

3. **Complications** include **bezoars** and **lead poisoning,** which can present as a variety of neurologic and psychiatric manifestations. Lead poisoning is extremely dangerous and is more common in areas of older homes with lead-based paint. Lead poisoning should be suspected in any child with an encephalopathy or who exhibits unusual behavior.

4. **Treatment** involves increasing the amount of stimulation for the child. (Most cities offer infant-stimulation programs.) Psychotherapy for the child and parents may be necessary. Of course, dangerous objects should be removed from the child's environment, and any nutritional deficiencies should be corrected.

B. **Rumination disorder** is a potentially fatal disorder that is most common in infancy and early childhood and is characterized by purposeful expulsion of previously ingested food followed by re-chewing of the food. This usually occurs when the child is alone or is attended only peripherally. On extremely rare occasions, the disorder may be seen among adults, usually with coexistent bulimia nervosa or mental retardation.

1. **Epidemiology.** Rumination disorder is rare and may be decreasing in incidence.

2. **Etiology.** Although theories abound, the disorder often occurs in families in which the parents are psychosexually immature and either distant or overstimulating. Food and chewing may take on a transitional quality for the child and soothe the infant when alone, much like a special doll or blanket.

3. **Treatment**
   a. **Dyad (parent–child) interactions should be observed.** Cues that the parent gives the child to encourage regurgitation should be interpreted and eradicated.
   b. **In-depth psychotherapy of one or both parents** is often needed.
   c. The **infant's nutritional status** should be followed closely.

C. **Feeding disorder of infancy or early childhood (failure to thrive)** is diagnosed when a child fails to gain or to maintain weight at age-appropriate norms. Usually, the third percentile for age-group is considered the threshold. Failure to grow in height sometimes accompanies this, but failure of head circumference growth occurs only in severe cases. In addition to the physical growth retardation, a characteristic emotional and behavioral constellation may be observed as well. This constellation is described within the *Diagnostic and Statistical Manual of Mental Disorders,* 4th edition (DSM-IV) category of **reactive attachment disorder of infancy or early childhood** and is characterized by disturbed and developmentally inappropriate social relatedness. This may take the form of either social unresponsiveness, withdrawal and inhibition, or excessive interpersonal familiarity and lack of appropriate social boundaries.

1. **Etiology**
   a. **Nonorganic failure to thrive.** Failure to thrive as a **psychiatric condition** has numerous causes and manifestations. The following list divides these causes by developmental phase but is not meant to be complete.
      (1) **Early infancy.** Before 8 or 9 months of life, a child is inactive and relies on parental feeding. Failure to thrive in this age range may indicate poor parenting* or troubled parent–child interactions.
      (2) **Late infancy.** After 8 months, failure to thrive may be secondary to anaclitic depression, poor parenting, or childhood psychosis.
      (3) **Toddler stage.** The negativism associated with the "terrible twos" can also apply to eating. Children may refuse to eat in the service of autonomy. Sometimes this negativism may develop earlier, as when parents frantically force food on a 1-year-old child.
   b. **Organic failure to thrive.** A variety of medical conditions can cause failure to thrive and should be evaluated. These include juvenile-onset diabetes mellitus, other endocrine disorders, and malabsorption syndromes.

2. **Treatment.** Any organic cause must be ruled out, and underlying medical disorders must be treated. Parent–child interactions should be evaluated carefully.
   a. **Teaching the parents to recognize and respond to the cues of their child** is in some cases adequate intervention.
   b. In other cases, the **child may need to be hospitalized** to observe if he can gain weight in a new environment.
   c. When parental neglect is present, **child protective agencies** must be involved both to ensure that there is adequate care of the child and that the services necessary to correct parental deficits are available. At times, custody of the child must be taken from the parents, and the child must be placed outside the home.

IV. CHILDHOOD PSYCHOSES

A. **Autistic disorder**

1. **Clinical data.** Autistic disorder is an illness in which the child is relatively unresponsive to other human beings, demonstrates bizarre responses to his environment, and has unusual language development. Autistic disorder most commonly begins before the age of 3 years. Autism is a symptom of several disorders (e.g., schizophrenia). As a symptom, autism refers to a preoccupation with the internal world of the individual to the exclusion of external reactivity.

---

* "Poor parenting" does not fairly encompass all parent–child interactional problems that contribute to this disorder. Eating problems in infancy may also be caused by a lack of synchrony between the parent and the biologic rhythms (e.g., hunger) of the child. The parent may misinterpret certain cues from the infant and miss other cues altogether.

    a. Autistic children often treat other individuals indifferently, almost as though they are inanimate objects.

    b. Language abnormalities include echolalia, pronoun reversals (e.g., use of the pronoun "you" when "I" is correct), mutism, qualitative abnormalities (e.g., a sing-song or monotonous quality), and general language delays.

    c. Autistic children have a great need for consistency in their environment and may decompensate if, for example, furniture is rearranged. The cause of this need for sameness is unknown.

    d. Social development is invariably abnormal.

2. Diagnostic criteria. See Table 10-1.

3. Epidemiology. Although the disorder has an even socioeconomic distribution, it is more common in boys.

3. Etiology. A cold, distant mother figure was thought to be responsible for the development of coldness and aloofness in the child (i.e., growing in an emotional vacuum leads to unrelatedness in the child). However, this theory has been replaced by the understanding that **organic rather than reactive pathology** underlies the disorder, although precise neuropathologic processes have not been determined. Genetic, congenital, immunologic, neuroanatomic, neurophysiologic, and biochemical aberrations have all been suggested.

4. Associated findings

    a. Abnormal auditory evoked potentials (i.e., tracings of the transmission of sound stimuli from the brain stem to the cerebral cortex) are seen.

    b. Imaging studies (e.g., computed tomography scans and magnetic resonance imaging) suggest possible **structural abnormalities**.

    c. Positron-emission tomography studies suggest possible **glucose utilization abnormalities**.

    d. Decreased nystagmus in response to vestibular stimulation occurs.

    e. Developmental distortions (i.e., qualitative abnormalities in development) above and beyond mere delays may occur.

5. Differential diagnosis

    a. Hearing deficits

    b. Visual deficits

TABLE 10-1. Diagnostic Criteria for Autistic Disorder

Social interactional deficits, such as impairment in:
    nonverbal communicative behaviors
    peer relationships
    taking the initiative in social interactions
    interpersonal reciprocity within relationships

Communicative deficits, such as:
    impairment in language development
    impairment in conversational skills
    use of repetitive or idiosyncratic language
    impairment in the development of imaginative or imitative play

Behavioral deficits, such as:
    consuming preoccupation with one, or a few, idiosyncratic areas of interest; otherwise, restricted breadth of interest in the surrounding environment
    excessive need for routine; ritualized behaviors; inordinate resistance to change
    stereotyped motor movements (e.g., hand flapping, rocking)
    preoccupation with parts of objects

    c. Mental retardation accompanied by global developmental delays (not focal social and language distortions and delays as in autism)

    d. Organic mental disorders (e.g., hepatic encephalopathy and congenital cytomegalovirus), which can mimic autism

    e. Tourette syndrome

    f. Fragile X syndrome

    g. Obsessive-compulsive disorder

    h. Childhood schizophrenia

    i. Elective mutism

    j. Other pervasive developmental disorders (e.g., Rett's disorder, childhood disintegrative disorder, Asperger's disorder)

6. Treatment

    a. A **highly structured classroom setting** is important to help autistic children focus their attention on learning and communication tasks. Pragmatics, daily living skills, and a functional curriculum may take precedence over conventional academics. Precautions should be taken to ensure that the environment remains stable.

    b. **Psychotherapy for both the child and parents** may be of value in cases in which parental factors are considered to be partly contributory. Psychotherapy may also be indicated when the family is having trouble coping with the stress of having an autistic child.

    c. **Medication is rarely of value unless a specific indication is present.**

        (1) Some hyperactive autistic children may benefit from stimulant medication (e.g., fenfluramine or methylphenidate).

        (2) Obsessional features may respond to clomipramine or fluoxetine.

        (3) Mood instability may be improved with **mood stabilizers** such as lithium, valproic acid, and carbamazepine.

        (4) Self-stimulating behaviors may improve with **opioid-antagonists** such as naltrexone.

        (5) Rarely are **low-potency neuroleptic medications** indicated except for acute stabilization of aggressive, self-injurious, or severely out of control behaviors.

        (6) **High-potency neuroleptic medications,** such as haloperidol, may benefit the stereotypical social withdrawal in certain autistic children.

    d. **Adjunctive therapies,** such as speech/language therapy, occupational therapy, and physical therapy, are frequently indicated.

7. Prognosis. Many autistic children develop grand mal seizures before adolescence. However, the prognosis for autistic disorder is better if the child has:

    a. A high intelligence quotient

    b. Reasonable language development

    c. Relatively mild symptomatology

B. | **Childhood schizophrenia**

1. Clinical data. Symptoms of childhood schizophrenia may include:

    a. Preoccupation with gory or grotesque fantasies

    b. Hallucinations (usually not prominent; visual hallucinations are more common in children than adults)

    c. Delusions (less common in children than adults)

    d. Propensity to digress, with poor attention span

    e. Responsiveness to individuals in the environment without consistent demonstration of sociability, reciprocity, or empathy

    f. Possible abnormal motor movements

    g. Unusual mannerisms

2. Diagnostic criteria. DSM-IV criteria are the same for children as for adults (see Table 2-1).

3. Etiology

    a. A genetic cause for childhood schizophrenia has not been as well delineated as it has for adult schizophrenia.

b. A **grossly chaotic upbringing** with constant exposure to aggressive and sexual themes (e.g., chronic violence in the family) could be contributory.

c. A **failure of repression** is also considered to be active in the disorder. For example, a child who is repeatedly exposed to violence may be unable to repress sexual and aggressive fantasies. The ability to repress such fantasies normally occurs by the age of 6 years.

d. Whether the prepubertal onset of schizophrenia in childhood represents an early onset within the same spectrum as the adult disorder or whether the prepubertal variant would be better described as schizophreniform disorder remains uncertain.

4. Treatment

a. Psychotherapy is very helpful. Family therapy may be indicated when disruption within the family is evident. When aggression and sexualized stimulation cannot be minimized within the home, out-of-home placement should be considered.

b. Psychiatric day treatment may be indicated when the child's symptoms preclude his ability to function adequately within a public school environment.

c. Antipsychotic medication (e.g., thioridazine at an orally administered daily dose of 1 mg/kg or haloperidol at an orally administered daily dose of 1–5 mg) may be necessary.

5. Prognosis. The prognosis for childhood schizophrenia is generally more favorable than for adult schizophrenia, provided adequate treatment and remediation of environmental deficits occur. Nonetheless, studies indicate that at least 50% of individuals with childhood schizophrenia persist with significant symptoms and deficits into adulthood. A family history of schizophrenia worsens the prognosis.

C. **Symbiotic psychosis**

1. Clinical data. Symbiotic psychosis is a disorder in which parents misperceive themselves as their child. The reciprocal is usually true also. Although this disorder usually occurs in mothers and their children, fathers occasionally are affected.

a. A loss of ego boundaries (i.e., the inability to distinguish oneself from others) is apparent.

b. Great anxiety at the threat of separation of the child from the parent is seen in both. Upon reuniting, the anxiety clears.

c. The overlap between parent and child can be manifested in almost any area (e.g., if parents diet, they assume that the child needs to diet).

d. Although this disorder is still observed clinically, it is not specifically accounted for within the DSM-IV, where it would be considered a psychotic disorder not otherwise specified.

2. Etiology. Parents who have **poor object relations** may see their child as an extension of themselves. **Borderline psychopathology** may predispose people to this disorder. Although the parent is the cause of the problem, the child usually manifests the symptoms (e.g., severe separation anxiety).

3. Treatment. Psychotherapy aimed at separating the child from the parent is needed. Sometimes parents may require support to help them permit the separation and development of autonomy in the child. In certain refractory cases, an actual separation through out-of-home placement may be necessary.

4. Prognosis. Symbiotic psychosis carries the best prognosis of all the childhood psychoses, probably due to the fact that its etiology is reactive and developmental rather than organically based.

V. **CHILDHOOD MOOD DISORDERS.** Biologic markers, which are still being investigated, are even less valuable in identifying childhood depressive disorders than in identifying adult disorders.

A. **Clinical data.** Depressive illness presents at all stages of development.

1. **Children between the ages of 7 and 30 months** demonstrate **anaclitic depression**. The cause is a lengthy separation (more than 1 week) from caregivers with whom they have established an attachment relationship. Symptoms include listlessness, anorexia, psychomotor retardation, and sad facial expressions. The treatment is restitution of the relationship.

2. Depressed **preschool children** often demonstrate behavioral difficulties, such as hyperactivity and aggression, more than older children. These symptoms are called **depressive equivalents**. Separation from caregivers or a poor sense of mastery over developmental tasks (e.g., toilet training) may be etiologic. Treatment should be aimed at changing the child's environment. Psychotherapy may help.

3. **Schoolchildren** may manifest the usual signs and symptoms of depression (e.g., vegetative signs, a depressed mood). Biologic vulnerabilities and a sense of helplessness or incompetence may play an etiologic role at this age. Treatment is psychotherapy aimed at helping the child feel a sense of competence in relation to her environment.

4. **Adolescents** also demonstrate the usual signs of depression, especially a pervasive sense of boredom and lack of future orientation. The incidence of depressive disorders increases in adolescence, with girls affected more frequently than boys. In children and adolescents, the depressive mood is commonly expressed as **marked irritability**.

B. **Diagnostic criteria.** DSM-IV criteria are the same for children as for adults (see Table 3-1).

C. **Treatment**

1. **Psychotherapy.** Insight-oriented models aimed at grieving past losses and at remediating early intrapsychic traumas have been used effectively in treating childhood mood disorders. Cognitive–behavioral models aimed at correcting cognitive distortions and reversing pervasive patterns of negativistic thinking have also been successful.

2. **Medication.** Although the research remains somewhat controversial, clinical experience suggests that **antidepressants** may be a useful adjunct in the treatment of depression in certain children and adolescents.
   a. Most often, medications are used to augment ongoing individual or family psychotherapy.
   b. Both **tricyclic antidepressants,** such as imipramine and nortriptyline, as well as the newer-generation selective serotonin reuptake inhibitors (**SSRIs**) such as fluoxetine, have been used effectively with children and adolescents.
   c. Parents must take the responsibility for administering the medication and for safeguarding the child and siblings from inadvertent overdosage.

D. **Associated mood disorders**

1. **Manic-depressive (bipolar) illness** may present in early childhood. DSM-IV criteria are the same for children as for adults (see Table 3-2).
   a. **Mood stabilizers,** such as lithium, valproic acid, and carbamazepine, have been used effectively in children and adolescents.
   b. **Hyperactivity** [attention deficit hyperactivity disorder (ADHD)] may be **mistaken for mania;** however, major mood changes are not seen in hyperactive children.

2. **Suicide** may be a complication of a mood disorder in childhood and adolescence, as well as in later developmental stages.
   a. The **incidence** of suicide is increasing in preadolescence and in adolescence (it has essentially tripled among adolescents over the past 30 years).
   b. **Treatment.** Depressed children should be carefully evaluated for suicidal ideation. When present, suicidal children may require psychiatric hospitalization for acute clinical stabilization and their own safety.

VI. TOURETTE DISORDER

A. **Clinical data.** Tourette disorder consists of recurrent, involuntary, purposeless motor movements accompanied by vocal tics (e.g., coprolalia, involuntary swearing, barking, and grunting). Motor tics may precede or follow the development of vocal tics. Psychological stress exacerbates the symptoms, but the cause, although unknown, is probably organic. Both ADHD and obsessive-compulsive disorder occur with increased frequency among patients with Tourette disorder.

B. **Diagnostic criteria** (Table 10-2)

C. **Epidemiology.** Tourette disorder is more common in boys. Onset is before the age of 21 years and often occurs in early childhood. Tourette disorder occurs in all socioeconomic classes and is considerably more prevalent than once believed. There is a spectrum of symptom severity, and previously undiagnosed cases with more mild symptoms are now being appropriately diagnosed.

D. **Treatment**

1. **Psychotherapy** is indicated when the tics cause psychological problems.

2. **Education** about the nature and course of the disorder for both the patient and the family is essential.

3. **Medical treatment** includes the use of the following:
   a. **Haloperidol** suppresses the tics.
   b. **Pimozide** is an effective neuroleptic medication; however, it may cause cardiac arrhythmias.
   c. **Clonidine** has also proved to be effective in some cases of Tourette disorder. Although highly sedating, clonidine does not lead to the dystonic and dyskinetic side effects of the neuroleptics.

VII. SLEEP DISORDERS

A. **Parasomnias** are sleep disorders that usually affect stages 3 and 4 of sleep, which predominate early in the sleep cycle. Thus, these disorders usually occur early in the night. Examples include the following:

1. **Somnambulism** (sleep walking) is exacerbated by psychological stress in some cases but is normal much of the time. Alcoholism unmasks somnambulism in adults.

2. **Somniloquy** (sleep talking) has little clinical significance; however, if somniloquy is present, more significant parasomnias may be present.

3. **Night terrors** are very common between the ages of 2½ and 5 years, affecting 30% of children in this age bracket. Terrors are sometimes exacerbated by stress.

TABLE 10-2. Diagnostic Criteria for Tourette Disorder

Multiple tics, including both motor and vocal tics
Frequent tics, nearly daily, for a year or more with no asymptomatic period of more than 3 months
Emotional distress and/or functional impairment as a result of the tics
Onset before age 18

    a. Night terrors should be distinguished from nightmares, which occur during rapid eye movement (REM) sleep and whose content is remembered as a bad dream by:

      (1) The inconsolability of the child during the event

      (2) The absence of recall of the content of the dream

      (3) The absence of recall of the event the following morning

    b. Treatment. Although seldom necessary, night terrors may be treated by agents that suppress deep sleep, such as **chloral hydrate** or **benzodiazepines**.

  4. Nocturnal enuresis (see VIII A 1) is due generally to stress or to slow central nervous system (CNS) maturation. The disorder dissipates with increasing age and is, therefore, self-limited.

B. **Narcolepsy** is characterized by REM-onset sleep.

  1. Manifestations

    a. The entire sleep cycle is affected, resulting in **excessive daytime drowsiness and sleep attacks**.

    b. Cataplexy is the loss of motor tone in response to an emotion (e.g., anger or excitement).

    c. On awakening, the patient may be transiently, but completely, paralyzed (**sleep paralysis**).

    d. Hypnagogic hallucinations are vivid auditory and visual hallucinations that occur at the onset or end of sleep.

  2. Treatment. Administration of agents that suppress REM sleep, such as psychostimulants and tricyclic antidepressants, provide some symptomatic relief for patients suffering from narcolepsy.

VIII. ELIMINATION DISORDERS

A. **Enuresis**

  1. Clinical data. The child with enuresis continues to urinate at inappropriate times and places after the time when he should have been toilet trained (i.e., between the ages of 2 and 4 years). The disorder is much more common in boys.

    a. Primary enuresis is that which has never been interrupted by a period of good bladder control.

      (1) Nocturnal enuresis is a parasomnia that occurs during stages 3 and 4 of sleep.

      (2) Diurnal enuresis occurs during the waking hours.

    b. Secondary enuresis develops after a period of at least 1 year of good bladder control. As in primary enuresis, the disorder may occur both during the sleeping and waking hours.

    c. The DSM-IV specifies that episodes occur at a frequency of at least twice weekly for 3 months or more. In addition, the condition is not diagnosed before the chronological age (or developmental age in developmentally impaired children) of 5 years.

  2. Etiology

    a. Organic disorders may cause enuresis. These include:

      (1) Systemic illnesses, such as:

        (a) Juvenile-onset diabetes mellitus

        (b) Sickle cell anemia or sickle cell trait

        (c) Diabetes insipidus

      (2) Central nervous system disorders, such as:

        (a) Frontal lobe tumor

        (b) Spinal cord lesion (e.g., spina bifida or spina bifida occulta)

        (c) Peripheral nerve damage

(3) Anatomic disorders, such as:
   (a) Posterior urethral valvular dysfunction
   (b) Proximal genitourinary malformations
(4) Urinary tract infections
(5) Delayed CNS maturation (after the age of 4½ years, as many as 10% of boys remain enuretic, frequently due to delayed maturation)

b. Psychological factors account for the majority of cases of secondary enuresis.
   (1) Acute stress can cause enuresis (e.g., the birth of a sibling, a family move, starting kindergarten).
   (2) Ambition. Enuresis sometimes occurs in very ambitious boys. Strength and quality of the urine stream may become equated with physical prowess. Micturition can then become conflicted, resulting in urination at inappropriate times.
   (3) Hostility can be expressed through the symptom of enuresis. Such an expression of hostility is nearly always unconscious: The child does not deliberately void at inappropriate times.
   (4) Family reaction to the enuresis sometimes causes more psychopathology than do the psychological causes of the enuresis per se. The family may encourage enuresis unconsciously. A possible vicarious pleasure for the parents in the child's enuresis may exist.
   (5) Preoccupation. Children who are too busy or preoccupied to use the bathroom may suffer from enuresis.

3. Treatment may be only sporadically necessary. Because enuresis is a self-limited disorder, sometimes no treatment is best. Parents should be reassured that the disorder is a time-limited, normal developmental variant (especially the primary nocturnal pattern) that will ultimately be outgrown.
   a. Probing diagnostic procedures to search for an organic etiology, unless the preponderance of evidence points to such, **should be avoided**.
   b. The parents should be assured that the child is not purposefully wetting (enuresis is usually beyond the child's control). **Remedial measures** include:
      (1) Reduction of fluid intake after dinner
      (2) Awakening the child to urinate after 1 to 2 hours of sleep
      (3) Bladder exercises (having the child hold urine during the daytime for progressively longer periods of time)
      (4) Use of special feedback devices that set off an alarm upon urination in bed
   c. Medication
      (1) Tricyclic antidepressant therapy can be effective. Imipramine, for example, should be administered in an after-school dose. Often, the desired effect can be obtained with considerably smaller doses (10–25 mg) than are required for an antidepressant effect. Antidepressants should be used judiciously, particularly in refractory or unusual cases (e.g., the parents are completely intolerant of the condition). Although initial symptom response to imipramine is common, breakthrough on that same dose may occur, resulting in the recurrence of enuresis.
      (2) Desmopressin, a synthetic antidiuretic hormone that is produced as a nasal spray, may also offer symptomatic improvement.
      (3) Because of the time-limited nature of the disorder, drug holidays should be evaluated at least every 6 months to assess the need for continuing pharmacologic intervention.
   d. The child should be treated for any psychological stress. In refractory cases, intensive **psychotherapy** may be indicated.

B. Encopresis

1. Clinical data. Encopresis is fecal incontinence beyond the period when bowel control should normally have developed. Most encopresis is unconscious and involuntary; only occasionally does it occur deliberately.
   a. Primary encopresis is that which has occurred continuously throughout the child's life.

b. Secondary encopresis develops following a period of at least 1 year of good bowel control.

c. The DSM-IV delineates two additional **subtypes:**
  (1) **With constipation and overflow incontinence**
  (2) **Without constipation and overflow incontinence**

2. Etiology
  a. Organic disorders. Hirschsprung disease rarely presents in older children as encopresis.
    (1) In this disorder, the functional obstruction is proximal to the rectal vault so that no fecal obstruction is palpable on digital examination.
    (2) In the encopresis variant with constipation and overflow incontinence, however, the children avoid evacuating their bowels and retain feces.
      (a) This results in a fecal impaction that is readily identifiable within the rectal vault.
      (b) In these children, stool is passed around the impaction, oftentimes in small amounts.
  b. Psychological factors
    (1) **Unresolved anger at a parent** sometimes is expressed unconsciously through fecal incontinence. The child consciously and unconsciously perceives that his stool has a negative impact on the family.
    (2) **Regressive wishes** may be expressed by soiling in undernurtured and emotionally deprived children.
    (3) Fecal smearing may be a **psychotic symptom,** especially if the child is older than 4 or 5 years of age.
    (4) As is true with enuresis, parents can get vicarious pleasure from their child's symptoms.
    (5) When **autonomy and control battles** focus on toilet training at the age of 2 to 3 years and when parents are too punitive and unyielding in their approach to the toilet training, conflicts over bowel evacuation develop in the child.

3. Treatment
  a. Correcting fecal impaction is necessary. A bowel regimen that consists of periodic cathartic administration to ensure that no impaction develops and to help regulate bowel control (e.g., administration of a bisacodyl suppository daily at the same time, immediately followed by placing the child on the toilet) may be of benefit.
  b. Behavior modification that reinforces continence is effective in some children (e.g., rewarding a child after a day of good bowel control or after evacuation in the toilet).
  c. Psychotherapy is usually indicated. Occasionally, encopresis is a symptom of psychosis. The underlying disease should then be treated.
  d. Family therapy is often also indicated.

IX. MASTURBATION

A. **Definition.** Childhood masturbation involves genital manipulation and fondling. It is a universal behavior, not a disease. Nonetheless, many parents complain to the physician about this behavior in their children. An open attitude on the part of the physician is important in allowing the parents to express concern. Any notions that masturbation may cause growth retardation, mental retardation, or any adverse physical consequence should be dispelled.

B. **Incidence.** Masturbation occurs in all children. It can develop before the age of 1 year. During the oedipal period (i.e., between the ages of 3½ and 6 years), there is heightened focus on the genitalia.

C. **Etiology.** Continuous masturbation may be a sign of severe understimulation, environmental deprivation, or of excessive sexual stimulation or sexual abuse.

    1. Other signs of self-stimulation (e.g., rocking, head banging, hair pulling) should be sought. The child should be enrolled in a stimulation program, and the situation should be followed up.

    2. Signs of child abuse should also be sought. A detailed history of the child's exposure to sexual stimulation should be elicited. A careful physical examination may be indicated.

X. THUMB SUCKING

A. **Incidence.** Thumb sucking is more common in girls and is normal at transitional periods in the child's life (e.g., at bedtime, at times of separation from the parents). When it persists into the grade-school years, it more likely suggests underlying individual or family pathology.

B. **Treatment** is not usually needed. If thumb sucking is chronic and occurs after the age of 3½ years, it can cause changes in dentition.

    1. An in-depth exploration of the child's relationship with the parents is usually indicated, as is **psychotherapy**.

    2. Thumb sucking in the older child can be a sign that the child is insecure or withdrawn. **Behavior modification** can be useful.

    3. Coating the thumb with astringent agents has been of limited benefit.

XI. SCHOOL PHOBIAS

A. **Definition.** School phobias are a fearful attitude toward and avoidance of school. In adolescence, they may herald the emergence of schizophrenia.

B. **Incidence.** School phobias most commonly occur when a child is first introduced to school (at age 4 or 5 years) and in early adolescence when children are required to shower at school after gym class. School phobias occur throughout childhood, however.

C. **Etiology.** School phobia is best considered a symptom. It is caused by a variety of conditions, including:

    1. Separation anxiety suffered by the child

    2. Separation anxiety suffered by the parent

    3. Malingering (e.g., the child has not completed a homework assignment)

    4. A legitimate cause of fear to the child at school (e.g., gangs, a cruel teacher)

    5. Vulnerable child syndrome

    6. Homosexual panic in an older child

D. **Treatment**

    1. Legitimate causes of fear should be evaluated for and eliminated when present. **The child should usually be sent back to school immediately.** Thus, school avoidance is not reinforced by staying home.

    2. Psychotherapy to treat the underlying disorder may be needed.

3. **Desensitization and other behavior therapy** modalities may be of benefit.

4. **Parental therapy** is necessary when the child is acting out the parent's anxiety about separating from the child.

5. Some cases are exceedingly refractory to treatment interventions and may even require **psychiatric hospitalization**.

6. **Anxiolytic medications,** such as tricyclic antidepressants, buspirone, and occasionally benzodiazepines, may offer acute symptom relief. In general, they are usually unnecessary on an ongoing basis.

XII. ATTENTION DEFICIT HYPERACTIVITY DISORDER (ADHD)

A. **Clinical data.** Key symptoms of ADHD include a short attention span, difficulty concentrating, impulsivity, distractibility, excitability, and hyperactivity.

1. **Hyperactivity** is defined subjectively as an increase in motor activity to a level that interferes with the child's functioning at school, at home, or socially.

2. It is important to note, however, that symptoms of **attention deficit disorder may exist with or without hyperactivity**.

3. The DSM-IV distinguishes **three subtypes** of the disorder based on this differentiation:
   a. ADHD; predominantly inattentive type
   b. ADHD; predominantly hyperactive–impulsive type
   c. ADHD; combined type

B. **Diagnostic criteria.** See Table 10-3.

TABLE 10-3. Diagnostic Criteria for Attention Deficit Hyperactivity Disorder

Symptoms of inattention, such as:
lack of attention to details
difficulty sustaining attention for prolonged periods
not listening
difficulty following through or completing tasks
disorganization
avoidance of activities that require sustained attention
tendency to lose personal belongings
marked distractibility
forgetfulness
Symptoms of hyperactivity, such as:
fidgetiness or squirminess
difficulty remaining in seat, or sitting quietly
developmentally excessive activity level
difficulty engaging in nonaction activities
talking excessively
Symptoms of impulsivity, such as:
blurting out answers without raising hand, or waiting for the end of the question
difficulty with "turn-taking" activities
frequent interruption or intrusion into others' conversations or activities
Presence of some symptoms before 7 years of age
Significant functional impairment as a result of the symptoms

C. Etiology

1. **Medication.** Sedative–hypnotics paradoxically cause hyperactivity in some children.

2. **Depression.** Sad feelings may be expressed by means of increased activity.

3. **Anxiety**

4. **Severe CNS disease.** A grossly abnormal CNS or a history of significant head trauma may cause hyperactivity.

5. **Constitutional hyperactivity.** Some children have a hyperactive temperament that is present from birth.

6. **An intolerant parent, teacher, or supervisor** may bring about factitious hyperactivity (i.e., the child is not truly suffering from increased motor activity).

7. **Specific learning disabilities** may be associated with hyperactivity.

8. Severe **language disorders**

9. There is an increased incidence of ADHD among children with **Tourette disorder**.

D. Treatment. Any underlying disorder should be treated (e.g., depression should be treated by means of psychotherapy, possibly in conjunction with antidepressant medication).

1. **Medications**
   a. **Stimulant medications** are effective (e.g., **methylphenidate** administered in a divided dose of 5–60 mg/day). Alternate choices include **dextroamphetamine** and **pemoline**. Growth curves should be followed on all children taking stimulant medication because appetite and growth suppression are the most common side effects.
   b. **Clonidine** has been shown to be an effective alternative to psychostimulants in many children. It may also be used effectively to augment psychostimulants in certain refractory cases. Its predominant side effect is sedation.
   c. **Antidepressants** such as **desipramine** and **bupropion** have been effective alternative agents in some children.

2. **Diet.** An alteration in the child's diet may be helpful, presumably because the emphasis on food alters a parent's relationship with a child in some meaningful way.
   a. Many parents of hyperactive children report that reducing the child's sugar intake reduces the hyperactivity.
      (1) These parents may pay more attention to their child, feel more in control of the problem, and spend more time with the child at mealtime as a result of changing the child's diet.
      (2) All of these secondary effects can be beneficial.
   b. No direct effects of diet on either the etiology or treatment of ADHD have been demonstrated, however.

3. **Behavior modification programs** are often beneficial. Despite the ADHD symptomatic deficits, children with this disorder must still be held accountable for their behavior and its consequences.

4. While **psychotherapy** is not the mainstay of treatment in this disorder, it may be a useful adjunct to a comprehensive treatment plan in certain children.

5. **Environmental engineering** is of great benefit in this disorder. Because children with ADHD do not readily adapt to change, or function well within highly stimulating environments, the environment around them should be constructed to minimize these deficits.
   a. Within the classroom, children with ADHD attend and concentrate better in the front row than in the rear.
   b. Study carrels are helpful because they block distracting stimuli.
   c. Children with ADHD function better with one-on-one instruction or small groups than in larger groups.

XIII. SPECIFIC DEVELOPMENTAL DISORDERS

A. **Clinical data.** There are a wide range of disorders that interfere with the child's ability to perform certain intellectual functions. Children may suffer from specific reading, processing, writing, mathematical, and language disabilities (e.g., developmental dyslexia).

1. These disorders are to be distinguished from both mental retardation and pervasive developmental disorders.

2. **Diagnosis** is established by documenting a mismatch between the child's performance on standardized measures of the skill in question and her intellectual capacity as measured by IQ testing.

3. The DSM-IV includes the following **categories and specific disorders**.
   a. **Learning disorders**
      (1) Reading disorder
      (2) Mathematics disorder
      (3) Disorder of written expression
   b. **Motor skills disorder** (developmental coordination disorder)
   c. **Communication disorders**
      (1) Expressive language disorder
      (2) Mixed receptive–expressive language disorder
      (3) Phonological disorder
      (4) Stuttering

B. **Differential diagnosis** of specific developmental problems includes a variety of psychiatric conditions.

1. **Depression**

2. **ADHD**

3. **School phobias**

4. **Other anxiety disorders**

5. **An interaction problem with the teacher**

6. **Childhood psychosis**

7. **Mental retardation**

8. **Pervasive developmental disorders**

C. **Treatment** is aimed at the underlying dysfunction. Learning disorders require academic remediation. The spectrum of services in this domain ranges from extra tutoring focused on the problematic academic skill (e.g., phonics tutoring for children with dyslexia) to placement in self-contained, special education classrooms for those with learning disorders.

1. **Motor skills disorder** may require occupational or physical therapy.

2. **Communication disorders** usually require intensive speech and language therapy.

XIV. PROBLEMS OF ADOLESCENTS. A variety of disorders increases in incidence during adolescence (e.g., anorexia nervosa, adult schizophrenia, depression). Specific problems of adolescent development are discussed here.

A. **Identity disturbances.** Adolescents struggle to achieve a stable identity. Certain problems result when this aspect of development breaks down.

1. **Identity diffusion.** An adolescent has a poor sense of himself and is easily swayed by the opinions of others.

2. **Peer-related disorders.** Some adolescents can be persuaded to do dangerous things (e.g., become sexually promiscuous, take drugs, drink alcohol, drive recklessly) in order to identify with their peer groups.

3. Problems with successfully resolving this developmental task may contribute to the development of **identity disorder, narcissistic personality disorder, and borderline personality disorder.**

B. **Adult sexual development.** In adolescence, adult sexual functioning is achieved, and sexual preferences are solidified.

1. **Homosexual behaviors** are found commonly in early adolescence. However, when they occur consistently throughout adolescence, it usually represents a true homosexual preference.

2. **Paraphilias.** The symptom expression found in exhibitionism, fetishism, frotteurism, pedophilia, sexual masochism, sexual sadism, transvestic fetishism, and voyeurism usually begins or heightens in adolescence.

3. **Pregnancy** may be the outcome of increased sexual promiscuity or may manifest from emancipation difficulties. For example, an adolescent who is struggling with separating from her family may become pregnant and turn the infant over to the parents for care. The infant, thus, replaces her and makes her emancipation easier.

4. **Sexually transmitted diseases,** including human immunodeficiency virus (HIV), are a risk of heightened sexual expression and activity during adolescence.

C. **Separation.** Adolescents negotiate emancipation from their family, and they redefine the parent–child and sibling roles and boundaries.

1. **Difficulty with emancipation** can be etiologic in a variety of clinical disorders. For example:
   a. **Schizophrenia.** Psychosis becomes evident in many schizophrenics when they first leave home.
   b. **Anorexia.** The battle over food is really a struggle for autonomy and independence in many anorectics.
   c. **Depression.** Separation and loss can trigger depressive feelings and even a major depressive episode in individuals so predisposed.

2. Difficult emancipation can lead to **mobilization of aggression** on the part of the adolescent, and intrafamily fighting ensues. Many adolescents feel that only through conflict will they be able to successfully emancipate.

3. **Incest** can develop to prevent a child from emancipating, and inappropriate sexual contact within a family sometimes signifies separation problems.

D. **Treatment.** Special problems develop in the psychotherapy of adolescents.

1. **Labile allegiances.** Adolescents love the therapist one day and hate her the next day.

2. **Labile moods.** Because adolescents are in great hormonal and psychological turbulence, unstable moods frequently result.

3. **Communication difficulties.** Adolescents may not be comfortable with verbal communication but are too old for communication through play.
   a. Some adolescents **communicate by means of their behavior** (e.g., reckless driving may signify anger or depression).
   b. **Obstinancy** may signify an emancipation problem because the child refuses to take responsibility for himself.

4. Overprotective parents or parents with indistinct parent–child boundaries may meddle in an adolescent's treatment. In most cases, adolescents should be seen at their own request, even if this is contrary to the wishes of the parents. When parents are involved in the treatment of an adolescent, the confidentiality of the relationship between the physician and the adolescent still is paramount. Parents should be notified, however, if the patient is:
a. A danger to himself
b. A danger to others
c. Gravely disabled and unable to care for herself or to exercise appropriate judgment on her behalf

XV. CHILD ABUSE occurs when the individuals in a child's environment retard his development by hurting the child.

A. Epidemiology

1. Child abuse may be **physical, sexual, or emotional. Significant neglect** should be considered equivalent to abuse.

2. Approximately **15% of children who come to the emergency room with obvious trauma** have been abused.

3. **Parents who were abused** as children are at greater risk for abusing their own children.

4. Parents who are not overtly abusive may be **silently participating** in the abuse by failing to protect the child from the abusive parent (e.g., a mother who is physically present within the home, yet who is "unaware" of years of ongoing father–daughter incest).

5. **Premature infants** are abused more often than full-term infants, which is probably due, at least in part, to poor bonding.

6. **Reasons** for the abuse of infants often differ from those for the abuse of older children.
   a. Abuse of older children may be associated with psychosexual development (e.g., a 3-year-old soils her pants and is beaten).
   b. Abuse of infants occurs more frequently because their parents are emotionally needy and feel that the infant is taking attention away from them.
   (1) In this case, role reversal is common as well. That is, the parent feels it is the duty of the child to meet their emotional needs—to make the parent feel whole and good about himself.
   (2) When the infant "demands" that her needs for basic care or nurture be met, conflict with the reciprocal "demand" by the parent results and a potentially abusive situation ensues.
   (3) Likewise, when the parent's esteem is threatened by the perception that they are not a good or effective parent (e.g., when the child cries), they are at increased risk for abuse of the child.
   (4) Therefore, periods of normal infant fussiness (e.g., when hungry, sleepy, in need of diapering) or times when the infant is physically ill become potential crisis points for abusive parents and their infants.

7. **Children with physical or developmental disorders** are at increased risk for abuse and neglect.

8. The abused child is often the **scapegoat** for the individual pathology of other family members or for family pathology.

9. It is **unusual for child abuse to begin after the age of 6 years,** with the exception of sexual abuse.

10. Abuse occurs in **all socioeconomic groups.**

B. Effects on the child

1. Occasionally, **emotional development may be precocious**.
   a. The expectation that a child function as "a parent" (role reversal) causes some children to develop quickly.
   b. Fear of being abused for mistakes can also lead to precocious development and to **perfectionism** as a personality trait.
      (1) The precocity, however, tends to be superficial and defensive.
      (2) The underlying desire to be validated as a child for age-appropriate attributes is usually also apparent.

2. Conversely, in some children, **development may be retarded** if the abuse is severe or enduring. In these cases, the destructive and deleterious impact of the abuse outweighs the child's ability to mount adaptive defenses against it.

3. **Physical injuries** are a constant risk.

4. **Emotional injuries** are an equally significant and consistent risk.
   a. These injuries may take the form of **low self-esteem and excessive guilt,** which derive from the irrational acceptance of responsibility for the abuse (i.e., "I am bad or unlovable," rather than "My parent has a problem").
   b. **Chronic depression** and full-blown **posttraumatic stress disorder,** where symptoms of the abuse are persistently reexperienced, may occur.
   c. Both **psychic numbing** and **chronic hyperarousal** are present.

5. There is a **risk of abusing future offspring** when the abused child grows up and identifies with his parents.

6. **Exposure to chronic violence** can increase aggression and antisocial behavior in the abused child.

C. Treatment

1. **Suspected abuse must be reported** to the county protective services. If the child's health or life is in jeopardy, he should be removed from the abusive environment. If there is no improvement within 1 to 2 years after diagnosis, severance of parental rights should be considered.

2. **Most abused children need psychotherapy.** Ultimately, the goal is to break what is often a multigenerational pattern of abuse within a family and to allow the child to grow into an adult who is capable of empathy, intimacy, and relational reciprocity in ways the previous generations were not. At times, the therapeutic relationship may be the first adult–child relationship that models a nonexploitive, noncontingent, emotionally available and empathically attuned focus on the needs and well-being of the child.

3. **Parents almost always need intensive, individual psychotherapy,** and often **marital therapy** as well.
   a. Parents may also benefit from **parent training classes,** which educate them about normal development, appropriate limits and boundaries, and nonexploitive techniques for discipline and behavioral management.
   b. It is often erroneously assumed that the knowledge base of parents far exceeds what it does in actual practice.

BIBLIOGRAPHY

American Psychiatric Association: *Diagnostic and Statistical Manual of Mental Disorders,* 4th ed. Washington, DC, American Psychiatric Association, 1994.

Emde RN, Harmon RJ, Good WV: Depressive feelings in children: A transactional model for research. In *Depression in Childhood: Developmental Perspectives.* Edited by Rutter M, Izard D, Reed P. New York, Gilford Press, 1986.

Garfinkle BD, Carlson GA, Weller, EB (eds): *Psychiatric Disorders in Children and Adolescents.* Philadelphia, WB Saunders, 1990.

Green M, Solnit AJ: Reactions to the threatened loss of a child: A vulnerable child syndrome. *Pediatrics* 34:58–65, 1964.

Klaus MH, Kendall JH: *Parent-Infant Bonding.* St. Louis, CV Mosby, 1982.

Lewis M (ed): *Child and Adolescent Psychiatry: A Comprehensive Textbook.* Baltimore, Williams & Wilkins, 1991.

Spitz RA: Hospitalism: An inquiry into the genesis of psychiatric conditions in early childhood. *Psychoanal Study Child* 1:53–74, 1945.

Steele BF, Pollock CB: A psychiatric study of parents who abuse infants and small children. In *The Battered Child.* Edited by Helfer RE, Kempe CH. Chicago, University of Chicago Press, 1968, pp 103–145.

Wiener JM (ed): *Textbook of Child and Adolescent Psychiatry.* Washington, DC, American Psychiatric Association, 1991.

DIRECTIONS: Each of the numbered items or incomplete statements in this section is followed by answers or by completions of the statement. Select the ONE numbered answer or completion that is BEST in each case.

1. A 22-year-old woman has just delivered a healthy boy by cesarean section under general anesthesia. When she awakens she is frantic because she has not bonded to her child. The physician should

(A) reassure the patient that bonding is a lengthy process
(B) suggest that the mother breast-feed to offset the effects of poor postnatal bonding
(C) return in 1 day to see if the patient's concerns have dissipated
(D) recommend psychiatric counseling aimed at helping the patient attach to her child
(E) none of the above

2. Which of the following statements about childhood schizophrenia is most accurate?

(A) A genetic linkage with the adult syndrome of schizophrenia has been established
(B) A failure of repression has been suggested etiologically
(C) Auditory hallucinations are prominent
(D) Antipsychotic medication is seldom indicated due to the age of the child
(E) None of the above

3. Anaclitic depression classically occurs between

(A) birth and 6 months
(B) 7 and 30 months
(C) 18 and 36 months
(D) 30 and 48 months
(E) none of the above

4. Which of the following statements about encopresis is most accurate?

(A) The symptom is usually deliberate
(B) The symptom usually derives from delayed nervous system maturation
(C) The symptom usually indicates underlying gastrointestinal pathology
(D) The symptom usually derives from an underlying psychotic disorder
(E) The symptom is never adequate to establish diagnosis in children younger than 4 years

5. Which of the following statements regarding learning disorder is most accurate?

(A) Subtypes of the disorder include reading, writing, mathematics, history, and humanities
(B) It is an equivalent but less pejorative term than mental retardation
(C) Achievement testing and intelligence testing reflect differential profiles among individuals with these disorders
(D) They fall within the broader spectrum of pervasive developmental disorders
(E) None of the statements are accurate

Questions 6–8

A 7-year-old boy is brought to the child psychiatrist by his parents on a referral by the school where the child is in the second grade. The boy does not have a discipline problem, but he frequently answers questions without being called upon and is often out of his seat without permission. His schoolwork is adequate, but the teacher believes he is capable of better. He has difficulty completing tasks and appears to spend much of the class time daydreaming.

6. Which additional piece of information would be most helpful in considering a differential diagnosis?

(A) A history of head injuries
(B) A history of neurologic symptoms
(C) A history of tics
(D) His medication history
(E) All of the above

7. Which of the following conditions would NOT be included in the differential diagnosis?

(A) Pervasive developmental disorder
(B) Anxiety
(C) Depression
(D) Attention deficit hyperactivity disorder (ADHD)
(E) All of the disorders should be included

8. Regarding treatment, the best advice to the family would be

(A) he has a diagnosable disorder so he should not be held accountable for his symptoms
(B) they should alter his diet immediately
(C) he needs intensive, probably long-term psychotherapy
(D) medications might be helpful
(E) they should probably not discuss his diagnosis with his school teacher as it might be stigmatizing

Questions 9–11

A 3-year-old girl is brought to the emergency department by her mother with a swollen and discolored forearm. Radiographs reveal an ulnar fracture. Her mother describes that the child had been jumping on the bed, lost her balance, and fell. The physician observes that the mother is apparently in her seventh or eighth month of pregnancy. He also observes that the child is quite thin and somewhat disheveled in appearance, and her hygiene is poor. When he asks if anyone else lives in their home, the mother acknowledges that her boyfriend does, and then hastens to state, "but he wasn't even home when this happened."

9. In addition to the radiographs, the medically necessary work-up would potentially include

(A) a complete physical examination
(B) a genital examination
(C) a detailed developmental history
(D) an interview with the child
(E) all of the above

10. Which statement best describes the physician's obligation to report the incident to the local child protective service agency?

(A) If the physician suspects that the injuries might derive from abuse, then the incident must be reported
(B) If the physician finds additional evidence of deprivation and neglect, then he must report it
(C) If the physician finds additional evidence of physical abuse, then he must report it
(D) If the physician finds additional evidence of sexual abuse, then he must report it
(E) If in addition to the physician's findings, the child alleges abuse, then he must report it

11. Which of the following is NOT considered a risk factor for child abuse and neglect?

(A) Chronic illness
(B) Developmental delays
(C) Developmental phases
(D) Provocative temperament
(E) Scapegoating

DIRECTIONS: Each of the numbered items or incomplete statements in this section is negatively phrased, as indicated by a capitalized word such as NOT, LEAST, or EXCEPT. Select the ONE lettered answer or completion that is BEST in each case.

12. Which of the following findings has NOT been demonstrated to support a neurologic etiology of autistic disorder?

(A) A high incidence of grand mal seizures
(B) Abnormal auditory evoked potentials
(C) Decreased responsivity to vestibular stimulation
(D) Enlarged ventricles on computed tomography scans
(E) A high incidence of mental retardation

13. Which of the following medications does NOT target specific symptoms of attention deficit hyperactivity disorder (ADHD)?

(A) Haloperidol
(B) Fenfluramine
(C) Clonidine
(D) Bupropion
(E) Methylphenidate

DIRECTIONS: Each set of matching questions in this section consists of a list of four to twenty-six lettered options (some of which may be in figures) followed by several numbered items. For each numbered item, select the ONE lettered option that is most closely associated with it. To avoid spending too much time on matching sets with large numbers of options, it is generally advisable to begin each set by reading the list of options. Then, for each item in the set, try to generate the correct answer and locate it in the option list, rather than evaluating each option individually. Each lettered option may be selected once, more than once, or not at all.

Questions 14–17

Match the following medications with the correct clinical indication.

(A) Enuresis
(B) Bipolar disorder
(C) Tourette disorder
(D) Attention deficit hyperactivity disorder (ADHD)
(E) Autistic disorder

14. Pimozide

15. Pemoline

16. Valproic acid

17. Desmopressin

Questions 18–21

Match the following childhood disorders with the most likely clinical etiology.

(A) Maturational delays
(B) Parent loss (loss of attachment figure)
(C) Parental pathology
(D) Adult-spectrum disorder
(E) Neuropathology

18. Autistic disorder

19. Feeding disorder of infancy or early childhood

20. Enuresis

21. Schizophrenia

1. The answer is A *[II A, B]*. Bonding and attachment are processes that occur over a lengthy period of time. Although many parents worry that a cesarean section interferes with this process, simple reassurance usually is helpful to them. Breast-feeding would not necessarily offset any sort of aberration in bonding and attachment. At first, many new mothers feel that their infants do not belong to them. This feeling can last several days. Returning to see the patient is a good idea but should be done 3 to 4 days later; however, conditions can warrant returning sooner. When the mother is severely depressed, anxious, or psychotic, she should be evaluated for psychiatric treatment and follow-up.

2. The answer is B *[III B 2]*. Childhood schizophrenia is a regression to a psychotic state after previous attainment of better mental functioning. Suggested etiologies include a grossly chaotic upbringing with constant exposure to aggressive and sexual themes with a subsequent failure of repression. A genetic cause is possible as well; however, it has not been as well delineated as it has for adult schizophrenia. Auditory hallucinations may be present but are seldom prominent. Antipsychotic medications may be helpful to the child, although children tend to respond less completely to antipsychotic medications than do adults.

3. The answer is B *[V A 1]*. Anaclitic depression is classically described as occurring after 7 months of life and before 30 months of life. During this phase of development, children are aware of who their primary caretaker is but do not yet have object constancy; that is, they lack the ability to maintain an image of their caretaker in the caretaker's absence. Therefore, they are vulnerable to lengthy separations (more than 1 week). Such separations from caretakers can result in a depressive syndrome that includes sad facial expressions, anorexia, apathy, and withdrawal from other individuals. The best treatment is to avoid prolonged separations. If that is not possible, a familiar individual or surrogate caretaker should be available to the child while the primary caretaker is away.

4. The answer is E *[VIII B]*. Soiling is only variably deliberate and is usually self-limited.

Whereas enuresis often derives from delayed nervous system maturation, this is not true for encopresis. Neither does it usually signify underlying gastrointestinal pathology. Although it may signify an underlying psychotic disorder within the child, this is not typically the case. DSM-IV specifies that the disorder is not assigned before the chronological age (or the developmental equivalent) of 4 years.

5. The answer is C *[XIII A]*. There are three subtypes of learning disorders: reading, writing, and mathematics. Although mental retardation is often euphemistically referred to as learning disorder, the term is used inaccurately at these times. Although learning disorders fall broadly among the developmental disorders, they are not subsumed within the pervasive developmental disorders, which are characterized by pervasive developmental deficits in language, social relatedness, and behavior. Diagnosis of learning disorders is established by documenting a mismatch between cognitive potential (as demonstrated on intelligence tests) and academic performance (as demonstrated on standardized achievement tests).

6–8. The answers are: 6-E, 7-A, 8-D *[XII C–D]*. Both major and minor nervous system dysfunction may underlie the symptoms of attention deficit hyperactivity disorder (ADHD) in certain children. Major pathology may take the form of a grossly abnormal central nervous system or of a history of significant head trauma. More minor nervous system dysfunction may take the form of nonspecific electroencephalograph changes and soft neurologic findings on examination. A history of tics is important both because Tourette disorder and ADHD are frequently comorbid conditions, and because tics may be a side effect from stimulant medications that are commonly used to treat ADHD. Certain medications, particularly sedative–hypnotics, may result in paradoxic excitation, which causes hyperactivity in some children.

ADHD is characterized by variable levels of hyperactivity along with impulsivity, distractibility, and attention and concentration deficits. Both depressed and anxious children may manifest the same symptom profile, albeit with differing underlying pathologic processes. Whereas many children with pervasive developmental disorders are also diagnosed with ADHD, the primary deficits in these disorders are pervasive abnormalities in language, social, and behavioral development. In this case, the vignette suggests no indication of pervasive developmental deficits.

Although the child has a diagnosable disorder, he still must be held accountable for his behavior and its consequences. Although many parents believe to the contrary, there is little empiric support for the notion that diet plays a role in this disorder, either etiologically or in terms of its treatment. Likewise, uncomplicated ADHD probably does not require psychotherapy, other than occasional behavioral interventions. Although stigmatization is always a risk of psychiatric diagnosis, ideally the school would be a partner in the therapeutic process both to implement behavioral programs, as well as to monitor overall therapeutic efficacy. Most cases of ADHD will be most effectively managed with medications, used at least adjunctively.

9–11. The answers are: 9-E, 10-A, 11-D
[XV C]. Although the child's injury might have been sustained exactly as described by her mother, the physician must wonder whether nonaccidental trauma is involved. Complete physical examination to look for other signs of abuse (e.g., bruises in various stages of healing, burns, bites, or abrasions) would be appropriate. If the index of suspicion is high enough, long-bone radiographs might be obtained to look for previous fractures. In addition to consideration of the potential for physical abuse, the physician must also be sensitive to the potential for sexual abuse. Consequently, a genital examination might be indicated as well. Developmental history is important insofar as frequently there is a history of problematic bonding between abused children and their parents. Likewise, children who deviate from the norm either physically or developmentally, are at increased risk for abuse. An interview with the child is essential. This should occur separate from the parent, and the child should be asked the source of her injuries. Questions should be otherwise nonleading, and in language appropriate to the developmental level of the child. Likewise, the responses of the child should be assessed in terms of their appropriateness to her developmental level.

Reporting laws across the United States require that reasonable suspicions of abuse and neglect must be reported. Physicians are

mandated to report under these circumstances and are civilly liable for failing to follow these reporting guidelines. Proof of abuse is not necessary. Neither is an inordinately high level of suspicion, or direct allegations made by the child. Rather, any reasonable level of suspicion must be reported.

Both chronically ill and developmentally delayed children are known to be at increased risk for abuse and neglect. Likewise, children in certain developmental phases (e.g., age-normal oppositionality, toilet training) may be at increased risk, particularly when parental impulse control is tenuous. Scapegoating is frequently observed in abusive families, in which case the abused child becomes the symptom bearer for pathology across the family. Provocation, however, should never be considered a risk factor for child abuse and neglect, as it implies that the child "earned" the abuse, at least in part. Always, abuse and neglect must be viewed as reflecting parental pathology.

12. The answer is D *[IV A 4]*. Autistic disorder is a neuropathic disorder that commences in early childhood (before the age of 3 years) in which the child demonstrates disturbed relatedness to other human beings, inappropriate responses to his environment, and delays and oddities in language development. Findings that support the neurologic etiology of this condition include abnormal auditory evoked potentials, a high incidence of grand mal seizures during childhood, decreased nystagmus in response to vestibular stimulation, and a high incidence of comorbid mental retardation. Enlarged ventricles on computed tomography scans have not been consistent findings in this condition.

13. The answer is A *[XII D 1]*. Both methylphenidate and fenfluramine are psychostimulants, and the efficacy of stimulants in ameliorating the hyperactive, impulsive, and distractable symptoms of attention deficit hyperactivity disorder (ADHD) are well documented. Clonidine, which is a centrally acting, α-adrenergic stimulant that is more commonly used in adults as an antihypertensive agent, has been found to be an effective treatment for ADHD both individually and as an adjunct to the psychostimulants. Bupropion, which is an antidepressant that may produce central nervous system (CNS) stimulant effects, has also been demonstrated to be of some therapeutic benefit, particularly in individuals with ADHD and depressive symptoms. Haloperidol offers no direct effect and may be of benefit only indirectly, secondary to sedation. Given the significant long-term side effects of haloperidol, along with the absence of any primary indication, seldom would it be an appropriate treatment for this disorder.

14–17. The answers are: 14-C *[VI D 3 b],* **15-D** *[XII D 1 a],* **16-B** *[V D 1],* **17-A** *[VIII A].* Pimozide, haloperidol, and clonidine have all been used to treat the tics of Tourette disorder. Pemoline, methylphenidate, and dextroamphetamine have all been used to treat the symptoms of attention deficit hyperactivity disorder (ADHD). Valproic acid, lithium, and carbamazepine are all effective mood stabilizers useful in bipolar disorder. Desmopressin, an antidiuretic hormone, is useful in managing the symptoms of enuresis; the tricyclic antidepressants may be useful as well. There is no primary pharmacologic treatment for autistic disorder. Pharmacologic intervention in this disorder is aimed at specific target symptoms.

18–21. The answers are 18-E *[IV A],* **19-C** *[III C],* **20-A** *[VIII A],* **21-D** *[IV B].* While once thought to derive from faulty parenting, autistic disorder has been clearly established as a neuropathologically based condition. Although feeding disorder of infancy or early childhood may derive from organic illness within the child, often it is secondary to parental pathology, and/or pathologic parent–child interactions (nonorganic failure to thrive). Most often, enuresis, especially the primary nocturnal subtype, is a time-limited condition deriving from nervous system maturational delays, which the child will ultimately outgrow. Although childhood schizophrenia remains poorly defined, data indicate that at least 50% of individuals with childhood schizophrenia persist with significant deficits into adulthood. This suggests that there is some continuity with the adult-spectrum schizophrenia disorder.

Chapter 11

Personality Disorders

James H. Scully

I. **INTRODUCTION.** Each of us has a repertoire of coping devices or defenses that allows us to maintain an equilibrium between our internal drives and the world around us. This repertoire is **personality—the set of characteristics that defines the behavior, thoughts, and emotions of an individual**. The characteristics become ingrained and dictate our life-styles.

A. **Personality traits** are generally viewed as resulting from development that has been influenced by culture and society as well as by the child-rearing practices of the individual family. In addition, recent studies in child development suggest that there may be genetically determined temperamental factors involved in the course of personality development. Certain genetic characteristics may make a specific behavioral response more likely to occur, thus leading to a specific personality style. When this stable pattern of response leads to problems, a personality disorder may be present. **A personality disorder is present when personality traits are inflexible and maladaptive, causing either significant impairment in social or occupational functioning or subjective distress.** Manifestations of a personality disorder are usually recognized by adolescence and continue into adulthood. However, symptoms may become less obvious in later years.

B. **Expression of symptoms.** Personality disorders are among the most common emotional disorders seen in psychiatric practice, particularly in the outpatient clinic. The patient's perception of the problem and the expression of symptoms, however, are different from those demonstrated in other psychiatric illnesses, making treatment difficult. Patients with personality disorders may complain of mood disturbances, particularly depression or anxiety. They may exhibit:

1. **Ego-syntonic symptoms,** whereby patients do not recognize that anything is wrong with them that needs to be changed. They view existing disturbances as being the result of the world being out of step with them.

2. **Ego-dystonic symptoms,** whereby patients may be experiencing internally distressing symptoms that are self-induced but are still unable to alter their behavior.

C. **Clinical picture.** Symptoms of personality disorders almost always affect other individuals. The symptoms involve work, play, and all relationships.

1. **Individuals with personality disorders have trouble in their work settings.** They have often had many jobs and work below their capacities.

2. **Social relationships are disrupted or absent.** Because individuals with personality disorders can be irritating and infuriating to those involved with them, the reactions to personality disorders by these involved individuals are often more pronounced than the disorder itself in the affected person.

3. **These patients may seek help as a result of a concurrent medical or surgical problem or because of a primary emotional distress.** In any case, these patients may elicit strong negative reactions in the physicians and other health care personnel who take care of them.

4. **In general, patients with personality disorders tolerate stress poorly,** and they seek help to alleviate the outside stress rather than to change their character. If stress is great, as it can be in those who are physically ill, patients may regress.

D. Biology

1. **Genetics.** Twin and adoption studies show strong genetic components to **personality traits**. Less is known about **personality disorder**.

2. **Familial associations.** There is increased risk for both Axis I and Axis II disorders (see Chapter 1) in families of persons with a personality disorder.

E. Diagnosis

1. **Comorbid Axis I disorders are common.** The majority of persons with personality disorder also have one or more Axis I disorder. It is sometimes difficult to diagnose a specific personality disorder when a patient has a mix of traits; however, **the *Diagnostic and Statistical Manual of Mental Disorders,* 4th edition (DSM-IV) allows for the diagnosis of more than one personality disorder if the patient meets the diagnostic criteria for several disorders**. Diagnosis of a personality disorder should be made carefully in a person who is reacting to a major environmental or social stress; for example, some young men develop maladaptive coping mechanisms in the military that they do not otherwise employ.

2. **Axis I disorders make the assessment of personality disorder more difficult.** For example, a diagnosis of personality disorder should not be made in a person with schizophrenia unless the personality disorder *clearly* preceded the onset of schizophrenia.

II. CLUSTERS OF PERSONALITY DISORDERS.

Eleven specific personality disorders are described in the DSM-IV. Because of the similarities in symptoms or traits, they are grouped into three clusters: The odd or eccentric group is cluster A; the dramatic, emotional, and erratic group is cluster B; and the anxious and fearful group is cluster C.

A. Cluster A. The **odd or eccentric group** includes the **paranoid, schizoid, and schizotypal personality disorders**.

1. Affected individuals use the **defense mechanisms of projection and fantasy** and may have a tendency toward psychotic thinking.
   a. **Projection** involves attributing to another person the thoughts or feelings of one's own that are unacceptable (e.g., prejudice, excessive fault-finding, paranoia).
   b. **Fantasy** is the creation of an imaginary life with which the patient deals with loneliness. A fantasy can be quite elaborate and extensive.
   c. **Paranoia** is a feeling of being persecuted or treated unfairly by others. Paranoid patients may feel that others are talking about or making fun of them.

2. Biologically, patients with cluster A personality disorders may have a **vulnerability to cognitive disorganization when stressed**.

3. **Schizotypal patients** have been found to have some of the same biologic markers seen in schizophrenic individuals, including low levels of monoamine oxidase (MAO) activity in platelets and disorders of smooth pursuit eye movements.
   a. It has been speculated that not everyone who has a genetic vulnerability to schizophrenia becomes psychotic, but some of these individuals may be diagnosed as having a schizotypal personality disorder.
   b. In families in which there is a history of schizophrenia, there is also an increased number of relatives with schizotypal personality disorder.

B. **Cluster B.** The **dramatic, emotional, and erratic group** includes **histrionic, narcissistic, antisocial, and borderline personality disorders**.

1. Affected individuals tend to use certain **defense mechanisms, such as dissociation, denial, splitting, and acting out**.

 a. **Dissociation** involves the "forgetting" of unpleasant feelings and associations. It is the unconscious splitting off of some mental processes and behavior from the normal or conscious awareness of the individual. When extreme, this can lead to multiple or disorganized personalities.

 b. **Denial** is closely associated with dissociation. In denial, the patient refuses to acknowledge a thought, feeling, or wish, but is unaware of doing so.

 c. **Splitting,** often seen in patients with borderline personalities, occurs when the patient divides individuals into all good and all bad and cannot experience an ambivalent relationship. The patient cannot even be ambivalent in regard to her own self-image.

 d. **Acting out** involves the actual motor expression of a thought or feeling that is intolerable to the patient; this can involve both aggressive and sexual behavior. Patients with these types of personality disorders may be biologically vulnerable to stress (i.e., a tendency to low cortical arousal causes them to easily overstimulate) and a wide variation of autonomic and motor activities. Thus, a psychobiologic pattern may develop, which increases the potential for acting out that is not associated with any particular anxiety.

2. **Mood disorders** are common in cluster B and may be the chief complaint.

3. **Somatization disorder** is associated with histrionic personality disorder.

C. **Cluster C.** The **anxious and fearful group** includes **avoidant, dependent, and obsessive-compulsive** personalities.

1. Affected individuals use **defense mechanisms of isolation, passive aggression, and hypochondriasis**.

 a. **Isolation** occurs when an unacceptable feeling, act, or idea is separated from the associated emotion. Patients are orderly and controlled and can speak of events of their lives without feeling.

 b. **Passive aggression** occurs when resistance is indirect and often turned against the self. Thus, failing examinations, clownish conduct, and procrastinating are aspects of passive-aggressive behavior.

 c. **Hypochondriasis** is often present in patients with personality disorders, particularly in dependent, passive-aggressive patients. Biologically, these patients may have a tendency toward higher levels of cortical arousal and an increase in motor inhibition. Thus, stressful stimuli may lead to high anxiety or affective arousal.

2. Twin studies have demonstrated some **genetic factors** in the development of cluster C personality disorders. For example, obsessive-compulsive traits are more common in monozygotic twins than in dizygotic twins. **Patients with obsessive-compulsive disorder are not at increased risk for obsessive-compulsive personality disorder and vice versa**.

III. **SPECIFIC CLUSTER A PERSONALITY DISORDERS.** These disorders—schizoid, paranoid, and schizotypal personality disorders—do not occur exclusively during the course of schizophrenia, which is a mood disorder with psychotic features, another psychotic disorder, or a pervasive developmental disorder. If criteria are met before the onset of schizophrenia, a premorbid condition exists [e.g., schizoid personality disorder (premorbid)].

A. **Schizoid personality disorder**

1. A pervasive pattern of detachment from social relationships and a restricted range of expression of emotions in interpersonal settings that begins by early adulthood and is

present in a variety of contexts, as indicated by at least four of the following, indicate a schizoid personality disorder:

a. Neither desires nor enjoys close relationships, including being part of a family
b. Almost always chooses solitary activities
c. Little, if any, **interest in having sexual experiences** with another person
d. Takes pleasure in few, if any, **activities**
e. Lacks close friends or confidants other than first-degree relatives
f. Appears indifferent to the praise or criticism of others
g. Emotional coldness, detachment, or flattened affect

2. The **prevalence** of schizoid personality disorder is unknown because these **patients rarely seek treatment**.

3. **Medical–surgical setting.** Illness brings these patients into close contact with caregivers, which is often seen as a threat to their equilibrium. Patients may intensify their aloofness and are likely to leave the hospital against medical advice if they are intruded on too much. Physicians should respect the patient's distance, should expect the development of trust to take a long time, and should not demand emotional reactions from the patient.

4. **Treatment.** Individuals with schizoid, paranoid, and schizotypal personality disorders do not usually seek treatment. If treatment is sought, the physician should be respectful but scrupulously honest in dealing with the patient. Individual psychotherapy is usually the only possible way to begin. However, if the patient can tolerate it, group therapy can be more successful.

B. **Paranoid personality disorder**

1. **Definition (DSM-IV).** The central features of paranoid personality disorder are a pervasive and unwarranted suspicion and mistrust of people, hypersensitivity to others, and an inability to deal with feelings. Individuals with this disorder are neither psychotic nor schizophrenic. Although many paranoid individuals are careful observers and are often energetic and capable, they routinely misinterpret the actions of others as deliberately demeaning or threatening.

2. **Symptoms.** Paranoid personality disorder is indicated by at least four of the following:
   a. The patient **suspects, without sufficient basis, that others are exploiting or deceiving him**.
   b. The patient is **preoccupied with unjustified doubts** about the loyalty or trustworthiness of friends or associates.
   c. The patient is **reluctant to confide in others** because of unwarranted fear that the information will be used maliciously against him.
   d. The patient **reads hidden demeaning or threatening meanings into benign remarks or events**.
   e. The patient **persistently bears grudges** (i.e., is unforgiving of insult, injuries, or slights).
   f. The patient **perceives attacks on his character or reputation** that are not apparent to others and is **quick to react angrily** or to counterattack.
   g. The patient has **recurrent suspicions,** without justification, regarding fidelity of spouse or sexual partner.

3. The **prevalence** of paranoid personality disorder is unknown. People with this disorder tend to group themselves in esoteric religions and pseudoscientific and quasipolitical groups. Groups of paranoid individuals who set themselves apart and see others as "the enemy" tend to provoke negative reactions from the outside, which reinforces their paranoid views.

4. **Medical–surgical setting.** Illness tends to exacerbate the personality style of paranoid patients. They tend to become more guarded, suspicious, and quarrelsome. They are frequently overly sensitive to slights and project their concerns onto others. They

complain and are suspicious. Physicians should be courteous and honest, and should respect the defenses of a paranoid patient. There is a need to be straightforward and explain everything. Physicians should not expect to be trusted and should not impose closeness on these patients but should remain professional and even a little aloof.

5. **Treatment.** Individuals with paranoid personality disorders, like those with schizoid and schizotypal personalities, rarely seek treatment. If treatment is sought, the physician needs to be respectful, but scrupulously honest. For example, if the patient finds something amiss, such as lateness for an appointment, the therapist should admit fault and apologize immediately. The goal of treatment is to help the patient understand that not all problems are caused by others.

   a. **Individual therapy** is usually the only possible way to begin.

   b. Occasionally, a patient can tolerate **group therapy,** but great care must be taken in the selection of patients.

   c. The therapist needs to avoid getting too close to the patient too quickly. Some patients may become agitated and threatened, which causes a hostile defensiveness. **Limits** then must be set.

   d. **Antipsychotic medications** can be used in small doses for short periods of time to manage agitation. However, the physician must explain the side effects.

C. | **Schizotypal personality disorder**

1. **Definition.** The central features of this disorder are pervasive patterns of "strange" or "odd" behavior, appearance, or thinking. These peculiarities are not so severe that they can be termed schizophrenic, and there is no history of psychotic episodes.

2. **Symptoms.** Patients with schizotypal personality disorder are indicated by a pervasive pattern of social and interpersonal deficits marked by acute discomfort with, and reduced capacity for, close relationships. Cognitive or perceptual distortions and eccentricities of behavior also exist. Patients with this disorder are indicated by at least five of the following:

   a. **Ideas of reference** (excluding delusions of reference)

   b. **Odd beliefs or magical thinking** that influence behavior and are inconsistent with subcultural norms (e.g., belief in superstitions, clairvoyance, telepathy, or "sixth sense"; in children and adolescents, bizarre fantasies or preoccupations)

   c. **Unusual perceptual experiences,** including bodily illusions

   d. **Odd thinking and speech** (e.g., vague, circumstantial, metaphorical, overelaborate, or stereotyped)

   e. **Suspiciousness or paranoid ideation**

   f. **Inappropriate or constricted affect**

   g. **Behavior or appearance that is odd,** eccentric, or peculiar

   h. **Lack of close friends** or confidants other than first-degree relatives

   i. **Excessive social anxiety** that does not diminish with familiarity and tends to be associated with paranoid fears rather than negative judgments about self

3. **Prevalence.** Several studies indicate that 3% of the population have this disorder.

4. **Medical–surgical setting.** The problems in treating a patient with schizotypal personality disorder and a medical or surgical illness are similar to those encountered with schizoid patients. Schizotypal individuals tend to put off caregivers. Illness threatens their isolation.

5. **Treatment.** If treatment is sought, the physician should be honest in dealing with the patient. The odd behavior of these patients can cause uneasiness in the physician, who must avoid all ridicule. There is more of a chance of success with group therapy than with individual psychotherapy. However, only certain patients can tolerate group therapy. The physician should not expect to develop a warm relationship and should respect the patient's need for psychological distance.

IV. SPECIFIC CLUSTER B PERSONALITY DISORDERS

A. Antisocial personality disorder

1. Individuals with this disorder have a **history of continuous and chronic antisocial behavior by which the rights of others are violated**.
   a. The **essential defect** is one of character structure in which affected individuals are seemingly **unable to control their impulses** and postpone immediate gratification.
   b. Antisocial personalities **lack sensitivity** to the feelings of others; they are egocentric, selfish, and excessively demanding and are usually free of anxiety, remorse, and guilt.
   c. Antisocial personalities have been termed **sociopathic and psychopathic**. They persist in lifelong habits of violating the laws and customs of the communities in which they live.

2. **Symptoms** of a person with a schizotypal personality disorder include:
   a. Currently **18 years or older**
   b. Evidence of a **conduct disorder** with onset before age 15
   c. A pervasive **pattern of disregard for and violation of the rights of others** occurring since age 15, as indicated by at least three of the following:
      (1) **Failure to conform to social norms** with respect to lawful behaviors as indicated by repeatedly performing acts that are grounds for arrest
      (2) **Irritability and aggressiveness,** as indicated by repeated physical fights or assaults
      (3) **Consistent irresponsibility,** as indicated by repeated failure to sustain consistent work behavior or honor financial obligations
      (4) **Impulsivity or failure to plan ahead**
      (5) **Deceitfulness,** as indicated by repeated lying, use of aliases, or conning others for personal profit or pleasure
      (6) **Reckless disregard for safety** of self or others
      (7) **Lack of remorse,** as indicated by being indifferent to or rationalizing having hurt, mistreated, or stolen from another person
   d. Antisocial behavior does not occur exclusively during the course of schizophrenia or a manic episode.

3. **Epidemiology.** In the United States, it is estimated that 3% of men have the disorder. The Epidemiologic Catchment Area (ECA) study suggests that lifetime prevalence for men may be over 7% and women 1%.

4. **Etiology.** The etiology of antisocial personality disorder is unclear.
   a. There is often a **family history** of antisocial personality disorder in both men and women. Both **environmental and genetic factors** play a role. A sociopathic father is a predictor of an antisocial personality whether or not the child is reared in the presence of the father. Family problems with alcoholism also increase the risk of antisocial behavior.
   b. Some antisocial behavior is precipitated by **brain damage secondary to closed head trauma or encephalitis**. In these cases, the proper diagnosis is **personality change due to general medical condition**. The causative factors are generally felt to be biologic.
   c. Other studies show that **inconsistent and impulsive parenting** are more damaging than the loss of a parent.

5. **Medical–surgical setting.** The emergency department is a common site of interaction between physicians and patients with antisocial personality disorder. Impulsivity may lead to fights, suicide attempts, or other injuries. Substance abuse is a common complication.
   a. These patients may be superficially charming when under stress and not cause any particular problems initially. However, they tend to be manipulative if given a chance and will chafe against the rules of the hospital.

b. Young patients with antisocial personality disorder have particular difficulty with the authority of physicians and tend to be noncompliant with treatment. They are likely to leave the hospital against medical advice when threatened and generally disrupt the hospital setting.

6. Treatment

a. Setting of **firm behavioral limits** is crucial, and, in general, **inpatient settings** are the only places where behavior can be controlled. Outpatient treatment usually is totally unsatisfactory because the patient flees treatment as soon as unpleasant affects are elicited.

b. Group therapy is more helpful than individual therapy because the patient sees it as less authoritative. Inpatient groups can confront antisocial behavior because the group is made up of experts at recognizing this behavior. Group treatment may involve therapeutic communities as well.

c. Medication to control aggression may be useful in patients with brain dysfunction. β blockers, selective serotonin reuptake inhibitors (SSRIs), and bupropion have been used.

d. Treating comorbid substance abuse is often necessary.

B. | **Borderline personality disorder**

1. Definition

a. Origination of term. The term "borderline" originated with the concept that this disorder was on the border between neurosis and psychosis. The disorder has also been called borderline schizophrenia, pseudoneurotic schizophrenia, and ambulatory schizophrenia, but it is now thought to be distinct from schizophrenia.

b. The **most important features** of the disorder are **instability of self-image, interpersonal relationships, and mood.** An identity disturbance is usually present and is manifested by an uncertainty about sexual orientation, goals, types of friends, and self-image.

2. Symptoms. A pervasive pattern of instability of interpersonal relationships, self-image, affects, and control over impulses beginning by early adulthood and present in a variety of contexts, as indicated by at least five of the following indicate borderline personality disorder:

a. Frantic efforts to avoid real or imagined abandonment

b. A pattern of **unstable and intense interpersonal relationships** characterized by alternating between extremes of idealization and devaluation

c. Identity disturbance; that is, persistent and markedly disturbed, distorted, or unstable self-image or sense of self

d. Impulsivity in at least two areas that are potentially self-damaging (e.g., spending, sex, substance abuse, reckless driving, binge eating)

e. Recurrent suicidal behavior, gestures, or threats, or **self-mutilating behavior**

f. Affective instability due to a **marked reactivity of mood** (e.g., intense episodic dysphoria, irritability, or anxiety usually lasting a few hours and only rarely more than a few days)

g. Chronic feelings of emptiness

h. Inappropriate, intense anger or **lack of control of anger** (e.g., frequent displays of temper, constant anger, recurrent physical fights)

i. Transient, stress-related paranoid ideation or severe dissociative symptoms.

3. Prevalence. This disorder may be present in 1%–2% of the population. The diagnosis is made twice as frequently in women. Of the individuals with this diagnosis, 90% also have one other psychiatric diagnosis, and 40% have two other diagnoses.

4. Etiology. Almost all theories related to the cause of the borderline personality have postulated problems in early development. **Severe abuse in childhood** (verbal, physical, and sexual) is a common finding. **Neurocognitive deficits** and **decreased serotonin** levels are also found.

5. **Medical–surgical setting.** When an individual with a borderline personality becomes ill, there is an increase of stress and the potential for an exacerbation of symptoms related to the personality.

   a. The illness can mean a threat to any emotional homeostasis that the patient has developed.

   b. **Splitting** is seen (see II B 1 c). The hospital staff may unconsciously take sides and, with the patient, see things as all good or all bad. This split often occurs between the physicians and the nurses. The intensity of the feelings stirred up by the patient may make medical treatment difficult.

6. **Treatment**

   a. **Psychological.** There are two general approaches to the psychological treatment of the borderline patient.

      (1) The **psychodynamic approach** aims to understand the underlying psychopathology. In general, standard long-term psychotherapy is difficult because the patient tends to regress, and the reactions of therapists are intense.

      (2) **Treatment oriented toward supportive reality** is confrontational rather than interpretational. The therapist helps the patient recognize the feelings that are being stirred up and their connection with behavior. The therapist sets limits and provides structure. This approach is more appropriate in the general hospital setting.

   b. **Pharmacologic treatment** is clinically important, although modest improvement in patient mood and behavior can be obtained with pharmacotherapy.

      (1) **MAO inhibitors** (e.g., tranylcypromine) have been effective in improving mood but not in affecting behavioral changes. **Fluoxetine,** an SSRI, has helped in the areas of impulsivity and self-injury.

      (2) **Carbamazepine,** an anticonvulsant, has been shown to decrease behavioral dyscontrol.

      (3) **Antipsychotic medications** in low doses for brief periods are also effective.

      (4) **Benzodiazepines** are usually contraindicated for most patients because they may cause disinhibition, and drug abuse problems are common.

C. **Narcissistic personality disorder**

1. **Definition.** Individuals with narcissistic personality disorder have a grandiose sense of their own importance, but they are also extremely sensitive to criticism. They have little ability to empathize with others. They are more concerned about appearance than substance.

2. **Symptoms.** Narcissistic patients have a pervasive pattern of grandiosity (in fantasy or behavior), need for admiration, and lack of empathy that began in early adulthood and is present in a variety of contexts, as indicated by at least five of the following:

   a. A grandiose sense of self-importance (e.g., **exaggerates achievements and talents,** expects to be recognized as superior without commensurate achievements)

   b. **Preoccupation with fantasies** of unlimited success, power, brilliance, beauty, or ideal love

   c. **Believes that he is "special" and unique** and can only be understood by, or should associate with, other special or high-status people (or institutions)

   d. **Requires excessive admiration**

   e. A **sense of entitlement** (i.e., unreasonable expectations of especially favorable treatment or automatic compliance with his expectations)

   f. Is **interpersonally exploitative** (i.e., takes advantage of others as a means to achieve his own ends)

   g. **Lack of empathy** (i.e., unwilling to recognize or identify with the feelings and needs of others)

   h. Is often **envious of others** or **believes that others are envious of him**

   i. **Arrogant;** demonstrates haughty behaviors or attitudes

3. **Prevalence.** The prevalence of this disorder is unknown. Although the diagnosis has been made more often in recent years, this is likely to be due to a greater interest in this disorder rather than to an increased prevalence.

4. **Associated features.** Depression or a depressed mood is common with this disorder. Painful preoccupation with appearance occurs. Features of other cluster B disorders are often present.

5. **Medical–surgical setting.** An individual with a narcissistic personality reacts to illness as a threat to his sense of grandiosity and self-perfection. There is usually intensification of characteristic behavior and either overidealization or devaluation of the physician. The patient expects special treatment. These patients tend to stir up negative reactions in caretakers. Feelings of both anger and boredom can be expected. This disorder is sometimes encountered in the physician, rather than the patient.

6. **Treatment**
   a. **Individual psychotherapy** is the treatment of choice, with an attempt at understanding the pain suffered by the patient with this disorder.
      (1) The therapist must deal with transitions from being overidealized to being devalued.
      (2) These transitions can be stormy, and they occur when the therapist has misunderstood the patient or has not been perfectly empathic.
      (3) It is important that the physician is not defensive about her mistakes.
   b. **Group therapy** in combination with individual therapy can be useful in helping the patient get feedback about the effect he has on others.

D. **Histrionic personality disorder**

1. **Definition.** People with this disorder are flamboyant, seek attention, and demonstrate an excessive emotionality. Their emotions are shallow and shift rapidly. Typically, they are attractive and seductive and, like the narcissistic person, overly concerned with their appearance. This disorder was formerly called "hysterical personality," but that term has been discarded because of the many meanings of "hysterical."

2. **Symptoms.** People with histrionic personality disorder have a pervasive pattern of excessive emotionality and attention seeking that began by early adulthood and is present in a variety of contexts, as indicated by at least five of the following:
   a. Is uncomfortable in situations in which she is not the **center of attention**
   b. Interaction with others often characterized as **inappropriately sexually seductive** or **provocative**
   c. **Insincere** (i.e., displays rapidly shifting and shallow expression of emotions)
   d. Consistently **uses physical appearance to draw attention** to oneself
   e. Style of **speech that is excessively impressionistic** and lacking in detail
   f. **Self-dramatization,** with a theatrical and exaggerated expression of emotion
   g. **Suggestibility** (i.e., easily influenced by others or circumstances)
   h. **Aggrandizes relationships**

3. **Prevalence.** The prevalence of histrionic personality disorder is not known with certainty. It is thought to be common and is diagnosed in women much more frequently than in men. Men with similar patterns are often diagnosed as narcissistic.

4. **Associated features.** As with all of the cluster B disorders, mood and somatization disorders, especially depression, are common.

5. **Medical–surgical setting**
   a. Patients may be seen as charming and fascinating by the physician, especially when they are of the opposite sex.
   b. An illness is often thought of by patients as a threat to their physical attractiveness. It may be seen as a punishment for their thoughts or feelings, and in men it may be seen as a threat of mutilation.

    c. Men may behave in an inappropriate sexual manner with female nurses and physicians. The sexual behavior may be a cover for deeper concerns about dependency. These patients learn that they can be taken care of by being sexually attractive, and this behavior is accentuated under the stress of illness. The physician should approach the patient as a professional and remind him that the roles are set. At the same time, it is important to remain noncritical.

6. Treatment
    a. Psychotherapy, either individual or group, is generally the treatment of choice for histrionic personality disorder. In general, the therapist helps the patient become aware of the real feelings underneath the histrionic behavior.
    b. Antidepressant medications, especially MAO inhibitors and SSRIs, have been useful in treating mood disorders associated with this personality type.

V. SPECIFIC CLUSTER C PERSONALITY DISORDERS

A. Avoidant personality disorder

1. Definition. Individuals with this disorder are timid and shy but do wish to have friends. They are distinct from schizoid patients. They are so uncomfortable and afraid of rejection or criticism that they avoid social contact. If given strong guarantees of uncritical acceptance, they will make friends. They are self-critical and have low self-esteem.

2. Symptoms. People with avoidant personality disorder have a pervasive pattern of social inhibition, feelings of inadequacy, and hypersensitivity to negative evaluation that began by early adulthood and are present in a variety of contexts, as indicated by at least four of the following:
    a. Avoids occupational activities that involve significant interpersonal contact, because of fears of criticism, disapproval, or rejection
    b. Is **unwilling to get involved with people** unless certain of being liked
    c. Restrains self within intimate relationships due to the fear of being shamed or ridiculed
    d. Preoccupied with worrying about being criticized or rejected in social situations
    e. Inhibited in new interpersonal situations because of feelings of inadequacy
    f. Believes that one is socially inept, personally unappealing, or inferior to others
    g. Is **unusually reluctant to take personal risks** or to engage in any new activities because they may prove embarrassing

3. Epidemiology. The prevalence is unknown. Little is known about sex ratios or familial patterns.

4. Associated features. Social phobias and agoraphobia may be present, but they are also separate disorders that need to be ruled out.

5. Medical–surgical setting. Unlike schizoid patients, avoidant patients may do well in the hospital. These patients are undemanding and generally cooperative. Their illness can allow them to be taken care of and establish relationships with the staff. They are sensitive to criticism and may misinterpret equivocal statements as being derogatory or ridiculing and withdraw emotionally.

6. Treatment
    a. Psychotherapy, either individual or group, can be useful. These patients respond to genuine caring and support.
    b. Assertiveness training may give these patients new social skills.

B. Dependent personality disorder

1. Definition. Individuals with dependent personality disorder are **passive.** They allow others to direct their lives because they are unable to do so themselves. Other people, such as a spouse or parents, make all of the major decisions of their lives, including where to live and what type of employment to obtain.

   a. The **needs of dependent individuals are placed secondary to those of the people on whom they depend** to avoid any possibility of having to be self-reliant. These persons lack self-confidence and see themselves as helpless or stupid.

   b. Some authorities believe that the presence of this disorder depends to a large extent on **cultural roles** (i.e., some groups of people are "expected" to assume dependent roles on the basis of certain criteria, such as gender or ethnic background).

2. **Symptoms.** A person with dependent personality disorder has a pervasive and excessive need to be taken care of, which leads to submissiveness, clinging behavior, and fear of separation. This behavior begins by early adulthood and is present in a variety of contexts, as indicated by at least five of the following:

   a. Is **unable to make everyday decisions** without an excessive amount of advice and reassurance from others

   b. **Needs others to assume responsibility** for most major areas of his life

   c. **Has difficulty expressing disagreement** with others because of fear of loss of support or approval (realistic fears of retribution should not be included here)

   d. **Has difficulty initiating projects** or doing things on his own (due to a lack of self-confidence in judgment or abilities rather than to a lack of motivation or energy)

   e. **Goes to excessive lengths to obtain nurturance and support** from others, to the point of volunteering to do things that are unpleasant

   f. **Feels uncomfortable or helpless when alone,** because of exaggerated fears of being unable to care for himself

   g. **Urgently seeks another relationship** as a source of care and support when a close relationship ends

   h. **Unrealistic preoccupation with fears** of being left to take care of himself

3. **Epidemiology.** The prevalence is unknown, but passive-dependent traits are common. The diagnosis is more frequent in women and youngest children.

4. **Associated features.** Children who have had a chronic physical illness or who have had separation anxiety may be at risk for this disorder in adulthood. Depression is common.

5. **Medical–surgical setting**

   a. Being sick usually means being taken care of, and one might expect that dependent individuals would be good patients. However, **illness may stir up intolerable feelings of fear of abandonment and helplessness for these patients**. There is a pull to regress to an earlier state of dependency, which may frighten the patients because of its intensity. Feelings of dependency increase. Generally, these patients become demanding and complaining when sick.

   b. **Physicians need to set limits.** It is important for the physicians, nurses, and other staff to get together to plan with the patient what kind of care is going to be given. For instance, it should be clear to the patient how often the nurse will come by to check on her. If this is not done early, the negative reactions that these patients stir up can lead to punitive behavior on the part of the caregivers.

6. **Treatment**

   a. **Psychotherapy** can be very useful in the treatment of dependent patients. The focus is on the current behavior and its consequences. The therapist should be careful when there is a challenge to a pathologic but dependent relationship. The patient may leave therapy rather than give up such a relationship.

   b. Behavioral therapies, including **assertiveness training,** can be helpful.

C. Obsessive-compulsive personality disorder

1. **Definition.** Individuals with this disorder are perfectionistic, inflexible, and unable to express warm and tender feelings. They are preoccupied with trivial details and rules and do not appreciate changes in routine. **Obsessive-compulsive disorder (OCD)** is an Axis I anxiety disorder that involves time obsessions and compulsions and should be

distinguished from obsessive-compulsive personality disorder. Individuals with OCD may not have the personality disorder, and individuals with the personality disorder may not have the anxiety disorder.

2. **Symptoms.** A person with obsessive-compulsive personality disorder displays a pervasive pattern of preoccupation with orderliness, perfectionism, and environmental and interpersonal control, at the expense of flexibility, openness, and efficiency. This behavior begins by early adulthood and is present in a variety of contexts, as indicated by at least four of the following:

   a. **Preoccupation with details, rules, lists, order, organization, or schedules** to the extent that the major point of the activity is lost

   b. **Perfectionism that interferes with task completion** (e.g., inability to complete a project because one's own overly strict standards are not met)

   c. **Excessive devotion to work and productivity** to the exclusion of leisure activities and friendships (not accounted for by obvious economic necessity)

   d. **Overconscientiousness, scrupulousness, and inflexibility about matters of morality, ethics, or values** (not accounted for by cultural or religious identification)

   e. **Inability to discard worn-out or worthless objects** even when they have no sentimental value

   f. **Reluctance to delegate tasks or to work with others** unless they submit to exactly his way of doing things

   g. Adopts a **miserly spending style toward both self and others** (money is viewed as something to be hoarded for future catastrophes)

   h. **Rigidity and stubbornness**

3. **Epidemiology.** This disorder is more common in men, although the prevalence is not known with certainty.

4. **Associated features.** People with this disorder have few friends. They are difficult to live with and tend to drive people away. They may do very well in jobs that require detail and precision with little personal interaction. Hypochondriasis may develop later in life.

5. **Medical–surgical setting**

   a. Illness may be **perceived by compulsive individuals as a threat to their control** over impulses. Generally, stress increases compulsive behavior with an intensification of self-restraint and obstinacy.

      (1) Patients become more inflexible than before, which may lead to complaints about the sloppiness of the hospital and imprecision of the care being given.

      (2) When these patients are critical of failure to meet their standards, physicians should avoid defensive, authoritarian rebuttal. There is a fear of losing control of a situation on the part of these patients, and this may lead to a struggle for control with their physicians.

   b. **Control should be shared with the patient in as many ways as possible.** The patient should be allowed to participate actively in the decisions and details of his actual medical care. This may include charting medication times, carefully calculating caloric intake, and monitoring fluid intake and output.

6. **Treatment.** In general, individuals with compulsive personalities recognize that they have problems, unlike those with the other personality disorders. These patients know that they suffer from their inability to be flexible, and they realize that they do not permit themselves to have good feelings.

   a. **Individual psychotherapy** can be helpful, but treatment is difficult because these patients use the defense of isolation of affect. **Group therapy may be more useful.**

   b. Therapy should **focus on current feelings and situations,** and excessive time should not be spent on examining the psychological etiology of the condition. Struggles for control should be avoided. Depression, when present, should be treated.

VI. **PERSONALITY DISORDERS NOT OTHERWISE SPECIFIED.** Patients may not always present with all the criteria for a specific personality disorder but still have clinically significant distress or impairment. This category also can be used when the clinician decides that a specific personality disorder not included in DSM-IV is appropriate.

A. For example, **passive-aggressive personality disorder** was included in DSM-III-R, but not in DSM-IV, because studies indicated the diagnosis was too situation-specific and described a cluster of symptoms more than a personality disorder.

B. **Depressive personality disorder** has also been considered.

DIRECTIONS: Each of the numbered items or incomplete statements in this section is followed by answers or by completions of the statement. Select the ONE numbered answer or completion that is BEST in each case.

1. When individuals with personality disorders are unable to see their role in the disturbances in their lives, the symptoms that develop are considered

(A) self-induced
(B) ego-syntonic
(C) ego-dystonic
(D) internal
(E) characterologic

2. The defense mechanism whereby an individual attributes to another individual thoughts or feelings of her own that are unacceptable is called

(A) fantasy
(B) splitting
(C) regression
(D) projection
(E) identification

3. Somatization disorder is associated most commonly with

(A) paranoid personality
(B) histrionic personality
(C) narcissistic personality
(D) dependent personality
(E) schizotypal personality

4. Twin and adoption studies demonstrate which of the following characteristics?

(A) Genetic factors do not affect personality disorder
(B) Axis I comorbidity is common
(C) Personality is too complex to measure biologically
(D) Cluster C disorders are inherited
(E) There is a strong genetic component to personality traits

5. Factors thought to be involved in the etiology of an antisocial personality disorder include

(A) closed head injury
(B) encephalitis
(C) an alcoholic father
(D) loss of a parent
(E) low socioeconomic status

6. A defense mechanism commonly used by persons with cluster A personality disorder is

(A) somatization
(B) dissociation
(C) denial
(D) paranoia
(E) acting out

7. The term "hysterical" has been dropped as a diagnostic label because

(A) it has become too pejorative
(B) it refers only to women
(C) it has been replaced by the term "conversion"
(D) it refers to a neurosis not a personality
(E) it has become too nonspecific

8. Which of the following disorders is thought by many to be strongly influenced by cultural roles?

(A) Avoidant personality
(B) Antisocial personality
(C) Dependent personality
(D) Borderline personality

9. A personality disorder that has been dropped from the DSM-IV because it has not met criteria as a specific, separate disorder and because it is thought to be situation-specific is

(A) depressive personality disorder
(B) self-defeating personality disorder
(C) borderline personality disorder
(D) sadistic personality disorder
(E) passive-aggressive personality disorder

10. A new feature added to criteria for borderline personality disorder is

(A) impulsivity, such as reckless driving
(B) chronic feelings of emptiness
(C) transient, stress-related paranoid ideation
(D) identity disturbance
(E) self-mutilating behavior

11. Persons who experience others as either all good or all bad and cannot experience an ambivalent relationship are exhibiting the mechanism of

(A) splitting
(B) denial
(C) dissociation
(D) projection
(E) isolation

12. A person with which one of the following personality disorders is less likely to seek medical care or psychiatric treatment?

(A) Dependent
(B) Antisocial
(C) Borderline
(D) Schizoid
(E) Obsessive-compulsive

13. Medication that has been useful in decreasing self-injury in patients with borderline personality disorder is

(A) alprazolam
(B) fluoxetine
(C) phenylzine
(D) diazepam
(E) clozapine

14. A patient with which one of the following disorders is most likely to handle the stress of hospitalization relatively well?

(A) Schizotypal
(B) Dependent
(C) Antisocial
(D) Borderline
(E) Avoidant

15. Men who exhibit the clinical features of which of the following disorders are often diagnosed as narcissistic?

(A) Antisocial
(B) Borderline
(C) Histrionic
(D) Dependent
(E) Schizotypal

DIRECTIONS: Each set of matching questions in this section consists of a list of four to twenty-six lettered options (some of which may be in figures) followed by several numbered items. For each numbered item, select the ONE lettered option that is most closely associated with it. To avoid spending too much time on matching sets with large numbers of options, it is generally advisable to begin each set by reading the list of options. Then, for each item in the set, try to generate the correct answer and locate it in the option list, rather than evaluating each option individually. Each lettered option may be selected once, more than once, or not at all.

Questions 16–23

For each patient description, select the appropriate personality disorder.

(A) Antisocial
(B) Avoidant
(C) Histrionic
(D) Schizotypal
(E) Dependent
(F) Obsessive-compulsive
(G) Paranoid

16. Patients tend to group themselves in esoteric religious and pseudoscientific groups

17. Patients exhibit clairvoyance and telepathy

18. Patients display behavior similar to that precipitated by brain damage

19. Patients persistently bear grudges and are unforgiving of insults

20. Patients believe that they are socially inept, personally unappealing, or inferior to others

21. Patients are easily influenced by other people or by circumstances

22. Patients have difficulty expressing disagreement with others because of fear of loss of support or approval

23. Patients fear losing control

Questions 24–28

For each characteristic listed, select the appropriate personality disorder.

(A) Paranoid
(B) Borderline
(C) Narcissistic
(D) Antisocial
(E) Schizoid

24. Patients take offense quickly and question the loyalty of others

25. Patients have a defective capacity to form social relationships

26. Patients fail to plan ahead and are impulsive (e.g., may move without a job)

27. Patients form relationships that lack empathy; they idealize or devalue others

28. Patients exude a sense of entitlement with the expectation of special favors but without assuming reciprocal responsibilities

1. The answer is B *[I B]*. Patients with personality disorders perceive their problem and express their symptoms differently from patients with other psychiatric illnesses. Patients with personality disorders often feel that the disturbances in their lives are caused by the outside world (rather than internally), the symptoms of which are called ego-syntonic. Symptoms of a personality disorder are caused by the characterologic style of the patient. Symptoms include feelings of anxiety, depression, and anger, but these symptoms do not meet the criteria for a specific Axis I psychiatric illness.

2. The answer is D *[II A 1 a]*. Projection is the defense mechanism whereby an individual attributes to another individual thoughts and feelings that are unacceptable. Fantasy is the creation of an imaginary life. Regression is a retreat to earlier defenses. Splitting is attributing only all good or all bad qualities to an individual. Identification is the unconscious assumption of aspects of another individual's personality.

3. The answer is B *[II B 3]*. Patients with histrionic personality disorder often have a concurrent somatization disorder. Patients with the other personality disorders in cluster B, which is the dramatic, emotional, and erratic group, may have a number of concurrent problems but not necessarily somatization disorder. All of the patients with cluster B disorder can be difficult when they become ill, however. Patients with dependent or passive-aggressive personalities may have hypochondriasis, which is a different phenomenon than somatization disorder.

4. The answer is E *[I D]*. Twin studies have shown a strong genetic component to personality traits, but it has been difficult to show the same influence regarding personality disorder under cluster C. Comorbidity has not been the focus of twin studies.

5. The answer is C *[IV A 4]*. Although the etiology of antisocial disorder is not clear, it is thought that one powerful predictor is a sociopathic or alcoholic father. Antisocial behavior has been associated with closed head injury and encephalitis; however, the proper diagnosis for these behaviors is an organic personality syndrome. Loss of a parent has not been associated with the development of antisocial personality, but inconsistent and compulsive parenting has. Although antisocial personality is associated with low socioeconomic status, this is not thought to be a cause but rather the result of this kind of behavior.

6. The answer is D *[II A 1 c]*. The cluster A group of personality disorders are considered odd and eccentric. They have a tendency toward paranoid thinking, projection, and fantasy. Somatization, dissociation, denial, and acting out are more commonly seen in cluster B disorders.

7. The answer is E *[IV D 1]*. "Hysterical" is a term that has many meanings in psychiatry and, thus, has lost its usefulness because of this nonspecificity. It has also been used pejoratively when applied to women. Conversion reactions were once called hysterical conversion reactions, referring to both neurosis and a personality disorder. However, it too was dropped because of the lack of specificity.

8. The answer is D *[V B 1]*. Some researchers in psychiatry feel that dependent personality disorder depends to a large degree on cultural roles (i.e., certain individuals or groups are expected to assume dependent roles in the culture based on their gender or ethnic background). To some extent, this may be changing, but it can still be observed.

9. The answer is E *[VI]*. Passive-aggressive personality disorder was listed in the DSM-III-R but was dropped from the DSM-IV because studies indicated it was too situation-specific. Persons who appeared to have the disorder in some situations did not exhibit the symptoms in other situations. Depressive, self-defeating, and sadistic personality disorders were never in the DSM-III-R, and borderline personality disorder was in the last and current editions.

10. The answer is C *[IV B 2]*. Transient cognitive disorders, such as dissociation and paranoid ideation, are new features found to help clarify the diagnosis of borderline personality disorder. Impulsivity, chronic feelings of emptiness, identity disturbance, and self-mutilating behavior have been listed as diagnostic features of borderline personality disorder in the DSM-III.

11. The answer is A *[II B 1]*. These patients "split" the good and bad aspects of a normal relationship because they cannot deal with the emotions of ambivalence. The same person may be "all good" at one moment only to become "all bad" at another time. Caretakers can sometimes begin to act toward the patient and each other in these stereotypical ways.

12. The answer is D *[III A 4]*. Patients with the odd or eccentric (cluster A) disorders tend to avoid other people and stay by themselves. Cluster B and cluster C disorders are more likely to be seen by physicians among their usual patients.

13. The answer is B *[IV B 6 b (1)]*. The selective serotonin reuptake inhibitors (SSRIs), such as fluoxetine, have shown modest effectiveness in decreasing some behavioral impulsivity and self-injury in borderline patients. Benzodiazepines, such as alprazolam and diazepam, are generally contraindicated because they may cause disinhibition. Monoamine oxidase (MAO) inhibitors improve mood but not impulsivity. Clozapine has not been studied in these patients.

14. The answer is E *[V A 5]*. Patients with avoidant personality disorder are undemanding and generally cooperative. A medical illness allows them to be taken care of, which may help their illness. Patients with schizotypal, dependent, antisocial, and borderline personality disorders all tend to have more problematic interactions with staff while hospitalized.

15. The answer is C *[IV D 3]*. Histrionic patients are flamboyant, and they seek attention and demonstrate shallow emotions. Originally, this was called hysterical personality disorder, and the diagnosis usually applied to women. Clinical features are similar to those in narcissistic personality disorder.

16–23. The answers are: 16-G *[III B 3]*, **17-D** *[III C 2]*, **18-A** *[II A 4 b]*, **19-G** *[III B 2]*, **20-B** *[V A 2]*, **21-C** *[IV D 2]*, **22-E** *[V B 2]*, **23-F** *[V C 2]*. Patients with the cluster A disor-

ders, paranoid and schizotypal personality disorders, are odd and eccentric. Paranoid persons tend to form into eccentric groups and hold grudges. Schizotypal people have odd thinking, such as clairvoyance.

Patients with the cluster B group of disorders, which includes histrionic and antisocial personality disorders, are dramatic and erratic. Histrionic patients are highly suggestible. Sometimes compulsive, antisocial behavior can be precipitated by brain damage.

Patients with the cluster C group of personality disorders display anxious and fearful features. Avoidant people fear that no one will like them because they are not "good enough." Dependent persons will do anything to keep from being left alone, and obsessive patients are fearful of losing control.

24–28. The answers are: 24-A *[III B 2 b]*, **25-E** *[III A 1 a]*, **26-D** *[IV A 2 c]*, **27-B** *[IV B 2]*, **28-C** *[IV C 2 c, d]*. Patients with paranoid personality disorder are suspicious about the motives of others and have a basic deficit in trusting others, so they easily take offense and question whether others are loyal.

Although all personality disorders cause problems in interpersonal relationships, people with a schizoid personality lack the capacity to form relationships.

Irresponsibility and the inability to consider the consequences of impulsive actions are the features of patients with antisocial personality disorder. Whereas all personality disorders tend to cause problems in the workplace, antisocial people have particular difficulty being reliable.

A hallmark of a person with borderline personality disorder is a pattern of unstable and intense interpersonal relationships. Splitting, in which people are experienced as all good or all bad, can be seen in other disorders but is most often seen in those with borderline personality disorder.

People with narcissistic personality disorder expect to be treated specially without actually having achieved merit. They feel entitled, and tend to exploit others. Whereas they need and seek admiration from others, they lack the ability to identify with others' feelings.

COMPREHENSIVE EXAM

QUESTIONS

DIRECTIONS: Each of the numbered items or incomplete statements in this section is followed by answers or by completions of the statement. Select the ONE lettered answer or completion that is BEST in each case.

1. Early in the psychiatric interview, it is most important for the physician to

(A) inform the patient of the fee
(B) obtain details of past psychiatric illnesses
(C) let the patient talk about what is bothering him
(D) ask the patient about legal issues associated with his problems

2. High-voltage, slow-wave activity on the electroencephalogram (EEG) is commonly present in

(A) dementia
(B) delirium
(C) schizophrenia
(D) alcohol withdrawal
(E) human immunodeficiency virus (HIV)

3. Echolalia is an example of

(A) psychomotor retardation
(B) an uncooperative attitude
(C) a speech impairment
(D) monotone speech
(E) a rapid rate of speech

4. Tactile hallucinations of insects crawling over the skin are called

(A) hypnagogic
(B) hypnopompic
(C) formication
(D) kinesthetic
(E) gustatory

5. The dexamethasone suppression test can be used to

(A) diagnose schizophrenia
(B) follow the treatment course in bipolar illness
(C) treat refractory depression
(D) follow the treatment course in depression
(E) diagnose the presence of depression

6. The most important reason to monitor lithium levels is

(A) to check on patient compliance
(B) because the toxic dose is similar to the therapeutic level
(C) because lithium is rapidly excreted from the body
(D) because lithium is a salt rather than a drug
(E) none of the above

7. Which of the following personality constellations has been found by researchers to predict reliably the development of schizophrenia later in life?

(A) Extreme dependency (e.g., sharing bedrooms with parents until late adolescence and experiencing panic away from home)
(B) Shyness, withdrawal, social awkwardness, and inability to form close interpersonal relationships
(C) A pattern of lack of socialization, including cruelty to animals, fire setting, and enuresis
(D) Overcompliance, overconformity, and high academic achievement
(E) None of the above

8. A 35-year-old man has been hospitalized for several years in a state hospital psychiatric unit. The state hospital treatment team works with the community mental health center to plan the patient's treatment and care after discharge. In addition, the community mental health program contains all of the elements of a comprehensive treatment rehabilitation system for the chronically mentally ill. Which of the following elements might reasonably be included in the patient's treatment plan for the period immediately after discharge from the state hospital?

(A) Help in finding an apartment in the community
(B) A psychosocial rehabilitation program beginning when the patient is still in the hospital and continuing through his community placement
(C) A case manager
(D) Participation in a psychoeducational-oriented group therapy system
(E) A regimen of long-acting injectable neuroleptics monitored by a psychiatrist in the mental health center

9. A 30-year-old Native American man from one of the plains tribes is brought to the emergency room by relatives. Several days ago he found out that his sister had been killed in an automobile accident. On examination, the patient said he has twice seen his dead sister who appeared to him and asked him to join her in death. The most likely diagnosis is

(A) schizophreniform disorder
(B) brief reactive psychosis
(C) schizophrenia
(D) organic mental syndrome
(E) none of the above

10. Which of the following statements is true of paranoid schizophrenia?

(A) The patient must demonstrate persistent delusions of a persecutory or suspicious nature but need not have other symptoms associated with schizophrenia
(B) Paranoid schizophrenic patients frequently demonstrate marked incoherence and loosening of associations
(C) Because of interference with social function, paranoid schizophrenic patients have a worse prognosis than residual or undifferentiated schizophrenic patients
(D) Paranoid schizophrenic patients are more likely to have increased numbers of neuropathologic, neuroradiologic, and neurochemical abnormalities than other types of schizophrenic patients
(E) None of the above

11. A psychiatric resident is assigned to care for a 30-year-old woman with a history of multiple hospitalizations for schizophrenia. Between episodes of the illness, the patient lives in an apartment and receives Supplemental Security Income. She has worked at odd jobs in the past but has not been able to maintain a job. The patient has just been released from the university inpatient psychiatric unit after a 5-day hospitalization. Appropriate approaches for the resident physician to take include which of the following?

(A) Increasing the patient's medication to buffer the stresses she will encounter when she returns to her home
(B) Establishing a relationship with the patient's case manager and learning about the patient from him or her
(C) Establishing a therapeutic relationship with the patient with the understanding that the psychotherapy will attempt to cure the schizophrenia
(D) Establishing a therapeutic relationship in which the therapist helps the patient overcome negative symptoms by pushing the patient hard to achieve the goals the patient has set for herself
(E) Because medical responsibility rests with the physician, the resident takes over the case from the treatment team at the community mental health center

12. A patient being treated on an inpatient unit has been taking neuroleptics for 5 days and is becoming increasingly fearful and agitated. The patient is taking haloperidol and 4 mg of cogentin per day. The most likely explanation for the problem is

(A) the patient is experiencing anticholinergic toxicity from the combination of haloperidol and cogentin
(B) the neuroleptic has stopped working as well as it did because of activation of liver enzymes and resulting reduction in circulating neuroleptic levels
(C) the patient's psychotic illness is following its natural course and the neuroleptic cannot keep up with the worsening condition
(D) the patient is becoming increasingly agitated from the effects of akathisia as neuroleptic levels in the patient's body continue to rise
(E) the patient has developed a medical condition affecting brain function and inducing a delirium

13. Atypical depression describes a subset of major depressive disorder with which of the following symptoms?

(A) Delusions and hallucinations
(B) Manic as well as depressive symptoms
(C) Overeating and oversleeping
(D) Worthlessness and guilt
(E) Initial insomnia

14. Grandiosity is best described by which one of the following statements?

(A) It is always delusional
(B) It is seen uniquely in mania
(C) It is typically seen in the depressed phase of bipolar I disorder
(D) It can contribute to treatment noncompliance
(E) It is always associated with flight of ideas

15. Cognitive therapy of depression is based on which of the following findings?

(A) Animals in a learned helplessness paradigm have features reminiscent of depression
(B) Depressed individuals often have a history of loss
(C) Stress commonly precedes episodes of depression
(D) An anger-turned-inward model seems to explain symptoms in many depressed patients
(E) Many depressed patients have inaccurate, negative ideas about themselves that can change with therapeutic work

16. Electroconvulsive therapy (ECT) is best described by which of the following statements?

(A) It often causes reversible memory problems
(B) It often causes permanent brain damage
(C) It is ineffective in psychotic depressions
(D) It is ineffective in patients who have failed antidepressant medications
(E) It is contraindicated for most patients with major depressive disorder

17. Lithium is best described by which one of the following statements?

(A) It is metabolized by the liver
(B) It is excreted by the kidney
(C) It has a wide therapeutic index
(D) It tends to cause weight loss
(E) It is more effective than valproate for mixed episodes in bipolar disorder

18. A symptom that suggests that a patient has major depressive disorder rather than normal bereavement is

(A) the presence of initial insomnia
(B) the presence of terminal insomnia
(C) functional impairment 3 months after the death
(D) weight loss
(E) guilty feeling about the death

19. Agoraphobia is best characterized by which of the following statements?

(A) It is caused by a specific trauma
(B) It is treated with β-adrenergic blockers
(C) It involves fear of height
(D) It is a symptom of schizophrenia
(E) It commonly accompanies panic attacks

20. Panic disorder is usually treated initially with which of the following drugs?

(A) Diazepam
(B) Buspirone
(C) Trifluoperazine
(D) Imipramine
(E) Secobarbital

21. Obsessions are

(A) intrusive thoughts or impulses
(B) anxious thoughts
(C) symptoms of unconscious conflict
(D) fears of heights
(E) psychotic symptoms

22. Effective medications for obsessive-compulsive disorder include

(A) lorazepam
(B) desipramine
(C) fluoxetine
(D) carbamazepine
(E) trifluoperazine

23. Management of a hospitalized patient who becomes hostile whenever he is asked about his illness or his personal life might include which of the following approaches?

(A) Telling him that his hostility is interfering with the doctor–patient relationship
(B) Helping him to see that his anger is really a sign of anxiety
(C) Trying to become friendlier
(D) Allowing him to determine the degree of interpersonal distance
(E) Providing unlimited visiting hours

24. A 30-year-old chronic schizophrenic patient taking an antipsychotic drug develops anxiety and increased psychotic symptoms. Psychological approaches to management might include

(A) reality testing
(B) expressive psychotherapy
(C) systematic desensitization
(D) cognitive therapy
(E) stop thinking

25. A 25-year-old man becomes anxious whenever he must work closely with an authority figure. Which of the following factors should be evaluated to assess his candidacy for expressive psychotherapy?

(A) Catastrophic thinking
(B) Social class
(C) Interest in self-awareness
(D) Problems with anger
(E) Family history

26. Appropriate management of phobias includes which of the following techniques?

(A) Systematic desensitization
(B) Expressive psychotherapy
(C) Panic control therapy
(D) Biofeedback
(E) Supportive psychotherapy

27. Appropriate indications for propranolol in the treatment of anxiety include

(A) stage fright
(B) panic attacks
(C) situational anxiety
(D) phobias
(E) posttraumatic stress disorder

28. A 26-year-old woman presents to the emergency room with shortness of breath, dizziness, and tingling in her fingers for which no organic cause can be found. The psychiatric diagnosis that would most immediately explain these symptoms is

(A) acute stress disorder
(B) mixed anxiety–depression
(C) caffeinism
(D) hyperventilation syndrome
(E) posttraumatic stress disorder

29. A few days after a mastectomy, a 45-year-old woman begins making seductive comments to her 25-year-old intern. She divorced her husband because he was seeing a younger woman. There is no history of psychiatric illness. Factors that could be contributing to her behavior include

(A) anxiety about her attractiveness
(B) schizophrenia
(C) stranger anxiety
(D) separation anxiety
(E) obsessive-compulsive disorder

30. Which of the following is the most accurate statement about vascular dementia?

(A) Agitation in vascular dementia is best treated with benzodiazepines
(B) Early signs of vascular dementia include memory loss, irritability, and difficulty concentrating
(C) Women are affected more commonly than men
(D) The condition is rarely characterized by sudden exacerbations or by remissions
(E) The condition is usually first evident in individuals over age 80

31. Which one of the following symptoms is the most distinguishing feature of delirium?

(A) Fever
(B) Memory impairment
(C) Personality changes
(D) Reduced clarity of awareness
(E) Tremulousness

32. A 54-year-old woman without previous significant mental problems undergoes surgery for repair of a hip fracture and becomes agitated and uncooperative on the second postoperative day. By the third postoperative day, she appears to be hallucinating and calls the nursing staff by the names of her children. She is febrile and tachycardic. Which one of the following is the most likely mental disturbance?

(A) Brief psychotic disorder
(B) Catatonia
(C) Delirium
(D) Dementia
(E) Panic disorder

33. Which of the following groups of symptoms reflects the most distinguishing features of symptomatic hypocalcemia?

(A) Cramping, tetany, and irritability
(B) Fever, dry mucous membranes, and agitation
(C) Lid lag, hyperreflexia, and apathy
(D) Muscular weakness, anxiety, and confusion
(E) Sweating, tachycardia, and slurred speech

34. A 51-year-old woman becomes increasingly depressed over several months and complains of fatigue, weakness, dry skin, and brittle hair. Which one of the following diagnoses is most likely correct?

(A) Dementia due to hypothyroidism
(B) Dementia due to niacin deficiency
(C) Mood disorder due to hypothyroidism
(D) Mood disorder due to niacin deficiency
(E) Mood disorder due to systemic lupus erythematosus (SLE)

35. A 35-year-old man complains of paresthesia, itching, and difficulty concentrating. His purified protein derivative test recently converted from negative to positive, and he is undergoing treatment. Which one of the following conditions is the most likely cause of his symptoms?

(A) Chronic tubercular meningitis
(B) Infection with human immunodeficiency virus (HIV)
(C) Methamphetamine abuse
(D) Multiple sclerosis
(E) Pyridoxine deficiency

36. A 49-year-old man with a long history of alcohol dependence and homelessness insists that he has pressing business and family obligations that require immediate discharge from the hospital. Which of the following is the most likely additional finding on mental status examination?

(A) Auditory hallucinations
(B) Depressive symptoms
(C) Manic symptoms
(D) Memory deficits
(E) Reduced clarity of awareness

37. Which of the following conditions is most likely to increase the risk for subdural hematoma?

(A) Alcohol dependence
(B) Systemic lupus erythematosus (SLE)
(C) Vascular dementia
(D) Complex partial seizures
(E) Hyperthyroidism

38. A 28-year-old man has episodes of a subjective sense of unreality and transient memory impairment, followed by several minutes of confusion. Which one of the following infectious agents is most likely responsible?

(A) Herpes simplex
(B) *Mycobacterium tuberculi*
(C) Prion (slow virus)
(D) *Streptococcus*
(E) *Treponema pallidum*

39. Chronic abuse of which one of the following substances is most likely to rapidly result in dementia?

(A) Amphetamines
(B) Cannabis
(C) Hallucinogens
(D) Inhalants
(E) Opioids

40. In contrast to most hallucinogens, phencyclidine is often associated with

(A) hallucinations
(B) anxiety
(C) aggression
(D) depersonalization
(E) piloerection

41. Which of the following statements best characterizes cocaine?

(A) It is safe when used in moderation
(B) Its withdrawal causes delirium
(C) It is used mainly by high socioeconomic groups
(D) It is usually used by itself
(E) It is highly addictive

42. True statements about marijuana include which of the following?

(A) It is not associated with withdrawal syndromes
(B) Intoxication causes hypertension
(C) "Bad trips" are treated with psychotherapy
(D) Tolerance develops to hallucinations
(E) It does not impair driving

43. Stimulant withdrawal may be associated with

(A) decreased appetite
(B) paranoia
(C) suicide
(D) insomnia
(E) piloerection

44. True statements concerning opioid dependence include which of the following?

(A) Dependence does not increase mortality
(B) Most addicts are introduced to narcotics by pushers
(C) Young adults frequently abuse opioids
(D) Illicit narcotic use develops in epidemics
(E) Opioids are most frequently used by themselves

45. A middle-aged woman complaining of insomnia has visited a number of physicians over the years. On the night of admission to the hospital for elective surgery, she becomes anxious and agitated. There is no evidence of trauma, bleeding, infection, or neurologic disease, but the patient develops postural hypotension and fever. Admission of use of which of the following substances would be likely to clarify the diagnosis?

(A) Physostigmine
(B) Haloperidol
(C) Disulfiram
(D) Phenobarbital
(E) Thiamine

46. A 50-year-old man is admitted to the hospital with complaints of flank pain of 1 day's duration. A stat urinalysis performed in the emergency room reveals blood in the urine. The patient says that he has never before been hospitalized for this condition. He claims that he is a physician from another state who lost his license because of drinking. He says that he was on the faculty of the medical school in that state, but lacks insurance because he has not worked in 2 years. The patient says that he has published articles, particularly in European journals. A resident rotating onto the service believes that this man was a patient in a hospital in another county where he was doing a rotation. The resident remembers that the patient was being followed up for kidney stones. Assuming that the resident is correct, the most likely diagnosis is

(A) conversion disorder
(B) factitious disorder
(C) somatization disorder
(D) malingering
(E) hypochondriasis

47. Which of the following is most likely to be a conversion symptom?

(A) A 25-year-old man with multiple emergency room admissions for complaints that initially sound like a myocardial infarction, but never with electrocardiogram (ECG) or enzyme changes suggestive of myocardial infarction

(B) A 35-year-old woman with general malaise, but with normal complete blood cell count, serum chemistry, urinalysis, and negative human immunodeficiency virus (HIV) and drug screens

(C) A 20-year-old woman who, after a boating accident, develops bilateral blindness

(D) A 70-year-old man who believes that he has metastatic cancer to all of his internal organs, but has normal examination and laboratory test results

(E) A 19-year-old male college student who comes into the emergency room very fearful, with complaints of bright-red urine and an otherwise normal examination

48. Ms. Jones is a 22-year-old woman who swallows sharp objects, such as Exacto knife blades. Sometimes the blades are wrapped in tape, and sometimes they are not. When she comes to the emergency room, she tells the physician what she has done, and says that she was trying to kill herself. Because radiograph results do not distinguish between a wrapped object and an unwrapped one, she has received multiple surgeries to remove the objects. She has a history of other self-mutilating acts, such as slicing her arms. The most likely diagnosis is

(A) major depression
(B) somatization disorder
(C) borderline personality disorder
(D) schizophrenia
(E) partial complex seizures

49. Which of the following disorders is thought to be especially related to obsessive-compulsive disorder?

(A) Somatization disorder
(B) Body dysmorphic disorder
(C) Conversion disorder
(D) Pain disorder
(E) Factitious disorder

50. A 33-year-old man is concerned about his semen. He believes that he found blood in it, and visits to the urologist do not reassure him that this is most likely a normal phenomenon of middle-aged men. For medicolegal reasons, the urologist will not tell him absolutely that this is not something more sinister. This man saw a friend die of testicular cancer a year previously. He repeatedly palpates his testicles to determine if anything has changed. His repeated examinations sometimes cause inflammation and swelling, which bring him back to the urologist. The most likely diagnosis is

(A) somatization disorder
(B) conversion disorder
(C) factitious disorder
(D) malingering
(E) hypochondriasis

51. Which one of the following statements is the most reliable biologic finding concerning homosexual men?

(A) Homosexual men display lower testosterone levels than do nonhomosexual men
(B) Homosexual men have smaller anterior hypothalamic nuclei than do nonhomosexual men
(C) Homosexual men have higher luteinizing hormone (LH) response to estrogen administration than do nonhomosexual men
(D) Rat models of homosexual behavior are the current, accepted standard for testing hypotheses about the biology of homosexuality
(E) None of the above

52. A 25-year-old male medical student presents with complaints of premature ejaculation. The problem is of sufficient severity that it is endangering a relationship with his partner, who believes that it is a sign of his "neurosis." The best treatment for this man most likely is

(A) long-term, insight-oriented psychotherapy to get at the base of his neurosis
(B) a course of thioridazine
(C) a behavioral approach
(D) treatment of his depression

53. A 28-year-old woman who has been placed on a new psychotropic medication begins to lactate. The woman is not pregnant, has not recently given birth, and does not have a disease that would cause lactation. Which of the following medications is most likely to cause lactation?

(A) Alprazolam
(B) Fluoxetine
(C) Diazepam
(D) Chlorpromazine
(E) Bupropion

54. A clinician would most likely have to break the confidentiality of the physician–patient relationship if a patient comes in for treatment of

(A) sadomasochism
(B) frotteurism
(C) pedophilia
(D) voyeurism
(E) homosexuality

55. A young woman with anorexia nervosa steadfastly refuses to eat. She is not yet in imminent medical danger from starvation, and she remains an outpatient. A logical approach at this point would be to

(A) break off treatment with the patient, refusing to treat her unless she agrees to eat
(B) set a critical weight for the patient below which she will be hospitalized if necessary and forced to gain weight
(C) insist that the patient increase her caloric intake or she will be hospitalized
(D) try to curtail her physical activities (e.g., running and dancing)
(E) none of the above

56. Which of the following prognoses is most accurate for anorexia nervosa?

(A) Most patients recover
(B) Most girls recover, but very few boys recover
(C) The earlier the onset in life, the better the outcome of the disease
(D) By the age of 30 years, 30%–40% of patients die

57. The treatment of bulimia nervosa is most accurately described by which of the following statements?

(A) Hospitalization is regularly indicated
(B) Adjunctive medications are regularly prescribed
(C) Individual psychodynamic psychotherapy is seldom adequate
(D) Group psychotherapy is usually the treatment of choice
(E) Mixed modality treatment appears to offer promising results

58. A 6-year-old boy presents with acute onset of hyperactivity of 1 month's duration. It is noted in the patient's history that the behavioral change followed a few days after the child's first grand mal seizure. The next step in the physician's evaluation should be to

(A) perform a sleep-deprived electroencephalogram (EEG) with N-P leads
(B) take a medication history
(C) prescribe a computed tomography (CT) scan of the head
(D) consult a pediatric neurologist
(E) add carbamazepine to the drug regimen

59. Personality disorders are almost always

(A) manifested during adolescence
(B) worse in old age
(C) free of genetic–biologic influences
(D) associated with good occupational functioning
(E) seen intermittently in adult life

60. An individual with a schizoid personality disorder may do well in which of the following circumstances?

(A) When hospitalized for a medical illness
(B) In social situations, such as dating
(C) If others reach out to the person affectionately
(D) If treated with antidepressants
(E) In jobs that require social isolation

61. The concurrent presence of a mood disorder is more likely in which of the following personality disorders?

(A) Schizoid personality
(B) Paranoid personality
(C) Borderline personality
(D) Avoidant personality
(E) Antisocial personality

62. Cluster A, the odd or eccentric group of personality disorders, includes schizoid, schizotypal, and

(A) histrionic personalities
(B) borderline personalities
(C) paranoid personalities
(D) antisocial personalities

63. In families with a history of schizophrenia, there is also an increase in the number of relatives with which of the following personality disorders?

(A) Schizoid personality
(B) Antisocial personality
(C) Paranoid personality
(D) Schizotypal personality

DIRECTIONS: Each of the numbered items or incomplete statements in this section is negatively phrased, as indicated by a capitalized word such as NOT, LEAST, or EXCEPT. Select the ONE lettered answer or completion that is BEST in each case.

---

64. Perceptual abnormalities include all of the following EXCEPT

(A) hallucinations
(B) depersonalization
(C) illusions
(D) perseverations

65. The sleep laboratory (polysomnography) has been useful in studying all of the following conditions EXCEPT

(A) seizure disorders
(B) impotence
(C) depression
(D) schizophrenia

66. The clinical laboratory is important in the diagnosis and treatment of mental disorders. Important functions include all of the following EXCEPT

(A) assessing the severity of psychiatric illness
(B) identifying biologic markers of psychiatric illness
(C) monitoring blood levels of psychotropic medications
(D) screening for other medical illnesses

67. Risk factors for the development of schizophrenia include all of the following EXCEPT

(A) poor ego functions as demonstrated by lack of self–object differentiation and an increased vulnerability to narcissistic injury
(B) an environment characterized by high levels of cultural, economic, and psychosocial stressors
(C) a birth in early spring in either hemisphere
(D) a schizophrenic biologic relative
(E) a history of herpes simplex or viral encephalitis

68. Common treatment goals for schizophrenic patients include all of the following EXCEPT

(A) continuity of care, such as treatment plans, are carried through over time and changes in therapists
(B) treatment should be administered in the least restrictive setting
(C) comprehensiveness entails integrating medical, psychological, and social needs of the patient into a coordinated treatment plan
(D) confrontation of the patient's resistance to changes in his environment should be systematic, frequent, and assertive
(E) psychosocial rehabilitation should teach the patient social and functional skills, which may have been lost in earlier phases of the illness

69. Case management of the schizophrenic patient involves all of the following EXCEPT

(A) advocacy for the needs of the individual patient
(B) planning the overall treatment program among diverse service and care providers
(C) developing insight into intrapsychic causes of psychotic symptoms
(D) advocacy for groups of schizophrenic and other chronically mentally ill patients
(E) linking different care providers to coordinate treatment

70. Trends related to hospitalization of patients suffering from schizophrenia include all of the following EXCEPT

(A) shorter hospitalizations with more limited treatment goals than previously
(B) increased hospitalization for functional skills assessment
(C) increased use of partial hospitalization by the private sector
(D) decreased use of partial hospitalization by the public sector
(E) decreased use of hospitals for milieu therapy

71. A 21-year-old patient with a history of two previous psychotic episodes, and known residual functional deterioration and interepisode hallucinations and delusions at a reduced level, is brought into the emergency room by police. The patient was found wandering naked, disoriented, and hostile several miles from his home. An initial work-up showed no localizing neurologic findings, and complete blood cell count, urinalysis, and sequential multiple analysis results are within normal limits, except for signs of dehydration and a mildly elevated white blood cell count. Other laboratory results are pending, including toxicology screen. When the patient becomes increasingly agitated, all of the following interventions may be appropriate EXCEPT

(A) use of intravenous high-potency neuroleptics
(B) use of intramuscular low-potency neuroleptics
(C) use of benzodiazepines by any available route
(D) use of intravenous droperidol to control agitation
(E) no pharmacologic intervention if toxicity is suspected

72. A clinician observes the interaction of a young male schizophrenic patient and his family. It is clear that the family feels that the patient's condition is the result of a moral weakness, and they feel he is to blame for this shameful state. The family appears angry with the patient, and they say negative things about him in his presence several times during the interview. The clinician might reasonably suggest the following for the group EXCEPT

(A) encouraging the family to join the Alliance for the Mentally Ill and to be active in that organization
(B) educating the family and patient about the illness of schizophrenia, emphasizing the things that the patient and family can do to control symptoms
(C) telling the family to share in the responsibility for the patient's illness, because of their role in creating the illness during the patient's development
(D) arranging to reduce the contact between the patient and family to a more tolerable level with the aim of reducing tensions
(E) involving the family in a psychoeducational program aimed at reducing levels of expressed emotion and negativity about the patient

73. A patient taking clozapine for 3 weeks develops a fever of 102°F and feels lethargic. The patient is referred to the clinic, although his last complete blood cell count was normal. The following are appropriate steps to take EXCEPT

(A) telling the patient to go home and monitor the fever for 24 hours because fever is a common finding when starting clozapine
(B) performing a stat complete blood cell count
(C) performing a complete physical examination
(D) taking a chest radiograph
(E) monitoring the patient in the emergency room for several hours

74. All of the following neurotransmitters are suspected of being involved in the pathophysiology of schizophrenia EXCEPT

(A) dopamine
(B) prostaglandin E_1
(C) ascorbic acid
(D) norepinephrine
(E) serotonin

75. Antidepressant drugs with a wide therapeutic index include all of the following EXCEPT

(A) fluoxetine
(B) nortriptyline
(C) trazodone
(D) sertraline
(E) venlafaxine

76. Medical conditions that can cause manic-like symptoms include all of the following EXCEPT

(A) autoimmune deficiency syndrome (AIDS)
(B) Wilson disease
(C) hyperthyroidism
(D) tuberculosis
(E) Cushing disease

77. Anxiety is a common symptom of all of the following illnesses EXCEPT

(A) hypoglycemia
(B) hyperparathyroidism
(C) pheochromocytoma
(D) porphyria

78. A 30-year-old man complains of dizziness, palpitations, derealization, and a sense of detachment that are not associated with any obvious stress. The differential diagnosis includes all of the following conditions EXCEPT

(A) partial complex seizures
(B) acute stress disorder
(C) panic disorder
(D) hypercalcemia
(E) hyperthyroidism

79. The relationship between anxiety and depression is characterized by all of the following statements EXCEPT

(A) many depressed patients are also anxious
(B) many patients with panic disorder become depressed
(C) the same treatments are effective for panic disorder and depression
(D) panic disorder and depression run in the same families
(E) depression and anxiety usually alternate in patients with both symptoms

80. All of the following drugs are contraindicated in patients who are intoxicated with alcohol EXCEPT

(A) diazepam
(B) phenobarbital
(C) disulfiram
(D) glutethimide
(E) haloperidol

81. One aspect or another of alcohol withdrawal can be treated with all of the following EXCEPT

(A) thiamine
(B) benzodiazepines
(C) caffeine
(D) hydration
(E) neuroleptics

82. A patient hospitalized for gastritis is found to have an enlarged liver. Appropriate blood tests would include all of the following EXCEPT

(A) hemoglobin
(B) blood alcohol level
(C) blood cultures
(D) gamma glutamyl transferase (GGT)
(E) toxicology screen

83. Anticholinergic poisoning is characterized by all of the following EXCEPT

(A) warm, dry skin
(B) mydriasis
(C) psychosis
(D) tachycardia
(E) coryza

84. General treatment approaches for patients with substance abuse and dependence include all of the following EXCEPT

(A) detoxification
(B) controlled use of the substance
(C) family therapy
(D) contingency contracting
(E) twelve-step programs

85. A 25-year-old woman is referred to a psychiatrist by a surgical colleague. He has requested that the woman be "cleared" by the psychiatrist before he is willing to undertake reconstructive surgery on her breasts. The surgeon is concerned that the woman's breasts are within normal limits for size and shape. However, the woman believes that they are grossly deformed, and she hesitantly admits that she believes that they are so deformed that she shuns social contact, and has never had a sexual relationship. She further admits that she spends several hours each day examining the breasts and trying to "train" them into the "correct" shape. In formulating the treatment plan, the psychiatrist might reasonably include all of the following EXCEPT

(A) gathering historical information about depression, psychotic symptoms, panic disorder, obsessive-compulsive disorder, and her perceptions of her physical health
(B) a trial of clomipramine
(C) a trial of fluoxetine
(D) an educational approach to the possible disorder affecting her
(E) interpreting her concerns as a fear of an inability to nurture

86. A patient suffering from a major depressive episode is likely to have all of the following EXCEPT

(A) increases in gonadotropins
(B) blunted thyrotropin-releasing hormone (TRH)–stimulated prolactin response
(C) blunted suppression of cortisol secretion with administration of dexamethasone
(D) increased interleukin-1b production
(E) abnormally low natural killer cell functions at some times of the day

Questions 87–88

87. A medical student taking a history from a woman on a medicine service for complaints of abdominal pain realizes that the patient meets the criteria for somatization disorder, given the history of lifelong ill health and numerous past complaints. The medical student should be active in pursuing the following historical areas EXCEPT

(A) current relationships with family
(B) history of sexual abuse
(C) blank spots in memory
(D) relationship of physical symptoms to life events
(E) childhood history of illness

88. The medical student is asked by the attending physician to generate a treatment plan for the woman in question 87. The best strategy for the medical student to propose is

(A) placing the patient on long-term benzodiazepine medications
(B) an immediate transfer to the psychiatry service
(C) a trial of neuroleptic medication to control the delusional aspects of the patient's illness
(D) scheduling appointments in the outpatient medicine clinic for periodic evaluations of the patient's new symptoms by the same attending physician
(E) a trial of monoamine oxidase (MAO) inhibitors

89. The hospital management of anorectic patients commonly includes all of the following EXCEPT

(A) restriction of privileges
(B) nasogastric alimentation
(C) locked seclusion
(D) weight monitoring
(E) ketone monitoring

90. Diagnostic findings consistent with anorexia nervosa include all of the following EXCEPT

(A) normal serum protein and albumin levels
(B) hyperkalemia
(C) normal serum cortisol
(D) bradycardia, hypotension, hypothermia
(E) hypercarotenemia

91. All of the following conditions are considered disorders of bonding and attachment EXCEPT

(A) autistic disorder
(B) hospitalism
(C) anaclitic depression
(D) vulnerable child syndrome
(E) child abuse

92. Methods of treating autistic disorder include all of the following EXCEPT

(A) a highly structured classroom setting
(B) behavior modification
(C) imipramine administration
(D) psychotherapy

93. Signs and symptoms found in the syndrome of hospitalism include all of the following EXCEPT

(A) apathy
(B) absence of bonding
(C) susceptibility to infection
(D) jaundice

94. A 35-year-old man with an obsessive-compulsive personality disorder is likely to exhibit all of the following symptoms EXCEPT

(A) perfectionism that interferes with performance
(B) compulsive checking behavior
(C) preoccupation and concern for rules
(D) indecisiveness
(E) stinginess with compliments

DIRECTIONS: Each set of matching questions in this section consists of a list of four to twenty-six lettered options followed by several numbered items. For each numbered item, select the ONE lettered option that is most closely associated with it. To avoid spending too much time on matching sets with large numbers of options, it is generally advisable to begin each set by reading the list of options. Then, for each item in the set, try to generate the correct answer and locate it in the option list, rather than evaluating each option individually. Each lettered option may be selected once, more than once, or not at all.

Questions 95–96

Match the clinical vignettes with the most appropriate diagnosis.

(A) Major depressive disorder
(B) Dysthymic disorder
(C) Bipolar I disorder
(D) Bipolar II disorder
(E) Cyclothymic disorder

95. A 34-year-old waitress sees her internist and complains of low energy. She describes it as a chronic problem, which was partly responsible for her dropping out of college many years before. She feels her life is going nowhere. She has tried over the years taking classes at a community college, but is unable to concentrate on the material. Her sleep and appetite are normal, and she denies ever feeling suicidal. She drinks about two beers each week and denies any illicit drug use. She is medically well. She had a period of 1 month last summer when she felt happy and optimistic, after getting a job at a new restaurant, but the good feeling soon faded.

96. A 53-year-old man is admitted for psychiatric treatment for the first time after ingesting a bottle of over-the-counter sleeping pills. His wife reports that he has been depressed and irritable during the 4 months since their youngest son died of autoimmune deficiency syndrome (AIDS). The man has been sleeping poorly, has lost about 20 pounds, and has lost interest in books and sports. He had been talking about death for 1 week, but his wife did not think he had the energy to attempt suicide. His previous psychiatric history is significant for several years of alcohol abuse in his twenties, and two periods that his wife said were "manic depressive." Symptoms during these two, month-long episodes, which occurred at ages 30 and 38 years, included driven behavior, entitlement, increased spending (he bought a new car when they were strapped for money), and decreased sleep. The man was able to continue his job as a real estate agent during these times and was even recognized by his agency for his long hours and increased sales.

Questions 97–101

Match each statement with the type of medication it describes.

(A) Benzodiazepines
(B) Antihistamines
(C) Barbiturates
(D) Neuroleptics
(E) Selective serotonin reuptake inhibitors (SSRIs)

97. May cause tardive dyskinesia

98. May impair memory when used as anxiolytics in the elderly

99. Type of withdrawal syndrome related to half-life

100. Effective for obsessive-compulsive disorder

101. High danger of tolerance, addiction, severe withdrawal syndromes, and death from overdose

Questions 102–106

Match each statement with the type of anxiety it describes.

(A) Posttraumatic anxiety
(B) Situational anxiety
(C) Separation anxiety
(D) Anxiety about dependency
(E) Anxiety about loss of self-esteem

102. It may be associated with fear of loss of control

103. It results in distress when the patient is alone

104. It is manifested by treating others in a condescending manner

105. It results from threatened awareness of an unconscious conflict

106. Its onset may be immediate or delayed

Questions 107–109

For each type of seizure, select the most likely associated disturbance of consciousness.

(A) Anxiety attacks
(B) Brief periods of inattention and unresponsiveness
(C) Loss of consciousness
(D) No loss of consciousness
(E) Vivid hallucinations

107. Absence (petit mal)

108. Myoclonic

109. Tonic–clonic

Questions 110–111

For each presentation below, select the most likely associated electroencephalogram (EEG) findings.

(A) Bilaterally synchronous spike and slow wave
(B) Diffuse generalized slowing
(C) Fast-wave activity
(D) Normal tracing
(E) Sharp, triphasic synchronous discharges

110. A 53-year-old man with a 4-month course of malaise, emotional lability, and gait disturbance progressing to dementia and myoclonus

111. A 15-year-old girl with brief episodes of unresponsiveness and chewing movements

Questions 112–116

For each commonly abused substance listed, select the medication that is used to treat dependence on or withdrawal from that substance.

(A) Desipramine
(B) Methadone
(C) Disulfiram
(D) Phenobarbital
(E) Diazepam

112. Tranquilizers and sleeping pills

113. Cocaine

114. Phencyclidine

115. Alcohol

116. Narcotics

Questions 117–121

Match the medical, physical, or psychiatric complication with the substance that usually causes it.

(A) Motor vehicle accidents
(B) Paranoia
(C) Nightmares
(D) Septic arthritis
(E) Echolalia

117. Heroin

118. Pentobarbital

119. Phencyclidine

120. Methamphetamine

121. Alcohol

Questions 122–125

Match the conditions listed below with the most appropriate medication.

(A) Thioridazine
(B) Imipramine
(C) Methylphenidate
(D) Phenobarbital

122. Childhood schizophrenia

123. Hyperactivity

124. Enuresis

125. Idiopathic grand mal epilepsy

Questions 126–128

For each description listed, select the personality disorder that is most likely to be associated with it.

(A) Dependent personality
(B) Histrionic personality
(C) Obsessive-compulsive personality

126. Illness is often perceived as a threat to physical attractiveness

127. Pleasure, but not sexual arousal, is derived from the suffering of others

128. Tasks must be performed in certain ways, but delegation of responsibility is all but impossible because of a fear that others will not perform well

1. The answer is C *[Chapter 1 I B 3]*. Early in the psychiatric interview, it is important for the physician to let the patient talk about what is bothering him. Only after this point should the interviewer attempt to find out other details, including how the patient feels about what has been happening. Details about previous psychiatric illnesses and about the legal issues associated with these problems, if present, are important as the interview progresses. Informing the patient of the fee schedule is generally not done at the beginning of the interview.

2. The answer is B *[Chapter 1 II C 1 (2)]*. High-voltage, slow-wave activity is characteristic of delirium when seen on the electroencephalogram (EEG). Delirium associated with alcohol withdrawal or age dementia, however, does not show slow-wave activity. As yet, no specific EEG abnormalities have been seen in schizophrenia.

3. The answer is C *[Chapter 1 II B 4 d]*. Echolalia is an example of a speech impairment. The patient repeats like a parrot what the interviewer says. This is not an example of psychomotor retardation, in which the patient says little, nor is it considered an uncooperative attitude. The tone and rate of speech are not abnormal.

4. The answer is C *[Chapter 1 II B 6 a (4)]*. Tactile hallucinations of insects crawling over the skin are called formication. Hypnagogic and hypnopompic hallucinations occur while either falling asleep or awaking from sleep. Kinesthetic hallucinations are feelings of movement when none occurs, and gustatory hallucinations are hallucinations of taste.

5. The answer is D *[Chapter 1 II C 1 d (1)]*. The dexamethasone suppression test can be used to follow the treatment response in patients who are depressed. It is not particularly useful in diagnosing the presence or absence of depression or schizophrenia. It is not a treatment for depression, and it is not useful in treating bipolar illness or following the treatment course in bipolar illness.

6. The answer is B *[Chapter 1 II C 2 a]*. Toxic levels of lithium are very similar to the therapeutic levels, and in some patients, they are the same. For this reason, it is important to monitor lithium levels. Although patient com-

pliance and lithium excretion can be checked, these are not the most important reasons for monitoring blood levels of lithium.

7. The answer is E *[Chapter 2 VI A 1–4]*. Research has failed to demonstrate the existence of the schizophrenic personality, particularly one that reliably predicts later development of schizophrenia. However, some studies have revealed significant histories in some schizophrenic patients of extreme dependency, shyness, withdrawal, social awkwardness, inability to form close interpersonal relationships, an asocial premorbid personality, and a pattern of overcompliance and conformity.

8. The answer is A *[Chapter 2 IX H 1–6]*. After a long period of hospitalization, most schizophrenic patients are lacking in skills required to locate an apartment and to live without supervision in the apartment. Such planning might create crises in the patient's life and would make him or her prone to rehospitalization. If graduated supervised residential care is available in this community mental health setting, a supervised residential placement would be much more appropriate in the transition to independent living. Although the use of long-acting neuroleptics may well be indicated because of anticipated medication compliance problems, an ideal treatment program would encourage the patient to assume as much responsibility of self-administration of medications as possible. All the other elements (i.e., a psychosocial rehabilitation program, a case manager, and psychoeducational-oriented group therapy) would be appropriate to good treatment planning after the discharge of the patient.

9. The answer is E *[Chapter 2 VI A; VII A, B 6, 7, C]*. The case describes a normal culture-bound experience for Native Americans from plains cultures. The physician should remember that assessment of psychotic symptoms by a clinician from one culture in a patient from another culture should not be attempted without specific knowledge of the patient's culture.

10. The answer is E *[Chapter 2 V A 3]*. According to modern diagnostic criteria, patients with paranoid schizophrenia may not have incoherence, marked loosening of associations, flat or grossly inappropriate affect, catatonic behavior, or grossly disorganized behavior. The prognosis for paranoid schizophrenia is better than that for other types, perhaps because of the late onset that is characteristic. Paranoid schizophrenia tends to be associated with fewer neuropathologic abnormalities and neurochemical findings than other types of schizophrenia. In contrast to other types of schizophrenia, paranoid schizophrenic patients retain good social functioning despite frequent interferences with relationships because of delusions.

11. The answer is B *[Chapter 2 VIII F 2].*
There is no reason to suppose that increasing the patient's medication from inpatient levels will be useful or helpful. There is no reason to assume that the patient's return to her home will be more stressful than the hospital, and increasing the medication without a clear indication may subject the patient to increased risk of tardive dyskinesia. It is highly unlikely that the therapist will cure the patient's schizophrenia with any known form of psychotherapy, and such a false promise may be legally actionable. Placing more stress on the patient by "pushing hard" for the patient to achieve possibly unrealistic goals produces increased risk for more psychotic decompensation. Finally, taking over the treatment is a common error. The resident cannot hope to take over the global functions of most community mental health center treatment teams. Rather, negotiating a working relationship with the treatment team may be in everyone's best interest.

12. The answer is D *[Chapter 2 VIII L 1 d (4)].*
This hospital course is not uncommon, and any of the answers is a reasonable hypothesis. However, by far the most common cause for increasing agitation while neuroleptic blood levels are increasing is akathisia. Unfortunately, when patients cannot describe their experience articulately, and respond to the extreme discomfort of this condition with increasing motor activity and complaints of psychotic symptoms, they often receive increasing doses of the neuroleptic, which of course make the symptom worse. It is unlikely that liver enzymes would be induced in this short a time period. Although it is possible that the patient is unusually sensitive to anticholinergic effects, high-potency neuroleptics and a moderate dose of an anticholinergic agent are unlikely to produce this finding.

13. The answer is C *[Chapter 3 III A 1 b].*
Atypical depression, which may respond more successfully to monoamine oxidase (MAO) inhibitors or selective serotonin reuptake inhibitors (SSRIs) than to other drugs, is so named because patterns of eating and sleeping are the opposite of those seen in most depressed patients. Rather than exhibiting insomnia and poor appetite, those patients sleep excessively and gain weight. Delusions and hallucinations occur in patients with major depressive disorder with psychotic features. When both manic and depressive symptoms are seen concurrently, the patient is said to exhibit a mixed episode. Worthlessness, guilt, and initial insomnia are all typical symptoms of major depression.

14. The answer is D *[Chapter 3 III A 2 a].*
Grandiosity, which may or may not be delusional, is a common feature of manic episodes. It is also seen in some other conditions, such as mixed episodes, hypomanic episodes, delusional disorder, and narcissistic personality disorder. It is not typically seen during the depressed phase of bipolar I disorder. Although grandiosity and flight of ideas are commonly seen in the same patient, this is not necessarily the case. Grandiosity can contribute to noncompliance (e.g., when the patient feels more knowledgeable than his physician).

15. The answer is E *[Chapter 3 IV D].* Cognitive therapy of depression, which has been found in controlled studies to be an effective treatment for many patients, is based on the observation that many depressed patients have inaccurate, negative cognitions, such as "I'll never succeed in anything." Teaching patients to identify and change these cognitions can result in significant symptomatic improvement. Learned helplessness supports a behavioral approach. The history of earlier loss in many depressed patients and the anger-turned-inward model reflect psychodynamic thinking. The relationship between stress and mood episodes has been associated with the kindling model of bipolar illness.

16. The answer is A *[Chapter 3 V B 3].*
Electroconvulsive therapy (ECT) is not commonly used as a first-line treatment for depression, mostly because of a bad reputation, which dates to its use decades ago. It is a safe and effective treatment for major depressive

disorder as well as several other illnesses, including manic episodes and some cases of schizophrenia. Confusion immediately after the procedure and memory loss, which usually normalizes within several months, are common side effects. ECT may be particularly effective for psychotic depression and is often used in patients who have failed trials of antidepressant medication. There is no evidence that ECT causes permanent brain damage.

17. The answer is B *[Chapter 3 V C 3].*
Lithium is an ion, usually administered as lithium carbonate, and is treated like sodium by many physiologic processes. It is not metabolized, and it is excreted renally. Any situation that results in sodium loss (e.g., diarrhea, low-salt diet) causes the kidney to retain both sodium and lithium, leading to possible toxicity. Similarly, lithium levels drop as a result of sodium excess, as the body rids itself of the sodium. Monitoring serum levels of lithium is important because the drug has a narrow therapeutic index. Toxicity can lead to seizures, confusion, and even death. Weight gain is a common side effect at therapeutic serum levels. Valproate, another mood-stabilizing drug, appears to be more effective than lithium in the treatment of mixed episodes of bipolar disorder.

18. The answer is C *[Chapter 3 III B 1 d (4)].*
Normal bereavement features many of the symptoms seen in a major depressive episode, including sleep disturbance, anorexia, weight loss, and guilty feelings. Although patterns and symptoms of grieving vary in different cultures, the person who has suffered a loss usually feels less sad and more functional with time. Persistent, severe symptoms 3 months after the death suggest that the loss has precipitated a major depressive episode and that treatment should be considered.

19. The answer is E *[Chapter 4 I B 5 a (2)].*
Agoraphobia is fear of being away from home in situations in which escape might be difficult or embarrassing or help unavailable if the patient became symptomatic. Agoraphobia is often but not always a complication of panic disorder. Specific traumatic circumstances produce circumscribed phobias, especially specific phobias. Systematic desensitization may be necessary to treat residual phobic avoidance after panic attacks have resolved.

20. The answer is D *[Chapter 4 III C 1].*
Antidepressants are clearly effective for panic disorder. The benzodiazepines and buspirone are usually used for generalized and anticipatory anxiety. Doses of diazepam that would be expected to be effective in panic disorder are difficult for most patients to tolerate. Neuroleptics are used for anxiety associated with psychosis or severe disorganization. Barbiturates and related compounds should not be prescribed for any form of anxiety or insomnia.

21. The answer is A *[Chapter 4 I B 4].* Obsessions are defined as persistent, intrusive ideas, images, or impulses that are recognized as absurd but cannot be forced out of consciousness. Although they create anxiety, obsessions differ from typical anxious thoughts in that they bear no relationship to actual circumstances and are extremely unlikely to actually occur. Older theories held that obsessions represented the emergence into consciousness of unconscious desires or impulses, but treatment based on this assumption is ineffective. Obsessive impulses to jump from heights may occur, but fear of heights is called acrophobia. By definition, obsessions are not psychotic symptoms because the patient is aware that they are unrealistic. Obsessions that a patient becomes convinced are true are called delusions.

22. The answer is C *[Chapter 4 I B 4; III C].*
Benzodiazepines and antidepressants with the exception of the serotonergic tricyclic antidepressant clomipramine are ineffective for obsessive-compulsive disorder. Carbamazepine may be a useful adjunct in the treatment of posttraumatic stress disorder and benzodiazepine withdrawal, but it does not help obsessions or compulsions. Neuroleptics like trifluoperazine are of no use in obsessive-compulsive disorder unless obsessions are delusional in intensity or are accompanied by tics or psychotic symptoms. Selective serotonin reuptake inhibitors (SSRIs) such as fluoxetine are the only medications besides clomipramine with reliable anti-obsessional properties.

23. The answer is D *[Chapter 4 I; II].* The most likely cause of the patient's behavior is fear of intimacy, and possibly loss of control. Becoming friendlier, giving him more access to people, and interpreting his secret fears will all increase this anxiety, as will attempts to control his behavior.

24. The answer is A *[Chapter 4 III A 1, B].* Supportive psychotherapy, which includes encouragement of reality testing, is the appropriate approach to an acutely ill patient with limited psychological resources. Expressive psychotherapy is used to treat some neuroses; systematic desensitization is a treatment for phobias; cognitive therapy helps depression and panic disorder; and stop thinking is a treatment for obsessions.

25. The answer is C *[Chapter 4 III A 1, 2].* Expressive psychotherapy may be helpful to patients whose unresolved conflicts are stimulated by an external event. This therapy will only be helpful if these patients can keep themselves from acting on impulses and strong emotions often stimulated by this form of treatment. Patients must be interested in gaining self-awareness. Social class, family history, and the presence of anger do not affect treatment response. Catastrophic thinking would be an indication for cognitive behavioral therapy.

26. The answer is A *[Chapter 4 III B, C].* Systematic desensitization teaches the patient to feel relaxed and in control, instead of anxious, in phobic situations. Panic control therapy may secondarily help agoraphobia if it is secondary to panic disorder, but it is not a primary treatment for agoraphobia. Biofeedback is a treatment for generalized anxiety. Expressive and supportive psychotherapies are useful for a variety of conditions, but not agoraphobia.

27. The answer is A *[Chapter 4 III C 8].* Propranolol reduces stage fright when taken shortly before a performance. Panic attacks and phobias should be treated with antidepressants or high-potency benzodiazepines. Situational anxiety is treated with benzodiazepines and behavioral techniques. Posttraumatic stress disorder is treated with carbamazepine or selective serotonin reuptake inhibitors (SSRIs).

28. The answer is D *[Chapter 4 I E].* Acute stress disorder, mixed anxiety–depression, caffeinism, and posttraumatic stress disorder all can cause hyperventilation, which is the most proximate cause of such symptoms as shortness of breath, dizziness, paresthesia, headache, weakness, and occasionally carpopedal spasm.

29. The answer is A *[Chapter 4 III C].* Concerns about attractiveness and self-esteem are not uncommon in patients who have had surgery that alters their appearance. The intern should also consider the possibility of delirium related to the surgery or the illness. Schizophrenia and obsessive-compulsive disorder are unlikely to develop at this time of life, and the patient does not have any symptoms specific to these disorders. Because the patient is exhibiting anxiety in the presence of a familiar caretaker rather than when she is alone, separation anxiety and stranger anxiety are unlikely to be present.

30. The answer is B *[Chapter 5 II B 9 b; IV C 4 b].* Subtle cognitive changes may be the first signs of progressive dementia. More obvious cognitive deficits, such as speech difficulties, apraxia, and disorganization, may follow. Agitation is one of the most problematic symptoms of vascular dementia, and benzodiazepines can exacerbate agitation by increasing cognitive impairment. More appropriate treatment is low doses of antipsychotic medication (e.g., 1–2 mg of haloperidol). Vascular dementia is more common in men, has a fluctuating course, and is usually first evident in the sixth decade.

31. The answer is D *[Chapter 5 II A 1 a].* Delirium presents with many cognitive and emotional symptoms, but reduced clarity of awareness and a short and fluctuating course most often distinguish it from other cognitive disorders (e.g., dementia, amnestic disorders). Physical findings are often present in delirium as a result of underlying general medical conditions but are not the most distinguishing features.

32. The answer is C *[Chapter 5 II A 2].* Delirium is characterized by the rapid onset of confusion and agitation. Hallucinations are common. The fever and tachycardia are evidence of a causative general medical condition. Brief psychotic disorder is less likely given the concurrent physical symptoms.

33. The answer is A *[Chapter 5 IV K 4 b].* Hypocalcemia is characterized by muscle cramping, tetany, paresthesias, and cognitive and personality changes. Seizures and delirium can supervene. Hypocalcemia is most often due to parathyroid pathology.

34. The answer is C *[Chapter 5 IV K 3 b].*
Hypothyroidism is characterized by depression, weakness, somnolence, dry skin, brittle hair, cold intolerance, and hoarseness. Dementia may supervene but only after a prolonged course of untreated illness.

35. The answer is E *[Chapter 5 IV I 4].*
Pyridoxine deficiency is characterized by dermatitis, neuropathies, and cognitive deficits. It usually occurs in association with drugs that act as antagonists, such as isoniazid. Isoniazid is the drug most commonly used to treat tuberculosis infection, which is implied in the question.

36. The answer is D *[Chapter 5 II C 2 b].*
The case is suggestive of alcohol-induced persisting amnestic disorder (Korsakoff psychosis), which is characterized by an extensive history of alcohol abuse, memory deficits, and confabulation. It results from the effects of untreated or repeated alcohol-related thiamine deficiency.

37. The answer is A *[Chapter 5 IV H 2].*
Alcohol dependence increases the risk for subdural hematoma by increasing the likelihood of head trauma and coagulopathies. This condition should be considered in the differential diagnosis of any patient with alcoholism and altered mental status because focal findings and headache are sometimes absent.

38. The answer is A *[Chapter 5 IV D 2].*
The symptoms are suggestive of complex partial seizures (temporal lobe epilepsy). Focal central nervous system (CNS) herpes simplex infection is most often seen in the frontal and temporal lobes and can cause complex partial seizures.

39. The answer is D *[Chapter 5 II B 8 d].*
Many inhalants produce rapid damage to cortical neurons, and abuse is associated with severe and sometimes irreversible cognitive deficits. The use of inhalants is especially common in the early adolescent age-group.

40. The answer is C *[Chapter 6 II D 2 a, b (1)].*
Hallucinogens produce autonomic arousal, increased temperature, hallucinations, anxiety, depersonalization, and paranoia, without clouding of the sensorium. Phencyclidine produces the additional effects of violent behavior and neurologic signs.

41. The answer is E *[Chapter 6 III C 2 a; VIII B].*
Cocaine was once thought to be a relatively benign drug used primarily by the rich. However, cheaper preparations, especially crack, and an increase in criminal behavior have made cocaine abuse and dependence a characteristic of all social strata. People often combine cocaine with sedating drugs like opioids and tranquilizers to "come down." Withdrawal from cocaine causes depression. Cocaine is so rewarding that it is highly addictive.

42. The answer is A *[Chapter 6 III D 1, 2 a, 3; III D; VII D].* Hallucinogens and marijuana are not known to produce physical dependence (i.e., tolerance and withdrawal do not occur). Intoxication may cause depersonalization, anxiety, hallucinations, and dysphoria, but not hypertension. Bad trips can be ameliorated by reassurance in a quiet setting and by benzodiazepines, if necessary. Tolerance does not develop to the psychotropic effects, but marijuana use is frequently associated with reckless driving.

43. The answer is C *[Chapter 6 III C].*
Increased appetite, fatigue, depression, and suicidal ideation may occur with stimulant withdrawal. Although nightmares may occur, the patient usually sleeps excessively after being deprived of the stimulant. Paranoia is a symptom of stimulant intoxication, not withdrawal. Piloerection is associated with opioid withdrawal.

44. The answer is D *[Chapter 6 VI A, B].*
The combined mortality rate from overdoses, infections, suicide, and murder is approximately 10/100,000. Although many adolescents and young adults experiment with a variety of drugs, hallucinogens, stimulants, tranquilizers, and sedatives are used regularly with much greater frequency. Most addicts are introduced to opioids by their friends rather than by pushers. Heroin abuse tends to occur in epidemics in which addicted individuals "infect" their friends. Many opioid users also use other drugs, especially stimulants, cocaine, and alcohol.

45. The answer is D *[Chapter 6 III A, B].* The history of insomnia treated by multiple physicians suggests that the patient probably has been receiving more than one sleeping pill. Because the complaint has been present for years, the patient may have received barbiturates, which were in widespread use before benzodiazepine sleeping pills were introduced. Some physicians continue to refill prescriptions for such sleeping pills, although the medications tend to lose their efficacy over several weeks. In view of the rapid onset of possible withdrawal symptoms, abstinence from a short-acting benzodiazepine or a barbiturate is suggested.

Phenobarbital would suppress withdrawal symptoms from any tranquilizer or sleeping pill. Neuroleptics (e.g., haloperidol) may reduce psychotic symptoms and agitation caused by organic brain disease, but they are not specific treatments for withdrawal syndromes. Physostigmine is used to diagnose anticholinergic delirium. Thiamine is an adjunct in the treatment of alcohol withdrawal, which could be a factor in this case, but it does not establish the diagnosis by suppressing withdrawal. Disulfiram precipitates alcohol withdrawal in people using alcohol.

46. The answer is B *[Chapter 7 II H].* If the man is going from hospital to hospital with this story, he may be putting blood from a fingerstick into his urine. The kidney stone complaint is important because it is not an unconscious symptom. The use of serial hospitalizations makes it likely that the patient role is his goal, rather than a secondary gain. This man could probably hold up his end of a health-related conversation because many people with factitious disorder are health care paraprofessionals. Because of his story of the medical school faculty, he may be classified as having Munchausen syndrome.

47. The answer is C *[Chapter 7 V B 1 b (8)].* The young man presenting with the myocardial infarction–like symptoms is most likely suffering from panic disorder. Adequate treatment for the panic disorder and education about the disorder are likely to stop the symptoms. There is no firm diagnosis of the symptom of general malaise in the 35-year-old woman, but it is not a conversion-like symptom. She may well have an organic disease that requires further investigation, or may have a major depression. The 70-year-old man is very likely suffering from a major depression, quite possibly with psychotic features. The college student is likely suffering from a college prank in which someone gave him pyridium. If he had psychiatric symptoms and abdominal pain, the clinician would also have suspected porphyria. The young woman's

blindness is not an unusual presentation, particularly if she does not remember seeing the people who died in the accident.

48. The answer is B *[Chapter 7 IV H 1 b].* This odd presentation is difficult to categorize. Because of the history of self-mutilation, it is unlikely that the patient's reported suicidal ideation is accurate. The history suggests that the goals of this behavior may be surgery and the patient role itself. However, this patient is not trying to conceal or disguise the behavior. It is unlikely that depression would cause such a symptom on its own. Although the symptom sounds psychotic, there is no other evidence of schizophrenia (e.g., hearing voices, ideas of reference, ideas of influence). The intentional nature of the patient's actions preclude somatization disorder. On the other hand, self-mutilation behaviors are relatively common in borderline personality disorder.

49. The answer is B *[Chapter 7 V E 3 c].* An easy way to remember the answer to this question is to consider the behavior of patients suffering from this disorder. People with body dysmorphic disorder may spend several hours each day contemplating the supposedly deformed body part. This can be thought of as in some ways analogous to the checking behaviors of obsessive-compulsive disorder. Although each of the others has a possible link to obsessive-compulsive disorder, it may be that they are more closely associated with major depression.

50. The answer is E *[Chapter 7 V D].* Although this man's actions cause inflammation to his testicles, the last thing he really wants to be is a patient suffering from the disorder he fears. This makes factitious disorder unlikely. He lacks the rest of the diagnostic picture required for somatization disorder. The man's symptoms do not involve a pseudoneurologic picture, and do not resemble a disease closely, except in his mind, and so do not fit criteria for conversion disorder. This man is probably not faking having seen blood in his semen, and any gain from the symptom is not evident. He may well have a major depression or an anxiety disorder of some sort, but these are not options in the question. The best answer is hypochondriasis.

51. The answer is E *[Chapter 8 II C 4 a].* There are no consistent biologic findings associated with homosexuality. Rat models, once used to explain homosexuality, have been abandoned because of a number of major methodologic concerns.

52. The answer is C *[Chapter 8 III A 6]*. Behavioral techniques (e.g., sensate focus) are proven effective for treatment of this condition. Insight-oriented psychotherapy has not been demonstrated to be effective for premature ejaculation, and the neurosis model of premature ejaculation was abandoned several decades ago. Thioridazine might be temporarily effective in delaying ejaculation, but it poses risks (e.g., tardive dyskinesia) and is unlikely to be useful after the medication is stopped. Premature ejaculation is unlikely to be associated with major depression.

53. The answer is D *[Chapter 8 III D 1 h (5)]*. In this case, the key point is that dopamine inhibits prolactin secretion. When dopamine effects are blocked, prolactin secretion increases. The drug that is most likely to block dopamine effects is chlorpromazine, which exerts its effects primarily by blocking dopamine. Alprazolam, fluoxetine, diazepam, and bupropion are much less likely to produce lactation. Sertraline, which is a selective serotonin reuptake inhibitor (SSRI) like fluoxetine, has been reported to produce galactorrhea. However, this is a less frequent problem with fluoxetine. Even in this context, chlorpromazine is many times more likely to produce galactorrhea. In contrast, bupropion is likely to reduce prolactin secretion.

54. The answer is C *[Chapter 8 III A 14–17, 19]*. Most states have laws requiring physicians and others to report known instances of child abuse, including sexual abuse. It is likely that the pedophile patient will report specific instances of abuse of a child, which forces the clinician to report to the authorities. In the case of homosexuality, there would be no reason to violate confidentiality. In the cases of frotteurism and voyeurism, the patient may have performed illegal acts, but the clinician is not required to report them. There may be a legal duty to report felonies being planned by the patient, but the patient rarely reports the intentions to the clinician. In the case of sadomasochism, clinicians may be under an obligation to prevent serious harm done to or by their patients. However, experienced sadists are unlikely to maim or kill. Inexperienced sadomasochists or those who express a desire to kill or seriously injure others may force the

clinician to take legal action (e.g., invoking a civil commitment procedure); however, the possibility of a clinician seeing one of these patients is quite rare. Pedophiles presenting to clinicians is much more common.

55. The answer is B *[Chapter 9 I F]*. The weight of a patient with anorexia nervosa should be monitored closely, and limits should be reinforced; that is, weight that is too low should result in hospitalization or curtailment of privileges if the patient is already hospitalized. Although increasing caloric intake would normally result in some weight gain, anorectic patients have learned that they can compensate for ingested calories by vomiting, exercising, or abusing laxatives. Likewise, decreased exercise would be met with vomiting, laxatives, or decreased caloric intake. It is too difficult to eradicate all of the weight-losing maneuvers; therefore, weight should be monitored.

56. The answer is C *[Chapter 9 I G]*. The earlier the onset in life, the better the prognosis. The longer the disease course, the worse the prognosis of anorexia nervosa. The prognosis for recovery for boys may be worse than it is for girls, but most girls do not fully recover. The death rate of the disease is listed as 5%–15%; death is usually due to metabolic or electrolyte abnormalities or suicide.

57. The answer is E *[Chapter 9 II F]*. No one modality of treatment for bulimia nervosa has proven to be universally efficacious. A treatment plan that offers combinations of several treatment modalities (i.e., pharmacotherapy, psychodynamic psychotherapy, and group psychotherapy) appears to be most efficacious. Hospitalization may be indicated for certain medical complications, concomitant suicidal ideation, or severely out of control bingeing and purging behavior. In most cases, however, patients with bulimia nervosa can be managed on an outpatient basis.

58. The answer is B *[Chapter 10 XII C 1]*. Grand mal seizures in children are frequently treated with phenobarbital. Barbiturates, like other sedative–hypnotics, may result in paradoxical excitation in children. In such circumstances, discontinuation of the medication results in resolution of the symptom of hyperactivity. According to the history of the young boy described in the question, the acute onset of hyperactivity would be less likely secondary to a primary neurologic condition than as a side effect to the sedative–hypnotic medication. Selection of an alternative anti-epileptic medication would be indicated.

59. The answer is A *[Chapter 11 I A]*. Personality disorders are stable, not intermittent, patterns of responses that lead to problems in functioning. They are usually recognized early, that is, by adolescence, and they tend to become less obvious in old age. There is evidence that certain genetic characteristics may make a specific behavioral response more likely to occur. Poor social and occupational functioning are characteristic of personality disorders.

60. The answer is E *[Chapter 11 III A 1]*. Individuals with a schizoid personality disorder have a defective capacity to form social relationships. When hospitalized, they may become distressed when intruded upon too much by health care professionals. They generally do poorly in social situations, such as dating, and men, in particular, are unlikely to marry. They do not respond to warm, tender feelings of others. There is no evidence that antidepressants improve this disorder. These individuals, however, may do well in jobs that require social isolation.

61. The answer is C *[Chapter 11 II B 2]*. The group of dramatic and emotional personality disorders (cluster B) is most often associated with concurrent mood disorders, such as depression. This is particularly true of borderline personality disorder. Schizoid and paranoid patients rarely come to the attention of the physician. Individuals with avoidant and antisocial personality disorders occasionally have a concurrent mood disorder but not as commonly as borderline personalities.

62. The answer is C *[Chapter 11 II A]*. Because of the similarities of symptoms and traits, the personality disorders are grouped into three clusters: A, B, and C. Cluster A includes schizoid, schizotypal, and paranoid disorders. These disorders are grouped together because affected individuals use the defense mechanisms of projection and fantasy.

63. The answer is D *[Chapter 11 II A 3]*. In families with a history of schizophrenia, there is also an increase in the number of relatives with schizotypal personality disorder, not schizoid, antisocial, or paranoid personality disorders. Not everyone who has a genetic

vulnerability to schizophrenia becomes psychotic, and it is thought that some of these individuals may be diagnosed as having a schizotypal personality disorder.

64. The answer is D *[Chapter 1 II B 6 a–c]*. Perceptual abnormalities involve the sensory nervous system and include hallucinations, which are false perceptions of sensory stimuli; depersonalization, which is altered perception of one's reality; and illusions, which are misinterpretations of true sensory stimuli. Perseverations are abnormalities of the thinking process, which are manifested by repetition of the same word or phrase over and over. They are not considered perceptual abnormalities.

65. The answer is D *[Chapter 1 II C 1 e]*. Polysomnography, the study of sleep in a laboratory, has been useful in studying medical problems associated with psychiatric symptoms, such as seizure disorders and erectile dysfunctions. Depression has also been studied because of the abnormalities of sleep associated with this illness. Schizophrenia, however, does not demonstrate changes that can be measured by sleep studies.

66. The answer is A *[Chapter 1 II C]*. The clinical laboratory is increasingly useful in diagnosing mental disorders. The three main functions include identifying biologic markers of psychiatric illness, monitoring blood levels of psychotropic medications, and screening for any other underlying medical or organic condition that may be causing psychiatric symptoms. Unfortunately, laboratories still cannot assess the severity of psychiatric illness.

67. The answer is A *[Chapter 2 III E, F; VI A–C; VII A 11 c]*. Although disordered ego functioning is believed by some clinicians to be frequently present in schizophrenia, there is no good evidence that disordered ego functioning in any way predicts the development of schizophrenia. In addition, interrater reliability difficulties in assessing disordered ego functioning would make this criterion very difficult to assess should systematic studies of this factor be undertaken. A birth in early spring, environmental stressors, a schizophrenic biologic relative, and a history of herpes simplex or viral encephalitis are factors that are known to be at least statistically associated with an increased risk for the development of schizophrenia.

68. The answer is D *[Chapter 2 IX A, E, H].*
Comprehensiveness and continuity of care are elements of a reasonable care plan not just for schizophrenic patients but for patients with any chronic illness. Treatment of the patient in the least restrictive treatment setting, which may involve placement in the community as opposed to inpatient hospitalization or voluntary as opposed to civil commitment status, is a common treatment goal. Psychosocial rehabilitation is a central feature in the reintegration of schizophrenic patients into the community, and there is increasing evidence that it may significantly improve the prognosis in long-term patients. Confrontation of schizophrenic patients to overcome their resistances to change is likely to produce exacerbations in psychotic symptomatology, particularly if this intervention is carried out with a high degree of affect on the part of the therapist. Thus, systematic confrontation of schizophrenic patients is not indicated in any reasonable treatment plan.

69. The answer is C *[Chapter 2 IX F 1–4].*
The role of a case manager as it is defined in most service systems does not involve sharing the role of the therapist. Furthermore, current therapy of the chronically mentally ill does not involve insight-oriented therapy but rather a supportive, educational, problem-solving approach. Planning, evaluation, linking, and advocacy are all portions of the routinely described duties of case managers. Acting as an advocate for groups of mentally ill patients is included in some definitions of case management, although it is a controversial role; however, class-specific advocacy is a more common and widely accepted role for case managers than insight-oriented therapy.

70. The answer is B *[Chapter 2 VIII B 1, 4 a].*
All of the following trends are correct except for the use of inpatient hospitalization for functional skills assessment. By definition, assessing functional skills is best performed in the patient's usual environment. In addition, it is unlikely that any third-party payor would approve hospitalization for this purpose, unless the patient had additional symptoms and problems.

71. The answer is B *[Chapter 2 VIII L].* This is a difficult question to answer, but one likely to confront the clinician in clinical emergency practice. If the physician assumes that the patient is suffering from an exacerbation of

psychotic symptoms secondary to schizophrenia, use of high-potency neuroleptics may be the most reasonable choice. If toxicity from a drug like phencyclidine is suspected, particularly low-potency neuroleptics should be avoided because of the danger of a hyperpyrexic state and death. If a toxic state is suspected, it may be quite reasonable to refrain from pharmacologic treatment unless the patient or staff is in danger. Benzodiazepines have been found helpful in controlling many cases of severe psychotic agitation by reducing the component of fear; however, benzodiazepines disinhibit violent behavior in some patients. Droperidol is used in some parts of the country to control acute psychotic agitation. This drug wears off in a few hours in case of hyperpyrexia or if the patient needs an electroencephalogram (EEG). Unfortunately, droperidol is not approved by the Food and Drug Administration (FDA) for this use, and poses a higher legal risk for clinicians. Although there is a "least correct" answer to this question, there is no best answer in all circumstances.

72. The answer is C *[Chapter 2 VII F 2].*
All of these strategies, if performed in a positive and educational manner, have promise to improve the patient's course, except C. Not only is there no evidence for the "schizophrenigenic mother," but blame to the family may harm the patient and family by complicating interactions within the family. Difficult as it may be to believe, some psychiatrists did pursue strategy C for years. One of the results of this practice was the formation of the National Alliance for the Mentally Ill, one of whose purposes was to help families band together to support each other in the face of these demeaning practices by the psychiatrists of the past.

73. The answer is A *[Chapter 2 VIII L 2 b (4) (a)].*
Although a febrile state is common in this phase of starting clozapine, and the patient's complete blood cell count results were normal the previous week, it is possible that the patient has experienced a rapid onset of agranulocytosis and a secondary infection. All of these measures except sending the patient home with no further work-up are reasonable methods for looking for infections. If the patient did have an infection, it might be rapidly progressive and involve meningitis. Therefore, having the patient in the emergency room for several hours to watch the patient's

temperature and state of consciousness is not an unreasonable precaution.

74. The answer is C *[Chapter 2 VIII B 1 a, c, d, f].* Dopamine systems are thought to be central in the pathophysiology of schizophrenia. All of the compounds listed in the question—prostaglandin E_1, norepinephrine, and serotonin—except ascorbic acid are currently thought to be neuromodulators of the dopamine systems in schizophrenia. There are no known therapeutic or physiologic influences of ascorbic acid in schizophrenia although there is massive public lore about its efficacy in a variety of conditions.

75. The answer is B *[Chapter 3 V B 3].* The selective serotonin reuptake inhibitors (SSRIs) [e.g., fluoxetine, fluvoxamine, sertraline, paroxetine] have a wide therapeutic index and are fairly safe from the possibility of overdose when taken alone. When combined with some other agents, they can be more dangerous. For example, the potentially lethal serotonin syndrome is seen when these drugs are combined with other highly serotonergic drugs [including monoamine oxidase (MAO) inhibitors]. Trazodone (a triazolopyridine) and venlafaxine (a selective serotonin and norepinephrine reuptake inhibitor) are also fairly safe from overdose. Nortriptyline, however, can be very dangerous in overdose. As with all of the tricyclic antidepressants, a quinidine-like effect can lead to fatal arrhythmias or heart block.

76. The answer is D *[Chapter 3 III B 3 d].* AIDS can produce manic symptoms by several mechanisms, such as when frontal lobe tumors (e.g., caused by toxoplasmosis) result. Wilson disease can present with psychiatric symptoms, including manic-like personality changes. Hyperthyroidism can cause anxiety, increased activity, and insomnia. Cushing disease can also cause symptoms that resemble mania. Tuberculosis is associated with depressive, rather than manic, symptoms.

77. The answer is B *[Chapter 4 I D 3, 4].* Hyperparathyroidism is more likely to cause depression than anxiety. Anxiety caused by hypoglycemia and pheochromocytoma may be accompanied by signs of increased adrenergic activity such as sweating and tachycardia. Porphyria can produce a variety of psychiatric symptoms, including anxiety.

78. The answer is D *[Chapter 4 I B, C].* Chronic physical or psychological symptoms caused by panic disorder may mask the subjective sense of dread, making diagnosis difficult. Partial complex seizures and hyperthyroidism are two of the medical disorders that can produce anxiety. Acute stress disorder is accompanied by prominent dissociation. Hypocalcemia rather than hypercalcemia is a cause of anxiety and its attendant symptoms.

79. The answer is E *[Chapter 4 I B 10 a; III C 2, 3].* Approximately 70% of depressed patients are also anxious, and up to one third of apparent anxiety disorders are caused by an underlying depression. There is evidence of familial vulnerability to depression, panic disorder, and mixed anxiety–depression. Approximately half of patients with panic disorder become depressed at some point, and at least 20% of depressed patients have panic attacks. In patients with both anxiety and depression, the symptoms tend to accompany each other rather than alternate. With the exception of bupropion, antidepressants are effective for both depression and panic disorder.

80. The answer is E *[Chapter 6 II A 3 a, B; V E 4].* Central nervous system (CNS) depressants such as diazepam, phenobarbital, and glutethimide augment the CNS depression caused by alcohol, although phenobarbital and benzodiazepines are used to treat alcohol withdrawal. Disulfiram induces nausea, vomiting, and malaise when combined with even small amounts of alcohol; patients should be cautioned against eating foods cooked in wine. Restraint is the safest way to control an agitated patient who is intoxicated with alcohol, but a high-potency neuroleptic (e.g., haloperidol) may be administered if the patient continues to struggle.

81. The answer is C *[Chapter 6 III A 1–4].* Thiamine is used to prevent depletion of thiamine stores when glucose is administered, which can precipitate Wernicke encephalopathy. Benzodiazepines reduce agitation and confusion and prevent seizures. Hydration and sedation are the mainstays of treatment of severe abstinence syndromes, and neuroleptics may alleviate alcohol hallucinosis that does not remit spontaneously. Caffeine is not useful in the treatment of alcohol withdrawal, and it does not hasten sobriety in alcohol intoxication.

82. The answer is C *[Chapter 6 IV D 1].*
The presence of gastritis and an enlarged liver raise the possibility of alcohol abuse. A hemoglobin determination would be a component of evaluation of possible gastrointestinal bleeding. Elevated gamma glutamyl transferase (GGT) is the most sensitive liver function test for alcoholism. Screening for additional substances of misuse is appropriate in view of the high frequency of mixed abuse. Blood cultures would be more appropriate to the work-up of an unexplained fever, especially in a patient who uses intravenous drugs.

83. The answer is E *[Chapter 6 II F 2].* Many over-the-counter preparations and psychiatric medications have anticholinergic properties. Delirium, confusion, psychosis, or memory loss accompanied by tachycardia, warm, dry skin, and dilated pupils should raise the suspicion of anticholinergic poisoning. An influenza-like syndrome is associated with withdrawal from anticholinergic drugs rather than intoxication with them. Intravenous administration of physostigmine temporarily reverses coma and fever, facilitating diagnosis, but it is not a useful treatment because of a short half-life and a high incidence of adverse effects.

84. The answer is B *[Chapter 6 V A, C].*
The first step in any effective treatment program is to withdraw the substance completely. Most patients can never again use the substance safely in any amount. Family members should be included in the treatment plan because they may have substance-use disorders themselves, or they may be sources of encouragement of abuse or support for abstinence. Contingency contracting is very effective when important contingencies such as keeping a job, marriage, or professional license can be identified. Twelve-step programs based on the Alcoholics Anonymous approach have been found to be very helpful.

85. The answer is E *[Chapter 7 V E 4].*
This woman meets the criteria for body dysmorphic disorder. There seems to be an exclusive focus on one body part and its supposed deformity. Gathering further history will help to rule out other psychiatric disorders that might account for her symptoms. An educational approach to the disorder may be necessary to convince the patient to try any of the treatments for the condition. The two medications are the best known treatments reported

in the literature. Confronting the woman with supposed fears about her inability to nurture is unlikely to be effective, and may be perceived as irrelevant or bizarre by the woman. Statistically, an insight-oriented approach is less likely to be effective than the others. This would be a singularly badly timed approach in any case, before a therapeutic alliance had been established.

86. The answer is A *[Chapter 7 IV E 1].*
Dysregulation of the hypothalamic–pituitary axis and alterations in T-lymphocyte function are seen in major depression, and may help to explain some of the increases in physical illness associated with major depression. To date, little research has been reported on gonadotropins in depression, although on the basis of clinical observations, they would be expected to decrease rather than increase if there is central inhibition of sexual function.

87. The answer is B *[Chapter 7 V A 2 c].*
This question highlights one of the major controversies in modern psychiatry. Patients with somatization disorder are more likely to have been both sexually abused and more suggestible than the average patient. All of the answers represent potentially fruitful areas of exploration. However, particularly with somatization disorder patients, too concrete suggestions and probing about a sexual abuse history may help to create false memories of the events. Rather, sneaking up on the issue by asking about blank spots in memory, such as whole periods lost in childhood, will allow the patient to eventually voice suspicions of having been abused. The medical student should be careful to be supportive and sympathetic, but not to be disproportionately interested in the sexual abuse history, in contrast to the other parts of the patient's life and experience. This is a medicolegal as well as a clinical issue.

88. The answer is D *[Chapter 7 V A 5 a].*
The medical student and attending physician agree that continuity of care is the most important aspect of the patient's care. At each scheduled visit, the attending physician will conservatively evaluate new symptoms, will attempt to keep the patient away from exploratory or non-indicated surgery, and will avoid giving the patient narcotics and other habituating medications. Any medication should be prescribed only in the context of an ongoing relationship with a single doctor to avoid "doctor

shopping" and multiple prescriptions of habituating medications. The neuroleptic medications should be avoided because they are unlikely to produce substantial benefit, yet run the risk of producing tardive dyskinesia. The benzodiazepines should be used with caution because of the propensity for somatization disorder patients to become habituated and to use them in greater than prescribed amounts. The monoamine oxidase (MAO) inhibitors should be considered only with adequate informed consent, after the attending physician knows the patient very well. The patient will likely reject the transfer to the psychiatry service, taking it as a rejection and evidence of lack of competence of the medicine service. The patient is likely to try to get another doctor to diagnose and treat her condition "adequately."

89. The answer is C *[Chapter 9 I F 2 b (2)].*
The treatment of anorexia nervosa is aimed at preventing the medical complications secondary to starvation and typically involves behavior modification. With this modality, the medical status of the patient is measured by serially monitoring changes in weight or a catabolic state manifested by ketonuria. As the condition of the patient becomes medically compromised, negative reinforcers, such as restriction of privileges, are invoked. Nasogastric alimentation is provided as needed to reverse the state of starvation either when the condition is life-threatening or when behavior modification approaches have failed. Overtly aggressive or threatening behaviors, requiring locked seclusion, are uncommon among anorectic patients.

90. The answer is B *[Chapter 9 Table 9-2].*
Serum protein and albumin levels in anorectic individuals tend to remain in the normal range until starvation is far advanced. Serum cortisol levels tend to remain normal or slightly high, possibly representing a loss or normal diurnal variation in cortisol secretion. A lowered metabolic rate, which is characteristic of anorexia, is manifested by bradycardia, hypotension, and hypothermia. Increased carotene levels are common among anorectic individuals and tend to distinguish anorexia from other causes of weight loss. Hypokalemia typically becomes a problem during the course of starvation.

91. The answer is A *[Chapter 10 II C 1–5].*
Although once postulated to be a result of a disturbed parent–child relationship, autistic disorder has now been shown to be a neurologic-based condition. Hospitalism is a disorder in which the child fails to establish any primary attachment relationship. Anaclitic depression is a disorder in which an attachment relationship has developed but is disrupted (usually by parent–child separation) during a sensitive phase of development. Vulnerable child syndrome is characterized by a parent–child bond that is intrusive and overprotective due to an exaggerated concern over the child's vulnerability. Child abuse has its roots in disturbed attachment relationships between parent and child in many cases.

92. The answer is C *[Chapter 10 IV A 6].*
Administration of imipramine is not effective for treating autistic disorder. Behavior modification is the most suitable treatment for autistic disorder. It aims to promote social behavior and relatedness, to maximize language skills, and to eliminate idiosyncratic behavior. A structured educational setting with a low student-to-teacher ratio and a constant environment are helpful. Psychotherapy may be helpful when the family is having trouble coping with an autistic child or when environmental factors have complicated the illness. Psychotherapy for the child may be indicated in those children with sufficient language skills and intellect.

93. The answer is D *[Chapter 10 II C 1 a].*
Hospitalism is an extreme example of failure of any affective relationship to develop. No bond is established between the parent and child. It can cause apathy and susceptibility to infection. It is not, however, associated with jaundice. The syndrome develops in infants and is associated with a high mortality rate. Treatment consists of providing the infant with a figure with whom to attach. If parents are unavailable, surrogate parents should be provided.

94. The answer is B *[Chapter 11 V C 1].*
It is important to remember that the obsessive-compulsive disorder (i.e., the anxiety disorder) is a different illness from the obsessive-compulsive personality disorder. Individuals with the obsessive-compulsive personality disorder seem to have perfectionistic and inflexible personalities. These individuals are often indecisive, stingy with compliments and preoccupied by trivial details, but they do not exhibit symptoms of the anxiety disorder, such as compulsive checking and excessive washing.

95–96. The answers are: 95-B *[Chapter 3 III B 2 a]*, **96-D** *[Chapter 3 III A 1; III A 4; III B 4]*. Dysthymic disorder is a chronic illness (duration of at least 2 years), which features symptoms similar to those seen in major depressive disorder without being severe enough to merit that diagnosis. Patients can have short periods during which they feel well, and the clinician must differentiate feeling well from feeling abnormally high, which might suggest a diagnosis of cyclothymia. Optimism about a new job sounds like a normal reaction, but it would be worth exploring it more fully. Although mild compared with some other disorders, dysthymia can be accompanied by significant social impairment, health problems, and substance abuse.

The patient who attempted suicide has current symptoms consistent with a major depressive episode (MDE). Although the symptoms follow the death of his son, the severity of the symptoms rule out either adjustment disorder or normal bereavement. His previous "manic depressive" symptoms are most consistent with hypomanic episodes because they featured typical manic symptoms yet were not severe enough to result in hospitalization or occupational impairment. A patient in a current MDE with a history of hypomanic episodes would be diagnosed with bipolar II disorder.

97–101. The answers are: 97-D, 98-B, 99-A, 100-E, 101-C *[Chapter 4 III C]*. The risk of tardive dyskinesia precludes the use of neuroleptics in most cases of nonpsychotic anxiety. Antihistamines are frequently used as anxiolytics because of the low risk of abuse, but they are not predictably effective, and anticholinergic side effects may impair memory in older patients. The time of onset and acuteness of benzodiazepine withdrawal syndromes are related to elimination half-life. Selective serotonin reuptake inhibitors (SSRIs) are the only antidepressants that are effective in the treatment of obsessive-compulsive disorder. The risks of tolerance, addiction, dangerous withdrawal syndromes, and fatal overdose make barbiturates inappropriate choices for anxiety or insomnia.

102–106. The answers are: 102-D, 103-C, 104-E, 105-B, 106-A *[Chapter 4 II A, D, E, H, K]*. Patients who are afraid of becoming too dependent on others are often also anxious about losing control. Patients who actually experience excess dependency are more likely to regress (i.e., adopt a psychological posture more appropriate to that of a child) and exhibit distress (separation anxiety) when they are left alone. Patients whose self-esteem is threatened by an illness or other circumstance may attempt to feel more important by treating others as though they were inferior. When a psychological conflict of which the patient has been unaware begins to emerge into consciousness, the resulting signal anxiety may elicit psychological defenses to remove the conflict from the patient's consciousness. Anxiety following a traumatic event may appear immediately, or it may be delayed.

107–109. The answers are: 107-B, 108-D, 109-C *[Chapter 5 IV F 4 a]*. Absence seizures are generalized seizures, usually occurring in childhood, which involve brief periods of inattention and unresponsiveness. Myoclonic seizures are characterized by focal or generalized muscle contractions without loss of consciousness. Tonic–clonic seizures are generalized seizures characterized by loss of consciousness, tonic–clonic limb movements, and incontinence.

110–111. The answers are: 110-E *[Chapter 5 IV D 3 b]*, **111-A** *[Chapter 5 IV F 4 a (2)]*. The history of rapidly progressing dementia and myoclonus is most suggestive of Creutzfeldt-Jakob disease, a slow virus central nervous system (CNS) infection that characteristically presents with electroencephalogram (EEG) findings of sharp, triphasic synchronous discharges. Associated visual impairment is common. The history of brief episodes of unresponsiveness and automatisms is most suggestive of absence (petit mal) seizures. These seizures most often occur in childhood and have EEG findings characterized by spike and slow-wave activity.

112–116. The answers are: 112-D, 113-A, 114-E, 115-C, 116-B *[Chapter 6 II D 3 b; III B 2; V E 4; VI C 1 b; VIII D 1]*. Detoxification from combinations of central nervous system (CNS) depressants can be safely accomplished with phenobarbital. Reliable patients dependent on one benzodiazepine can usually be withdrawn with gradual dose reduction. Imipramine, desipramine, and maprotiline seem to reduce cocaine craving and possibly cocaine-induced euphoria. Bupropion and amantadine may also be useful in this regard. Diazepam is used to treat seizures and severe agitation associated with phencyclidine intoxication. Disulfiram helps to decrease the risk of impulsive drinking because the patient has to stop the drug several days before drinking to avoid an alcohol–disulfiram reaction. Methadone maintenance is effective in preventing relapse of opioid use.

117–121. The answers are: 117-D, 118-C, 119-E, 120-B, 121-A *[Chapter 6 II B, C; V D; VI B; VII A]*. Heroin injected into joints when veins are inaccessible, as well as metastatic complications of intravenous use, can lead to septic arthritis. Rapid eye movement (REM) rebound manifested as nightmares follows missed doses of drugs that suppress REM sleep, such as the barbiturates. Phencyclidine intoxication produces a variety of neurologic and catatonic signs and symptoms. Chronic amphetamine use may produce a schizophrenia-like psychosis, which may become chronic. Use of alcohol is the most common cause of traffic fatalities.

122–125. The answers are: 122-A *[Chapter 10 IV B 4]*, **123-C** *[Chapter 10 XII D 1 a]*, **124-B** *[Chapter 10 VIII A 3 c]*, **125-D** *[Chapter 10 XII C]*. Childhood schizophrenia is a psychotic disorder of childhood. Low doses of antipsychotic medication, such as thioridazine, may be helpful. It should be kept in mind, however, that these medicines can cause serious side effects.

Methylphenidate is used to treat attention deficit hyperactivity disorder (ADHD). Hyperactivity may be a symptom of ADHD. Side effects may include anorexia, growth retardation, tics, and excitation.

Imipramine may be used for the treatment of enuresis. It has anticholinergic properties, and it affects the central nervous system, both of which may be therapeutic in this condition. Side effects can be serious, the lethal dose ratio is low, and cardiac arrhythmias can develop. Consequently, imipramine should not be considered a first-line treatment for enuresis.

Phenobarbital treats grand mal seizures. This drug, like other sedative–hypnotics, can cause paradoxical excitation and hyperactivity in children. When this occurs, it may necessitate a change of anticonvulsants.

126–128. The answers are: 126-B *[Chapter 11 IV D 1]*, **127-C** *[Chapter 11 V C 1–2]*, **128-C** *[Chapter 11 V C 1–2]*. Patients with a histrionic personality disorder are constantly seeking praise and reassurance and tend to be vain and overly concerned with their appearance. Illness can be seen as a threat to their physical attractiveness, as punishment for their thoughts and feelings, and occasionally, as a threat of castration.

Patients with an obsessive-compulsive personality disorder, which must be distinguished from obsessive-compulsive disorder, have a need to be in control. Illness is perceived by these patients as a threat to their control, particularly over their own impulses and feelings. These individuals tend to be inflexible and perfectionistic. They are preoccupied with details and rules and do not appreciate changes in routine. They are often reluctant to delegate work to others because they cannot control it, but because of their perfectionism, they are unable to complete the task themselves.

Index

Note: Page numbers in italics denote illustrations; those followed by *t* denote tables; those followed by Q denote questions; and those followed by E denote explanations.